"It surely ranks as the best popular piece I have ever read on the subject. It was easy to read, and extremely accurate in its descriptions of what a newcomer to a routine obstetrical service might expect. I would have thought only someone with years of living through it could get it down so well. Ms. Walton's insight is amazing. In other words, it tells it like it is. It's all there. I shall be recommending it highly to my patients and urging them to read it."

—Dr. Donald Sloan, Assistant Clinical Professor and Director, Division of Psychosomatics, Department OB-GYN, New York Medical College

---

"The logical reaction upon walking into a dark room is to turn on the lights. Even familiar things can be frightening in the dark. The goal of childbirth eduction is to turn on the light, to prepare the couple for anything that might happen and give them the tools to cope with it. The education also helps the couple to be intelligent consumers of the medical care they are paying for. By knowing what is possible and how to obtain proper medical support and cooperation, couples can make childbirth a positive and exciting experience."

Vicki Walton

HAVE IT YOUR WAY

An Overview of Pregnancy,
Labor and Postpartum,
Including Alternatives
Available in the Hospital
Childbirth Experience

Vicki E. Walton

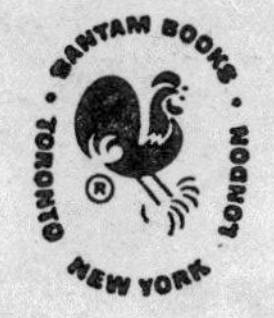

This low-priced Bantam Book has been completely reset in a type face designed for easy reading, and was printed from new plates. It contains the complete text of the original hard-cover edition.
NOT ONE WORD HAS BEEN OMITTED.

HAVE IT YOUR WAY

A Bantam Book / published by arrangement with Henry Phillips Publishing Company

PRINTING HISTORY

Henry Phillips edition published June 1976
2nd printing . . . . . . April 1977
Bantam edition / August 1978

ISBN 0-553-11421-2

Published simultaneously in the United States and Canada

Bantam Books are published by Bantam Books, Inc. Its trademark, consisting of the words "Bantam Books" and the portrayal of a bantam, is registered in the United States Patent Office and in other countries. Marca Registrada. Bantam Books, Inc., 666 Fifth Avenue, New York, New York 10091.

PRINTED IN THE UNITED STATES OF AMERICA

were reflected in their attitude in the delivery room when the doctor was not to arrive on time. This attitude is the beautiful theme that flows throughout this book—flexibility.

Writing a complete text on prepared childbirth is a task in itself. To include personal experiences and provoke thought for the consumer and vendor establishes a unique approach to the literature available for the expectant couple. Should the reader be frightened by the number of pages contained herein, then s/he can give it to a more scholarly friend as a gift and purchase Segal's *Love Story* and/or Bach's *Jonathan Livingston Seagull* for simplicity and brevity.

Just as Tolstoy wrote *War and Peace* for a broad view of love and history, and did not expect the reader to memorize his classic novel, so Ms. Walton's text is not to be considered as a last and final word on all aspects of childbirth. Its contents, however, are in keeping with the multitudinous advances in obstetrics and neonatal medical care. The references to fetal monitoring is an example of the author's honest approach to a controversial innovation.

She alludes to my personal thoughts. Machines are only extensions of our senses. They should not replace clinical judgment. For some reason, recently there seems to be less enthusiasm for the "great" innovations, and the lack of enthusiasm comes from a not-too-small and not-too-quiet multitude of parents-to-be who are less interested in fetal monitoring and in putting electrodes on their babies' scalps.

These parents prefer to be left alone as much as possible. They would even have the baby at home, maybe even unattended, if they thought that someone would put electrodes on their unborn child without giving reason or indication. What they really want is just a quiet, clean environment; a place to lie down and to have a baby without being harassed, and to be surrounded by people who love them and who care about them. Perhaps the goal of the doctor should be to assist a man and a woman in delivering a wanted and loved baby from a healthy and emotionally happy woman who is educated and prepared for the experience.

Somewhere between routine elective inductions, routine episiotomies, routine forceps deliveries, routine postpartum care, routine anesthesia, routine clamping of the cord at the moment of delivery and routine fetal monitoring, and even routine circumcision—somewhere between all of these routine things and the very dangerous unattended home delivery, somewhere between these two ends of the spectrum is an important median and balance that we must and will strive to attain.

It is the striving forward from the cold science, statistics, and routinism toward the understanding of human needs on an individualized basis that will bring us to the balance. What is important is to give skill and recognize complications without ignoring the dignity of the patient. What is the answer to the problems between consumer and vendor? I think that the answer is the re-evaluation of our obstetrical customs in the United States by both consumer and vendor. Demands on the established routinism and strong efforts to make birth at the hospital as normal, home-like, and inexpensive as possible must be made. To my fellow vendor, I say: start to consider childbirth as a physiologic experience instead of a pathologic event.

Besides examining customs of other countries which have lower infant mortality rates, it is time that we start to encourage medical schools to develop nurse-midwife programs. We all know, or should know, that well-trained nurse-midwives allow the obstetrician more time to handle the complicated obstetrics cases. I strongly urge the consumers and vendors to lift their voices high and demand legal reformation of training and licensing of nurse-midwives.

I am opposed to unattended home deliveries, and to those attended by only a paramedic who has good intentions, but is poorly-trained. Ninety per cent of all births are uncomplicated, and only ten per cent are difficult or tend to be complicated. But that ten per cent is damned important if you happen to be one of them. That ten per cent can mean 125 years of life; 75 years for the baby and 50-odd years remaining for the mother. That is too valuable to be left in the hands of poorly-trained paramedics who mean well but who do not know enough to know that they do not know very much.

The author's experiences and recommendations as a consumer are clear—shop well. Spend more time looking for an obstetrician and a hospital than considering which television or car or toothpaste to buy.

In the final analysis, be it this book or any other fine text on childbirth, you do not learn how to ride a Honda by reading the manual.

Bruce S. Steir, M.D.

Thank You

Without the help and encouragement of family and friends, the book would have never been possible. My mother, Bertha Johnson; my aunt, Viola Brewer; my parents-in-law, Henry and Ruth Walton; and my sister-in-law, Pat Walton, have all offered special encouragement at one time or another that provided a push in the right direction.

The following people read the manuscript: Penny Simkin, R.P.T., childbirth educator and Vice President of the International Childbirth Education Association; Judy Clark and Kathleen Britton, both instructors for Preparing Expectant Parents; Michael Kazaras, M.D., pediatrician; Bruce S. Steir, M.D., obstetrician; and Karin and Kent Besaw, future parents. Lunelle Chapin, journalism teacher at Lincoln High School in Seattle, kindly edited the manuscript. Without the many helpful and discriminating comments that these people made, the finished book would not be what it is.

John J. Bonica, M.D., F.F.A.R.C.S., Professor and

Chairman of the Department of Anesthesiology and Director of the Anesthesia Research Center and Pain Clinic at the University of Washington in Seattle, reviewed the medication chapter for factual accuracy. His time and contributions are greatly appreciated.

The cover and the inside illustrations were drawn by my friend, Lucy Rigg. Her considerable talent has added a great deal to the total appearance and value of the book. I am thankful to her.

I must also thank those parents who allowed me to include their birth stories. Their personal accounts have added much to the total scope of the book. Thank you, too, to the scores of parents whose short comments appear throughout.

To Sandy Steffes, I would like to extend a special thanks, for she is the one who introduced us to the fascinating world of childbirth when I was pregnant with our first child. Her exciting and able instruction helped make my birth experiences positive and rewarding.

And thank you to my three little ladies—Alisa, Ami and Tria. My life would have very little meaning without them.

And to my Philip. Thank you for everything.

Vicki W. Walton
Seattle, Washington
April 1977

Table of Contents

Charts and Illustrations

Have It Your Way!

Childbirth in America has been folded, spindled and mutilated. In many cases the most beautiful process in life is nothing but a routine hospital "procedure." People who are perceptive enough to realize that the birth of a baby belongs to parents, rather than to the medical personnel serving them, must bring the focus in childbirth back to where it belongs—on the mother, on the father, on the baby and on the family that the birth is creating.

This book is written with the intention of helping you make your birth experience the best it can be. It is not about home births. It is about how to have a happy, satisfying, humanistic birth in a hospital situation. It is about how to take the "procedure" out of your birth experience.

I am not totally against home birth, but at this time, qualified medical aid is not available in many areas of the United States to assist with home deliveries. I believe very strongly that professional medical care during pregnancy and birth is essential for a safe experience. If couples know what questions to ask, and what alternatives are available in hospital birth, they will be much more successful in bringing the "home" into the hospital experience.

Sprinkled throughout the text are comments made by parents about their own birth experiences. The quotations were not written specifically for inclusion in this book; the comments were selected from birth reports in the hope that they would illustrate how prepared parents feel about various aspects of their own experiences.

The photographs are of our second baby's birth and immediate postpartum period. As this book went to press, the only books we would find with really good birth photographs were books directed toward home birth. I wanted to offer expectant parents the alternative of seeing what a hospital birth can be like.

I hope you enjoy the book, but much more, I hope you gain something from it that will help you have the best, most meaningful experience possible when your baby is born.

Childbirth American Style

It's easy to summarize the traditional view of childbirth in America. We've seen it countless times on movie and television screens. It goes something like this:

****

LIGHTS. CAMERA. ACTION.

Young couple enters hospital. Father appears panic-stricken as he searches for someone to do something. Spots admitting desk. While Father completes the necessary forms, Mother tells him the "pains" are getting worse. He writes faster. Humorous dialogue usually ensues. The last we see of Mother is when an orderly whisks her away in a wheelchair.

Shot of delivery room door.

Shot of Fathers' Waiting Room. Father is watching television with a rather glazed look on his face. Camera zooms on overflowing ashtray. Camera pans several paper coffee cups.

Shot of delivery room door.

Shot of nurse entering Fathers' Waiting Room. Father jumps to feet. He sinks back when she says (very patiently), "Not you, Mr. Jones."

Shot of delivery room door.

Shot of Father pacing nervously in Fathers' Waiting Room.

Shot of delivery room door. Add a baby's cry.

Shot of nursery window. Nurse holds up bundle of baby. Father looks very, very proud.

****

That's what we have been raised to believe the birth of a baby is like. However, there are several major things wrong with that concept of childbirth and the roles it forces parents and medical personnel to accept.

In the first place, the mother and the birth are locked away behind closed doors. Hospital doors, no less. Viewers (and the father) are left to imagine for themselves what might be happening to her behind those sterile doors. Our imaginations have a lot to work with. Rightly or wrongly, most people associate hospitals with pain, needles, operations and all sorts of other not very nice things. The utter disappearance of the mother serves to reinforce the myth that birth is mysterious, extremely painful, and something no one really has any control over. This hospital mystique firmly implants the notion that childbirth is an illness and must be treated as such.

In the second place, the father is treated like an outsider at the birth of his own baby. The separation of the couple supports the ridiculous theory that the father's part in the childbirth process is completed as soon as the egg is fertilized. In actuality, the father has not only a right, but a responsibility, to participate actively in the birth of his child.

It is best for the baby to be surrounded by a responsive family circle from the very beginning. A woman who has been subjected to the indignities, heavy medication and feelings of helplessness associated with traditional childbirth is in no condition to respond positively to her child, if at all, at the moment of birth.

And it is impossible for the father to respond to the baby if he is Out There Somewhere in the Fathers' Waiting Room. Meeting one's child for the first time through the heavy glass of a nursery window can't possibly produce the feeling of closeness that active participation in the birth can bring. Father participation and support during childbirth can strengthen both parent-parent bonds and parent-child bonds.

Childbirth, by its very nature, is a creative and positive experience. Yet most women who have given birth using traditional methods associate fear, pain and loneliness with childbirth. It is unfortunate so many people equate those negative feelings to a process which, if approached in a knowledgeable, informed way can produce feelings of dignity, confidence and joy. A birth shared by two people who care for each other is a growing experience.

It must be stated, however, that these women have good cause to remember their own experiences in such a negative light because the fear, pain and loneliness are natural by-products of the way they experienced their own labors and births. Extensive psychological and physiological explanations could probably be advanced, but actually the reasons can be stated very briefly. They simply took the Ostrich Approach to childbirth.

According to legend, the ostrich believes that what it can't see can't hurt it. Even though the ostrich is a big, powerful and fast bird, it reputedly hides its head in the sand instead of using its strengths to combat enemies. An astonishing number of women feel the same way about childbirth; what they don't know can't hurt them. I'm not sure how successful this negative approach is for the ostrich bird, but it is known to be notoriously unsuccessful for the human woman in labor.

The fear comes from not knowing what to expect during the birth process. Labor is a strange, new set of sensations. A hospital is an unfamiliar environment. When a woman does not understand what is happening within her own body, nor what to expect of her physical surroundings, she is consequently fearful. This fear causes the entire body to tense—the muscles to tighten up—against the uterine contractions. With this tenseness, the sensation of pain is multiplied immeasurably. Total relaxation coupled with helping one's body function most efficiently and concentrating on something other than feelings of discomfort, can reduce pain sensations considerably.

The source of the loneliness is obvious. In an Ostrich birth, the father, the one whose love and support a laboring woman needs the most, is relegated to the Fathers' Waiting Room. Why shouldn't she be lonely? Her main source of love, encouragement and strength is Out There Somewhere instead of next to her offering support.

The huge majority of Americans seems to accept the movie view of childbirth as their own. That's unfortunate. Actively sharing the birth experience in dignity and caring can be tremendously satisfying to both partners. Meeting the challenge of childbirth together can strengthen a family at a time of great change. A great deal of mutual respect can be developed during the process.

It may be a concern for the population explosion, or it may be a concern for family economics, but people are having fewer children these days. Chances are good you'll only have one or two babies in your lifetime. Do you want to experience childbirth in the traditional American way (the Ostrich Approach) or would you like something more dignified and satisfying for yourself, your family and your baby?

Childbirth the Prepared Way

Natural childbirth is really a misnomer. The general public accepts the term to mean simply childbirth without medication, and such a definition frightens most people, particularly pregnant women! People tend not to look beyond the incomplete "no medication" definition to see what is really involved. What this book and numerous childbirth education groups all over the country really are advocating is "prepared" childbirth. Educating the mother and father during the pregnancy prepares them for the labor, delivery and postpartum experience; thus the term "prepared childbirth" is really much more accurate than "natural childbirth."

The logical reaction upon walking into a dark room is to turn on the lights. Even familiar things can be frightening in the dark. The goal of childbirth education is to turn on the light. It shows the prospective parents what will happen during the total birth process. It shows them what to expect and how to manage their own birth experience. It is an alternative to the Ostrich Approach.

It is sad that some women reject the entire idea of childbirth education because "I could never make it without anesthetics, so what's the use of taking the class?" They don't realize what the real goals of childbirth education are. These women get stopped by the thought of no medication and look no further. They shut their eyes and start burying their heads in the sand. They become Ostriches.

To many, the mere thought of little or no medication during childbirth brings to mind women who are very, very brave. A lot of people think women who "had natural childbirth" or those who used prepared techniques spent hours "biting the bullet" and enduring great pain. What they actually did was spend hours of intense concentration doing the hardest work they had ever done. Labor is called labor because it is very hard work.

Often, apparently because of her training, the support of her coach, and her own self-image, the prepared woman does not feel the need or desire for medication during her labor and delivery. However, that is not the primary goal of childbirth education. The goal is to prepare the couple for anything that might happen during the childbirth process, and give them the tools to cope with it. The education also helps the couple to be intelligent consumers of the medical care they are paying for. In short, childbirth education seeks to make couples aware of the options available to them. By knowing what is possible and how to obtain proper medical support and cooperation, couples can make childbirth a positive and exciting experience.

Why reject all knowledge of the childbirth process because one may eventually want medication? Training helps a woman to enjoy a more comfortable labor whether or not she eventually chooses medication. Anesthetics cannot be given before a certain point in labor anyway, and having all the tools possible to cope with early labor can help a great deal. If the point comes when the mother, the father and the doctor feel the use of medication is advisable, that's acceptable. However, the parents have the responsibility to know what risks to both the mother and child are involved when medications and anesthetics are administered. Childbirth education classes offer this sort of information.

Specific methods of prepared childbirth differ to some degree, but all rely heavily upon educating the prospective parents. During the prenatal education, the couples learn about all aspects of the childbirth experience. Couples receive instruction in what to expect during a normal pregnancy, labor and delivery; complications and possible variations from the normal patterns; fetal development; what medications can be used at each point during labor and delivery; and how to deal with medical personnel to best accomplish a common goal in a manner suitable to all. Frequently the classes also cover related subjects such as prenatal nutrition, postpartum experiences and breastfeeding.

Couples are taught effective methods of breathing and relaxation for use during labor and delivery. Women are even taught ways to make pushing during the expulsive phase of labor more effective. Fathers are taught how to help the mother during the labor experience; they are taught how to recognize the progress of labor, thus enabling them to function as an effective link of communication between the mother and the medical personnel assigned to care for her in the hospital. An important outcome of childbirth education is the realization by the father that his support and involvement at the crucial time of childbirth can be a decisive factor in how his partner perceives the experience and views him in his role as a father. Fathers are definitely not mere spectators in prepared birth.

Prepared women find the dignity and active participation in some or all of the childbirth process to be extremely helpful to their own self-image and their baby's health, as well as beneficial to their relationship with the baby.

THE SKEPTICS

Childbirth education is a routine part of pregnancy in many countries. Until a thorough program of prenatal education becomes commonplace in America, skepticism will slow the progress of our childbirth educators. The woman who chooses to seek out information about her pregnancy, labor and delivery experience may encounter such skepticism on four major fronts: the father of the baby, relatives and friends who have given birth using the Ostrich Approach, relatives and friends who have never given birth, and (sadly) some medical people.

The Father

The father's opinion is the most important of the four. A woman can always change doctors and ignore friends, but she needs the father's support, because he is an important part of the process. Working through all aspects of the childbearing experience together can bring couples closer and add strength to the relationship. However, if the male partner feels his most important function on his child's birth day is to distribute cigars, it's easy to understand why. He is operating in a framework manufactured by Ostriches. He has probably been raised to believe the birth is not his concern; that it is exclusively "women's work." He has been molded by many years of television and peer pressure.

Even though his role as labor coach and supporter is integral in the prepared methods of childbirth, few fathers are excited (at first) about the prospect of attending childbirth education classes. Most men have a real concern that they may be the only man in a room filled to overflowing with pregnant women. Once a man realizes that that's not the case, and that the class offers him something concrete, something he can use at a specific time, he usually becomes more comfortable with the idea of learning about childbirth.

An important aspect of prepared childbirth is making the man aware of the vital part he plays in the process; it's his baby, too. Most men readily accept an active role in birth when they realize how important their support and participation are to the mother. Men who have accepted their role in the childbearing process are among the most enthusiastic supporters of preparation. No matter how busy fathers are, they realize after taking the classes that their time has not been wasted.

In cases where the father is either unavailable to participate (e.g., away in the service) or absolutely refuses to do so, a substitute labor and delivery coach can be utilized; however, it must be emphasized that the father is the best qualified for the role of labor coach. If it is necessary to choose a substitute coach, do so carefully. A person with whom you share a close, caring relationship would be the best choice. A parent, sister, brother or friend could be appropriate, provided you have the proper relationship. The person who is planning to serve as your coach should attend the classes with you.

Most prepared fathers accompany their partners into the delivery room as well as into the labor room, but some men balk at this. Television conditioning may have something to do with this, but peer pressure is probably even a bigger influence. Men actually get hassled about delivery room plans by their friends ("You're not really going to watch that, are you?"). It is a certainty that none of the men who ask that question in incredulous tones were prepared fathers themselves. They were Male Ostriches. Some probably even feel subconsciously guilty about abandoning their own women during childbirth. Delivery is the culmination of months of waiting and hours of close teamwork by the prepared couple. In addition to the fact that the woman needs his presence in the delivery room as much as in the labor room, it is definitely the most exciting, fulfilling and rewarding event in the childbirth experience. It is, after all, the goal of the whole process. Missing the birth is like not reading the last chapter of a mystery.

Men who do choose to go into the delivery room enjoy the experience. Some are absolutely fascinated by the process and by the realization that they helped bring about this miracle. Fathers who go into the delivery room spend a lot of time later encouraging other men to do the same thing. On the other hand, fathers who do not choose to attend the birth frequently wish they had the decision to make again.

Relatives and Friends Who Have Given Birth Using the Ostrich Approach

Women who have had children using traditional methods involving heavy or total anesthetization sometimes have almost violent reactions when they talk about childbirth education. The most typical comment is something like, "I don't want to know a thing about it, just knock me out!" Listen politely, but don't take them too seriously. They are merely equating childbirth education to their definition of natural childbirth (suffering without anesthetics). Remember that they have actually been a part of the Ostrich Approach.

Even though you don't need to hear them, nor want to hear them, women will probably insist on telling you about their own Ostrich experiences (often in gory detail). Reading, and talking to couples who have used prepared techniques are effective ways to dilute the negative influence that the gory stories of suffering can produce. In response to a really persistent purveyor of doom, tell her you'd rather not discuss it further now, but that you'd be happy to compare experiences after you've had the baby.

Do remember, when dealing with this sort of woman, that she probably did have a rotten experience in childbirth. Her lack of knowledge, coupled with her fear, simply produced a tense, painful situation. And she probably had to go it alone, with no support from her partner. Your experience has nothing to do with hers; nor does your present experience have anything to do with a bad experience you may have had in the past. Approaching childbirth in an intelligent manner always helps.

Relatives and Friends Who Have Never Given Birth

These women try to project their own fears onto you. Surely you don't need their fears; you probably have enough of your own. They've spent a lot of time watching television births and talking to Ostriches. So have you.

You may get some interesting comments if you ask women whether they would like to be "knocked out" just before the wedding ceremony, and awakened several hours after the ceremony with no recollection of what happened in between. The only way they could be certain who it was they married is by looking to see who has a matching wedding band.

Medical People

Lots of doctors thrive, financially and egotistically, on the Ostrich Approach. In an unprepared birth the doctor is the central figure. In a prepared birth, all the doctor has to do is monitor the woman's progress and offer encouragement during labor as long as things progress normally. When the time for the actual birth arrives, s/he coaches the woman, tells her when to push, and "catches" the baby. S/he is not the powerful, omnipotent being that a doctor is in an unprepared birth. In an unprepared birth when the woman cannot push her baby out, the doctor must pull it out. Many doctors can't accept the fairly minor role accorded them during a prepared birth.

Some doctors understand and support a woman's desire for individuality, dignity and active participation in her birth experience. These same doctors realize the benefits to the baby of being pushed out instead of pulled out. Find one of these doctors. If you discover your doctor prefers a more traditional approach than you'd like, you are free to change doctors at any time during your pregnancy, until the day you deliver. However, if you choose your medical caretakers carefully in the beginning, you'll have no need to change in midstream.

BUILDING CONFIDENCE

You have enough to worry about without letting the skeptics chip away your confidence. It's normal to be frightened. No matter how much you may hear in class, this is still a new experience to you. You, too, have watched all of those television programs and talked to all of those Ostriches.

Concentrate on talking to couples who have used, or are planning to use prepared childbirth techniques. They are terrific morale builders. Couples who have had both unprepared deliveries and prepared births are especially enthusiastic about the prepared techniques. Seek them out.

I became interested in "natural" childbirth after witnessing the birth of a baby where the mother was asleep. It seemed so wrong for this mother to miss completely the birth of her baby.

With the birth of this baby, after taking the classes and sharing the experience with Tom, I had a feeling of elation I never experienced with my other two births, and I find it difficult to describe my emotions.

I remember being very afraid, even though I knew what was going to happen. But as soon as everything started, the fear went away. I was so busy remembering what to do and trying to stay awake, that there was not time to be afraid. It is nothing like the "screaming movie terror" Hollywood has produced.

Whether they choose to employ the techniques learned during labor and delivery is a decision only the couples can make; however, just knowing what is happening to the body and the aids available is of tremendous value. Not all daddies feel they belong in the delivery room, but I feel that parenthood is a shared experience.

He wasn't wild about the idea of being in the delivery room, but told me to find out more about the classes if I wanted to. As the months went by, the

more I thought about it, the more I decided I wanted to attend the classes for my own benefit so I would know what was happening inside me during labor. The thought of labor scared me because I had always heard it was very painful . . . As the doctor repaired the episiotomy, Allan and I watched every move Michelle made and everything the nurse did to her. We realize now that prepared childbirth is the only way to have a baby and are preaching the method to all our family and friends.

We enjoyed the classes very much, but Rich was afraid he just couldn't go through with being in the delivery room. It did hurt me that he felt he couldn't do it, but I made up my mind that I would absolutely leave it up to him. If he wanted to join me for delivery, I would be thrilled, but if he felt he couldn't do it, I felt that after our classes I could do it by myself if I had to. Rich and I hadn't talked any more about whether he would come into the delivery room, but as I went in I looked over my shoulder and there he was in a hospital gown and mask. He told all of our friends about the experience and even offered some encouragement to some fathers who were, like himself, pretty skeptical about the childbirth experience.

Childbirth is the most fantastic experience that has ever happened to us. We would not have missed it for anything.

Peter's involvement and the satisfaction we experienced in sharing the birth of our child is beyond expression.

When I know what to expect, I always feel more secure in a situation.

It is a glorious feeling to know that I gave birth to my child in complete awareness and control. John was present and able to witness the beauty of the birth of his child in an atmosphere of exuberant joy rather than one of agony and fear.

The birth of our baby was one of the most rewarding moments of our lives and we wouldn't trade the experience for anything. I feel that everyone should attend childbirth education classes even if they plan to have medication. Knowing what's happening gives you a greater insight into the birth of the child.

Even though I didn't have an unmedicated birth, I am so thankful for the experience and knowledge that the childbirth education classes gave me. This was our third child and I never realized all of the fascinating things that happen to a woman throughout her pregnancy and labor.

It was long, hard and a painful experience, but the three of us shared it and no one can take that away from us. We also feel very strongly that it strengthened our marriage.

I wanted my coach with me at all times but I did keep telling him to "shut up" and "leave me alone." He knew I didn't really mean these things. He kept on encouraging me, kept me breathing right, and reminding me to relax. A few times I couldn't stay on top of the contractions, but his encouragement kept me going.

We wish to thank our childbirth instructor and our doctor for enabling our family to be truly together from the very beginning.

My childbirth experience was extremely satisfying! The classes were very beneficial and I can't imagine how we could have had such an experience without them. The sharing we partook in during the classes, labor and delivery is continuing on as we care for our new daughters (twins).

We enjoyed the classes and the closeness we were able to experience in preparing for and participating in the birth of our son.

It was the most beautiful experience that Jesse and I could ever have together. Having prepared for childbirth, we can now look back and know and understand everything that happened during our baby's journey to the outer world. Although the mystery of such a miracle still lies above our comprehension, we were able to be there to greet our baby fully conscious and ready, awake and aware.

I felt this was a great experience, particularly because of our sharing it. We both have much more confidence in handling the baby, too, because it was a family experience.

The whole birth experience was really neat. Gordon was so excited and happy that he couldn't eat for two days. He is really glad that he could be in the delivery room.

My first labor was 36 hours long and I was only 18. I was alone in the labor room, not knowing what was going on and poor George was out in the Fathers' Waiting Room. After about 7 or 8 hours, they asked him to go home, saying it would be a while before I'd give birth. I didn't see George until the next day, and then only for 5 minutes. After giving birth to our first daughter I felt as if I'd been through the war and lost! I made sure with my second pregnancy that we would be together and that we would be prepared parents.

Methods of Childbirth Preparation

Read, Lamaze and Bradley are the best known methods of childbirth preparation in this country. The oldest of the methods are Read and Lamaze, and it is these that are the most widespread in America. In addition to Read, Lamaze and Bradley, Sheila Kitzinger, Erna Wright and Margaret Gamper have all been extremely active in the childbirth education movement, and their influence is being felt throughout the field.

All of the techniques use special breathing and relaxation and all attempt to educate the participants about the physiology of childbirth. The methods differ mainly in the specific breathing patterns, and the specific comfort-producing behaviors taught to couples for use during labor. All prepared childbirth philosophies have the common goals of making the birth experience personally satisfying and safe.

Many classes do not maintain a strict interpretation of any one method. Instructors often adapt the methods, drawing upon each for what she feels will best serve the needs of her particular students.

GRANTLY DICK-READ

Grantly Dick-Read of Great Britain is the acknowledged pioneer of prepared childbirth. He is the originator of the term "natural childbirth" which, unfortunately, is still used popularly to define unmedicated birth, whether or not the woman has received any childbirth training. Dr. Read himself did not object to the use of medication or anesthetics in obstetrical conditions where the mother or the child was in danger. He merely contended that women who are adequately prepared, earnestly supported and unafraid have a greatly reduced need and desire for medications.

In 1933, Dr. Read began to question the necessity of pain during childbirth after attending the delivery of a woman who refused the chloroform mask, the common form of pain relief during childbirth at the time. Dr. Read was understandably confused—no one had ever refused his offer of chloroform before. As he left, he asked her why she had refused. Her answer started his deep inquiry into the causes and preventions of pain in childbirth. Her answer was simply, "It didn't hurt. It wasn't meant to, was it, Doctor?"

Dr. Read began to observe that the most peaceful women, those who were the least fearful of childbirth, had the least painful births. He came to believe that the mystical qualities of birth and the joy would transcend the discomfort in childbirth if it were not for the pain-producing fear attendant in the majority of births in civilized societies. He identified the fear-tension-pain cycle in childbirth.

According to this theory, the fear of pain will actually cause true pain because of pathological tension. Once the fear-tension-pain cycle is established, it perpetuates itself. The fear causes true pain which in turn causes fear of more pain. In addition to being an obvious hazard to the possibility of a positive experience in childbirth, the cycle, if severe and persistent enough, can be dangerous to the mother and baby. When circulation of blood is restricted due to prolonged tension of uterine muscles, oxygen supply is diminished. Excessive intra-uterine pressure caused by uncontrollable fear and tension, coupled with the restricted oxygen supply, can cause severe fetal distress.

From his extensive inquiry into the part fear plays in childbirth, Dr. Read developed a program of preparation which consisted of educating the expectant mother about pregnancy, labor and delivery, relaxation, physical conditioning, and controlled breathing. The education was designed to alleviate the fears, thus stopping short the fear-tension-pain syndrome. Dr. Read's methods of relaxation were designed to counteract physical tension occurring during labor and delivery as well as reduce the degree of pain felt. The physical conditioning attempted to prepare the body for the work of labor in the belief that the pain threshold is lowered when the body is not in peak condition. Dr. Read taught methods of abdominal breathing for use during uterine contractions in an effort to reduce the amount of pressure exerted upon the uterus, thus freeing the uterine muscles to work more efficiently. This more efficient functioning could lead to shorter labors as well as decrease the amount of possible pain.

Emotional support for the woman from the father, as well as medical personnel, was important to Read's theories, but he did not utilize the labor coach as extensively as most present methods do.

The Read method tends to be too vague for many women, and teaches women a rather passive demeanor to use in labor. This lack of concrete action, coupled with skepticism from the medical community, probably accounts for the fact that the Read method did not spread rapidly. Read's observation of childbirth as a natural physiological function and theories involving the reduction of pain through the removal of fear were useful as preludes to the acceptance of later methods of preparing childbirth which gave the couple more concrete training for the birth experience.

FERNAND LAMAZE

The most widespread method of preparation is the Lamaze method. This method, with numerous adaptations, is the one most widely used in the United States. Fernand Lamaze, a French obstetrician, visited the Soviet Union in 1951 and observed women giving birth using Pavlovian techniques.

Ivan Pavlov was a Russian physiologist whose theory of conditioned reflex helps to explain how the brain responds to stimuli. His landmark studies proving that dogs can be taught to respond to artificial stimuli are a basis of modern psychology. It is a natural reflex for a dog to salivate when presented with food. Pavlov repeatedly rang a bell at the same time he presented food to the dogs. Eventually the dogs would salivate upon hearing the bell ring, even when no food was presented. This reaction is called a conditioned response because the response was learned; normally a dog would not salivate upon hearing a bell ring. The repeated coupling of the food and the bell caused the dogs to salivate in response to an artificial stimulus.

Even though the object was obviously not to train a laboring woman to salivate to the sound of a bell, Lamaze felt the Pavlovian theory of conditioned response could be applied effectively to childbirth. The untrained reaction to a powerful uterine contraction is to resist the power of the contraction by tensing first the surrounding muscles, and ultimately the whole body. This tension and resistance causes the discomfort to magnify and expand. Training and practice can teach a woman to respond in a different, more efficient way to the contraction. This new response—relaxation and lack of tension—is not the "natural" reaction, it is not the instinctive method of response; it is the conditioned response.

Lamaze returned to France with the impressions, theories and knowledge gained in the Soviet Union and developed a method that more suited his own patients' needs. In addition to the use of conditioned response, Lamaze advocates the use of visual, mental and physical distraction as a method of pain limitation during labor. The distraction comes in the form of breathing patterns, use of a focal point during contractions, and effleurage. Effleurage is a light massage performed on the laboring woman's abdomen by either the mother or her coach; this massage can be physically soothing and comforting to a woman as well as being an effective distraction.

Distraction methods are used because active concentration on a planned distraction serves to block out painful stimuli the brain may otherwise record.

Lamaze childbirth techniques involve the use of a labor coach. The pregnant woman and her coach devise a workable system of stimuli and responses for use during labor and delivery. The trained woman will respond to her coach's commands; these may be physical, oral or visual. Her conditioned reflex will be the necessary relaxation and lack of tension. In France this coach is usually a trained female called a monitrice. In the United States the father assumes this role in most prepared births. In this capacity, the father is able to help his partner direct her birth experience through use of commands and support. Through this teamwork the birth becomes a shared experience.

The Lamaze method of childbirth preparation is a psychoprophylactic approach to the birth experience. As such, it prepares the couple physically, psychologically, emotionally and intellectually for the birth process.

During the training period the correct responses are practiced, and when a woman goes into labor, she consciously uses the appropriate relaxation and breathing techniques. Use of the term "learned" or "automatic" response is sometimes used in place of "conditioned" response.

ROBERT A. BRADLEY

Robert Bradley is a Denver obstetrician who has developed a method of childbirth preparation he calls Husband-Coached Childbirth. His method began with an interest in the Read method, but he's made some important modifications. Bradley, like Read, believes in the power of serenity in making birth a pleasant, positive experience. The role of the father-coach in helping to create and maintain such serenity during the entire childbirth experience, including the pregnancy, is of extreme importance in the Bradley method.

Bradley does not find serenity and excitement to be incompatible. He actively promotes the excitement inherent in birth. He has found that when couples are properly prepared and accept the physiology of childbirth as natural, they are able to participate fully in the birth and, consequently, in the excitement surrounding the birth.

Bradley is firmly convinced of the positive value of the father's active participation throughout the birth process. His method is based upon imitating the instinctual behavior of mammals in labor. Mammals instinctively relax during labor and appear to experience no pain during the birth. Because he is advocating behavior and practices which are apparently instincts throughout the animal world, Bradley calls his techniques "true natural childbirth."

Bradley advocates a prenatal preparation program consisting of childbirth education; exercise; his own specific breathing and relaxation techniques; and thorough preparation of the father. Bradley stresses the value of the father's support and guidance to the laboring woman. He encourages each father to use his own intimate knowledge of his partner to help her achieve the common goal of a self-directed birth. Because he knows her so well, and can communicate in such special ways, the father can be a much more potent, positive influence during the crucial process of childbirth than can unfamiliar medical personnel.

Choosing Childbirth Education Classes

Education is at the very heart of prepared childbirth. Originally, childbirth education focused almost entirely on the actual period of labor and delivery. The trend now is to broaden class content to encompass a more total view of the childbirth experience. The emotional aspects of pregnancy and parenthood, infant care and feeding, and examination of postpartum adjustments are some of the additional areas covered in this expanded view of childbirth education.

Today the three basic components of childbirth education are factual information about pregnancy, labor and delivery; physical conditioning, relaxation techniques and breathing patterns; and information about breastfeeding, postpartum experiences and infant care.

Childbirth education is available from a wide variety of sources. Some of the more common sources are:

1. Classes offered by non-profit groups that exist solely to promote and teach childbirth education
2. Classes taught by private instructors trained to teach expectant parents
3. Classes offered by public service groups such as the Red Cross and YWCA
4. Classes offered by hospitals
5. Classes offered by doctors for their patients
6. Books and films

The quality, quantity and focus of the childbirth education received can greatly affect a couple's preparation for and perception of the birth experience.

Because of the predominance of the Ostrich Approach, very few American women know much about childbirth until they are pregnant. Even then many do not actively seek information. Often all a woman knows about the birth itself, even as her own delivery approaches, is what she has heard from other women (quite often women who have had extremely negative experiences in childbirth). This lack of qualified instruction and factual information usually leads to a feeling of fear on the part of the pregnant woman. Contrary to the belief of some, merely having had a baby does not automatically qualify a woman to give definitive information about "what it is like."

Qualified childbirth educators are individuals who have received special training in teaching expectant parents and are able to give extensive factual information based upon medical science, observation, specialized reading and (usually) personal experience. Most are dedicated to presenting the childbirth experience in a positive, but objective light. Hopefully the presentation of such information will not only help the couple during labor and delivery by reducing fear of the unknown, but will also make the pregnancy and postpartum experiences more pleasant

Factual Information About Pregnancy, Labor and Delivery

Understanding the reasons for physical and emotional changes during the pregnancy period can help couples become more comfortable with themselves and each other during this time of change. This comfort and knowledge can lead the couple to explore their own feelings and come to the realization that what they are experiencing both individually and as a couple is common. Numerous physical and emotional changes throughout the birth experience are inevitable.

Tremendous adjustments of all sorts must be made during the pregnancy period. Most of the changes and adjustments are interdependent. Some of the physical changes lead to emotional stresses. For example, aside from the changes in simple physical mobility and capability that the woman must make, she may have to cope with the feeling that she is no longer attractive to her partner. The father, in turn, must deal with woman's increased needs for reassurance while he is also adjusting to the changes in her appearance. Some parents do not have to deal with this particular problem; some men and women feel pregnant women are very beautiful.

Some of the stresses are purely emotional. Both parents are coping with the jumble of feelings and emotions that approaching parenthood is bound to produce. It is common for prospective parents, even those who desperately want children, to have second thoughts during the pregnancy. Changes in lifestyle, to some degree, are almost certain after the birth. A baby is a big and permanent responsibility. If expectant parents do not deal with the realization that some things will change during the expansion from couple to family, the parents will probably have a much harder time accepting the inevitable changes that a baby causes. The wants, needs and demands of a tiny baby are not tiny.

Being able to identify and discuss concerns about the baby, each other and the relationship can strengthen the relationship during a critical time of change. Such a strengthened relationship can offer the baby a much more secure family unit, a unit better able to handle the stresses of parenthood and parental responsibility.

A major stress, particularly for the mother, is the fear that the baby will not be normal and healthy. Disturbing dreams and thoughts about the possibility of deformity and death (both fetal and maternal) are quite common. Open expression of these feelings can provide a great deal of comfort and reassurance.

Very seldom are we free to experience something and react spontaneously. No matter what the event, we have probably formed some sort of impressions before we are able to touch the happening ourselves. These preconceived notions come from a myriad of past talk, sensory perceptions, dreams and expectations. All of these serve to color our perception of an event. Childbirth is an experience which is especially clouded by half-truths, misconceptions, and fear. For years we have heard uterine contractions called "labor pains," so it's logical for a pregnant woman to assume labor must be painful. Most babies are born in hospitals; hospitals are for sick, incapacitated people. In short, we have been led to "know" that childbirth is a painful, incapacitating thing that happens to us. How positive an attitude can a woman be expected to have when she's been conditioned to believe all of that? And why should any man want to be involved in watching such "ugly, inevitable things" happening to the woman he loves?

Factual information about the process of labor and delivery can lead couples to understand that they can both be active participants rather than passive receptors during the birth of their child. The dignity of a self-controlled childbirth experience cannot be overstressed. Knowing what is happening within her own body can increase a woman's self-respect as well as enable her to help things happen more efficiently.

Learning about hospital equipment and procedures ahead of time can help a couple to know what to expect when they enter the hospital.

Labor and delivery information focuses on correcting false impressions, calming fears and re-conditioning couples to accept childbirth as a natural, healthy physiological process.

Physical Conditioning, Relaxation Techniques and Breathing Patterns

Labor and delivery are physically stressful experiences. As with any other physical endeavor, the body in good condition, with the proper muscles prepared, will function more efficiently than an out-of-condition body. Good muscle tone and correct posture can make the entire birth experience, from early pregnancy through postpartum, more comfortable.

Muscle support and proper posture can help to relieve backache and other discomforts common to pregnancy. A woman in good physical condition will tire less easily during labor; the extra energy available and the trained response of proper muscles both contribute to making her pushing more effective during the expulsive phase of labor.

Breathing techniques serve two basic purposes: leaving the uterine muscles undisturbed so they can complete their job most efficiently, and giving the woman something to concentrate on, thus reducing the sensation of discomfort she may feel during the contractions. Clinical observation in several countries indicates that the precise pattern of breathing a laboring woman uses is not of crucial importance; it is her intense concentration on the breathing patterns, not the patterns in themselves, which serves to reduce the awareness of pain. Many physicians and childbirth educators, including Dr. Pierre Vellay, an early advocate of childbirth education, contend that the ability to relax is the real key to pain relief; the breathing techniques act as a distraction from the pain stimuli.[1]

Concentration on breathing rather than on the uterine contraction can be compared to a host of everyday activities. When you smash your thumb with a hammer, it hurts a great deal until you can get your mind on something else. When you start watching television, reading a book or talking to someone, the pain subsides. Even emotional pain reacts this way. If a lonely person concentrates constantly on his loneliness, he will soon become an extremely lonely person —he will turn inward and be so filled with his own misery that he will lose the ability to communicate with others.

Information About Breastfeeding, Postpartum Experiences and Infant Care

Even though breastfeeding is obviously the most natural way to feed an infant, many American women have difficulties, both physical and emotional, concerned with breastfeeding. The female breast is considered an absolute symbol of sexuality in our culture, and it is often difficult for a woman or man to accept it as anything else. Babies are small and helpless and pure. Some people have a hard time associating the innocence of the child to the sexuality of the breast. Some women are overly concerned about the prospect of nursing the baby in public. Information about breastfeeding, including its physical and emotional advantages, is most helpful to the expectant couple. Men, too, have misgivings about their partner breastfeeding the baby.

Facts and discussion can help prospective parents sort out their own feelings, and help them make an informed choice based upon solid reasoning rather than on how Aunt Mary or the next door neighbor fed her babies. Factual information and sharing of personal experiences can help couples choose the method of infant feeding that most readily fits into their own lifestyle.

Postpartum, the period following the birth, can be a jolting experience. It can be compared to the day after your birthday. Much of the fun of getting a present is the wondering what it is. The not knowing is exciting—there is something to look forward to. After you open the big gold box with the shiny red ribbon, some of the excitement is bound to disappear, no matter how much you like what was inside. Aside from this loss of day-to-day anticipation and excitement, new parents have many adjustments to make.

Frank discussion of the situations that may be encountered, and the feelings that may be felt during the postpartum period will help new parents make the transition from couple to family as smoothly as possible. Parents are not nearly so likely to be overwhelmed when they are aware ahead of time of the problems that might develop.

When to Take Classes

In most instances, childbirth education classes are designed to be taken during the last 9 to 12 weeks of pregnancy. This timing usually assures that the couple will complete the classes before delivery, yet will not be finished with the classes so far in advance of labor that they become bored with the exercises and breathing techniques and quit practicing them. Even though the classes are usually taken this late in the pregnancy, it is good to check earlier regarding sources in your area. Some areas have a real shortage of childbirth education teachers, and classes fill up fast.

CHOOSING CHILDBIRTH EDUCATION CLASSES

In some areas of the country there is only one source of childbirth preparation classes; in others numerous classes are offered by a variety of sources. When there's a choice, it should be made carefully. The particular method of preparation is not so important as the depth of the preparation. Many factors can influence the quality and quantity of education received.

Class size is an important consideration. Classes should be small enough to provide a feeling of intimacy, but large enough to allow a wide variety of input. One of the most valuable aspects of childbirth classes is the feeling of camaraderie that expectant couples share. Problems, fears, hopes and dreams connected with birth are similar whether the income level is $5,000 or $20,000. Pregnant tummies from Maine to California can make sleeping difficult.

Discussion of common problems and concerns can lead to imaginative and useful suggestions. The common bond between expectant parents can produce an atmosphere of mutual support. However, the desirable feeling of intimacy won't develop as readily in a group that is too large. It's impossible to say absolutely what the optimum class size is, but 5 to 9 couples seems to be a good size.

The classes can provide an important opportunity for couples to express their own fears. Until they have used the breathing and relaxation techniques in an actual labor/delivery situation, most couples are skeptical of the effectiveness. They have the attitude that it all sounds good, but they aren't sure it will really work. Expression of these concerns to an Ostrich can be unsettling. Ostriches usually waste no time exposing the "absurdity" of "natural childbirth"; and it is difficult to argue with Ostriches who have "been through it" and "know what it's like." Honest discussion about fears, concerns and questions within the supportive environment of the childbirth preparation class can serve to build confidence in the methods.

The student-teacher ratio should be favorable enough so that each couple receives a fair amount of individualized attention. Assistants are utilized in some classes to help achieve this end, but students should still receive attention from the primary instructor during each session. The breathing and relaxation techniques are not difficult, but they are new to most couples and require concentration to learn. Daily practice is recommended for the expectant couples, so it is important that they are practicing correctly. Individualized attention during class can correct mistakes and help couples develop confidence in their abilities.

Fathers (or some other labor coach) should be encouraged to attend classes with the mother. The instruction should be geared not only to giving information relevant to the mother's conduct during labor and delivery, but to helping the labor coach to develop effective behaviors to help the mother. Even though the basic assumption as evidenced throughout the course should be that the woman will be accompanied at least during labor by a coach of her choosing, women who have no coach should not be excluded from the classes. Childbirth education instructors should be able to supply labor coaches to women who need them. The ideal labor coach is a person with whom the mother shares a warm, caring relationship; but if necessary, another person can substitute. Continuous support and coaching of the laboring woman is essential to methods of prepared childbirth.

Find out how many hours of instruction are offered in the series. Classes usually meet once weekly for 6-10 weeks. Each session is typically 2-3 hours long. If a particular series of classes meets for a total of only 12 hours, most of that time will have to be spent on breathing and relaxation techniques and information that relates directly to labor and delivery in order to adequately prepare couples. Classes that meet for 16 or more hours can usually afford to spend more time discussing postpartum experiences, breastfeeding and related subjects without sacrificing labor/delivery preparation. The number of hours given here is only a guideline; obviously some instructors make better use of time than others. But do remember that the basic function of the childbirth preparation class is preparation for the labor and delivery experience. Related information and discussion is helpful, indeed extremely desirable, but shouldn't be given at the expense of adequate preparation for the directed birth experience.

Rehearsal of the physical techniques and methods usually constitutes approximately one half of the total class time. The breathing and relaxation techniques are most successful when the couple is totally knowledgeable about them, and practice is essential.

The need for detailed factual information is met in most classes; however, feelings, attitudes and emotional adjustments are sometimes ignored. Again, essential practice and rehearsal time shouldn't be sacrificed, but the psychological aspects of the birth experience should be included in the program of instruction if it is at all possible within the time framework.

In most cases, the cost of the classes probably shouldn't be the deciding factor of which course to take. The price of the series doesn't necessarily correlate with the quality of instruction offered. The most expensive classes are not always the best classes; nor are the least expensive classes always the poorest. But, then again, a class shouldn't be chosen simply because it is the least expensive one available. Careful examination of the course content, the instructor's qualifications and the sponsoring organization is the best way to choose a childbirth education class that will meet your needs.

If the cost of a particular series of classes proves to be a serious problem, most groups offer some sort of financial aid (e.g., partial payment, installment payment, free tuition) to hardship cases. The military CHAMPUS program and some public and private health programs will cover the cost of childbirth education for expectant parents.

The cost of childbirth education, and people's reaction to it, is interesting. Before the birth, most couples consider childbirth education a luxury, an unnecessary expense. After the birth the same couples normally consider the class fee an essential expense and spend a great deal of time convincing their pregnant friends to spend money on childbirth education classes.

The childbirth educator must be totally knowledgeable about her field. Because her function is as an educator rather than as a medical advisor, it is not necessary for a qualified instructor to be a Registered Nurse (R.N.) or a Registered Physical Therapist (R.P.T.). Certainly medical training is a good base, but not the only base. Many nurses have had very little obstetric experience beyond a basic obstetrics class, and both medical and non-medical personnel should complete an extensive childbirth study program before teaching classes to expectant parents.

The study program should be designed to familiar-ize the teacher trainee with all aspects of the childbirth experience, with emphasis on the "normal" pregnancy, labor and birth. The training should include information about methods of prepared childbirth, the reproductive anatomy, fetal and placental development, basic nutrition, physiological changes of pregnancy, physical changes associated with pregnancy, labor progression, labor complications, medications, breastfeeding and the newborn baby. This is all factual information.

In addition to knowing facts, she must know "how" to teach, how to discuss and deal with the many emotions that students bring to the childbirth education class. She must be able to present information to her students in a way that will help them choose what is right for them; not in a way that dictates what she thinks is "right." She must be familiar with the hospital procedures her students will probably encounter. She must know about what alternatives her students' doctors encourage and discourage. She must care about her work, care about her students, and be enthusiastic.

The childbirth educator is not trying to replace qualified medical care, nor usurp the doctor's authority. She is not in the business of dispensing medical advice. She is not teaching a do-it-yourself how-to-have-a-baby course. She is teaching about the physical and emotional processes of childbearing and making the couples aware of alternatives available in their childbirth experience. This teaching complements the qualified medical care the patient should be receiving.

Many expectant couples are more comfortable with, and have more confidence in, an instructor who has herself given birth. The confidence level rises even further if she has used prepared childbirth techniques and can speak from "experience." Since breastfeeding is covered fairly extensively in many childbirth education classes, it may be desirable if the instructor has successfully breastfed a baby.

The instructor can make a great deal of difference in the couple's perception of the birth experience and in their perception of themselves as related to the total childbearing and parenting experience. Trust in an instructor can instill a good deal of confidence in the techniques and bring the couple closer together in the birth process.

Non-profit childbirth education organizations have been spreading across the nation since the early 1950's. These groups usually have well-trained teachers and uniform, well-developed teaching materials. In most of the non-profit organizations much of the personpower is provided by volunteer efforts. Many of the groups sponsor public information meetings, film showings, speakers' bureau presentations, newsletters and outreach programs entirely with unpaid volunteers. As a rule the instructors and only a handful of the administrators are paid for their work. Volunteers are usually parents who have completed the group's classes and who are enthusiastic about what childbirth education did for them. Even the people who are paid, including the instructors, normally don't make a very good salary.

Despite the volunteer and semi-volunteer help, class fees must be enough to cover expenses such as postage, printing, office supplies, telephone, films, visual aids for instructors, teacher-training programs, and many more miscellaneous expenses. If it appears the class fee is too high, obtain an accounting of where the money goes in the organization. And do remember to check class size.

Established non-profit groups may have a working rapport with the medical community in your area. If the group has a good reputation, and the couples who have taken classes are usually well-prepared, the hospital staff will probably be more inclined to let students of that group accept more responsibility for their own experience. This is not to say the couple will receive less meticulous medical care; it is to say they may be allowed more freedom and greater privacy in directing their experience.

Classes offered by private instructors can be preferable to others in that they are often smaller, more intimate classes. The private instructor has probably had some contact with her students individually before the first class starts, so an atmosphere of support and friendship sometimes develops more quickly. Private instructors frequently work mostly with one or two doctors, and as a result have a very good working relationship with those doctors. A woman who works on her own has usually collected a variety of materials and developed her own, taking what she likes best from many sources. When she is teaching privately it is easy for her to incorporate new materials and information immediately into her class structure. This is usually not feasible in larger, more "committeed" organizations; material to be distributed in class must often pass an education committee, a parent committee, an instructor committee, etc., before it can be made available to students. Research is constantly being done in the childbearing and related fields, and the most up-to-date information can make birth experiences better and better.

The private instructor can afford to be more outspoken than can an instructor for a large group. She has only herself and her students to serve; she doesn't have to please a broad group of parents, group administrators and other instructors.

Private instructors will probably be harder to find than the other sources of childbirth education. Fewer students means less money for large circulation publicity, less word-of-mouth publicity, and less community involvement. However, fewer students also means more individual attention for students both during class time and during the postpartum period.

Private instructors are not bound by local organization teacher qualifications, so it is more important to ascertain the individual's personal qualifications. A competent, well-trained instructor will be happy to discuss her background in childbirth education with prospective students. In addition, she'll often supply the names of several of her former students as references.

Many private instructors are affiliated with national childbirth education organizations, so have extensive support with respect to teacher materials and visual aids.

National public service organizations, such as Red Cross and the YWCA, have many programs designed to improve health care and health awareness. Some offer classes for expectant parents as a part of their broader programs. As a rule the classes are free to the public, or are offered at a very nominal fee. The Red Cross class, for example, offers information about labor and delivery; nutrition; breast care; the baby's needs; bathing the baby; and the first year of the baby's life. For years these classes have been a good place to learn how to bathe, dress and care for a newborn infant. Recently the Red Cross has included what they call "adapted" breathing techniques in the 12-hour course. With the addition of the breathing techniques, the course is moving in the direction of becoming a true birth preparation course. However, for couples who are truly concerned about being adequately prepared for the period of labor and delivery, a class which covers exercise, relaxation and breathing techniques in much more detail is highly recommended. The expectant parent course is one of many programs offered by the Red Cross; it is not the only focus of the group as it is for the non-profit childbirth group.

Many hospitals offer courses to couples who plan to deliver at that particular hospital. How much information regarding the pregnancy and birth is given in the classes varies greatly from hospital to hospital. Some classes exist only as a short orientation to the hospital, and some are full-blown childbirth preparation classes. These courses are very good for acquainting couples with the exact routines they will encounter in their hospital.

Seeing the admitting area, the labor and delivery rooms, the nursery, and the other facilities can make the surroundings seem more familiar when the couple arrives in labor. Couples can ask questions about the

s which will be followed when the
s admitted. They can find out what
work can be completed in advance.
what access the laboring couple will
s, blankets and extra pillows. The
le to question the labor and delivery
ertain what attitudes exist toward
h, thus giving the couple some idea
y will receive during labor.
maternity care that aren't routinely
pital aren't stressed in classes offered
information may be geared toward
nt hospital procedures. Due to mul-
s, hospital courses are sometimes not
y could be.
uld probably be taken as an orienta-
d, but whether to depend upon them
on for the birth experience depends
eteness and bias of the particular
at classes offered in hospital facilities
fered by the hospital. In some cases
ups or instructors are merely using
each their own classes. In this case the
ely a location, not an "influencing"
factor.

Some doctors, albeit very few, have an organized class for their prenatal patients. These classes fall in much the same category as the classes offered by hospitals; they are very good for acquainting couples with the doctor's customary procedures and preferences. Sometimes, even though the course may be very complete and give good training in relaxation and breathing techniques, the material may serve to legitimize the doctor's routine care rather than offer access to innovative alternatives in maternity care. If a doctor is very supportive of family-centered maternity care and prepared childbirth, this situation may not present a problem. S/he is probably offering many alternatives to patients, and the classes may serve to point out these alternatives. The bias of the classes, however, as dictated by the doctor's routine practices and desires, should be considered.

If the doctor is working with a nurse-midwife, she would usually be the one who teaches the prenatal classes. In this instance, it is very likely she would be following the couple through labor as well as teaching the childbirth preparation classes. Her familiar presence can provide a great deal of comfort for the laboring couple. If the doctor is utilizing a nurse-midwife, the chances are the maternity care is patient-directed enough that the prenatal classes s/he offers are not designed to legitimize procedures, but have truly been developed to serve prenatal patients.

IN ADDITION TO CLASSES

The most widely used source of knowledge about anything, including childbirth, is books. Many, many books dealing with childbirth have been written. Reading is particularly good during the early months of pregnancy to make the whole thing seem "real" before the pregnancy is physically obvious. All childbirth education classes, no matter how extensive, are limited by time. Carefully selected books can complement the course of instruction and add new dimensions to the information received in class. The reason books must be carefully selected is that Ostriches, as well as people interested in childbirth education, write books. Some books on the shelves have been written by doctors who thrive on the Ostrich Approach. Most people, consciously or subconsciously, seem to accept what is on the printed page as Truth. Reading a book written from the Ostrich perspective can be as destructive to self-confidence as listening to an Ostrich who "knows" that prepared childbirth methods "positively don't work."

For a current list of books related to the childbearing field, contact the ICEA Supplies Center and request a copy of **Bookmarks. Bookmarks** is free and contains capsule descriptions and prices of all books that the ICEA Supplies Center handles.

HOW TO FIND CHILDBIRTH EDUCATION CLASSES IN YOUR OWN AREA

Doctors, clinics, hospitals and community service organizations usually can direct people to childbirth education classes in the area. Sometimes libraries and community colleges can be helpful, as can women's groups. National organizations that are concerned with childbirth education will be happy to furnish names and addresses of non-profit childbirth education groups as well as private instructors across the nation. These groups can also recommend physicians and health care facilities that are sympathetic to the prepared childbirth and family-centered maternity care movement. The names and addresses of some of these national organizations are listed in Appendix C.

Choosing Health Care

Several methods of health care are available to the pregnant woman; each has its own particular advantages and disadvantages. Personal preferences, financial status and even geographic location must be considered as appropriate care is selected. Location plays a part mainly because of availability of services. Large cities, for example, usually have a wider range of services and combinations of services than rural areas. However, no matter where you live, you may be pleasantly surprised at what options might surface when you really start looking.

As you explore the alternatives available in health care, remember to choose what is best for you; what you really want. It is your baby. Medical care is essential, but the form it takes can vary greatly. The particular methods and personnel should be carefully chosen with your individual needs in mind.

Throughout the childbirth experience, including pregnancy and postpartum, teamwork and trust are important. Make your choices accordingly. This section is an attempt to acquaint you with some available services. There are others available in some parts of the country, but most are variations of the services described herein.

PRIVATE PHYSICIANS

The most common source of prenatal care in America is the private doctor. Most private physicians practice either alone or in partnerships that range from two to possibly four or five doctors.

The doctor's support is extremely important in a prepared delivery. It is unfortunate, but some doctors view the prepared couple as a bother. Apparently it is easier to treat every woman in labor exactly the same. For instance, when you order a Big Mac at McDonald's, you get two all-beef patties, special sauce, lettuce, cheese, pickles, onions on a sesame seed bun. Everyone gets two all-beef patties, special sauce, lettuce, cheese, pickles, onions on a sesame seed bun. The person who comes in and wants a Big Mac without the special sauce really disrupts the routine. If you want your birth experience to be an original creation instead of a Big Mac, be sure that your doctor will take the time and effort to hold the special sauce.

Several different types of doctors deliver babies either frequently or occasionally. Which one you choose will probably depend upon your lifestyle, your geographic location and the individual physician involved.

The obstetrician-gynecologist (OB-GYN) specializes in prenatal care, delivery and the diseases specifically related to the female organs. In addition to the obvious benefit of the obstetrician's specialized knowledge and experience, there is another important advantage for the couple planning a prepared birth. An obstetrician delivers many more babies than any other type of doctor; therefore s/he has probably worked with a larger number of prepared couples. As a result, s/he may know more about helping the couple direct their own childbirth experience than doctors who deliver babies less frequently. This is a Rule of Thumb rather than a Truth. The obstetrician examines the baby briefly at birth, and may perform circumcision, but that is the only infant care s/he handles.

The general practitioner (G.P.) is an all-purpose sort of doctor. S/he is the family doctor, the Dr. Welby. A G.P. cares for the whole family, including the newborn baby. The goal is to treat the whole individual as a part of a family unit. When s/he discovers a potentially serious medical problem, s/he may refer the patient to a specialist in the appropriate medical discipline. Some G.P.'s refer all pregnant women to obstetricians for the duration of the pregnancy; others refer only high-risk pregnancies.

Because the G.P. cares for the whole family, it is sometimes easier for this kind of doctor to view childbirth as it relates to the total life relationships of the patient. This broad view can enable the G.P. to appreciate the desire for a shared birth experience and can lead him/her to offer the necessary support.

It is not so important which kind of doctor you choose as what kind of personality and life view s/he has. Given the history of obstetrics in America, it is easy for a doctor to make the whole birth the doctor's show instead of allowing the delivering couple to take center stage.

The doctor is an important part of the childbirth team. As such, s/he will be closely involved in medical decisions regarding your birth, so be sure you find a doctor who will discuss options with you, and consider your wishes before s/he acts. Draw on your doctor's wealth of experience and knowledge, but be informed enough about the childbirth process yourself to know what options are available. Know enough to be able to discuss, and possibly suggest, alternatives that may produce a more humanistic, satisfying experience. Some of the alternatives that are available will not even be mentioned unless you bring them up. Your doctor is much more likely to seriously consider your wishes if you appear to be knowledgeable and interested.

If you are already seeing a particular doctor, a simple way to find out how s/he sees her/his role in your childbirth process is to ask specific questions about any aspect of childbirth. Some doctors will take the time to answer as if you were an intelligent, thinking individual. Some doctors, on the other hand, will either overtly, or by attitude pat you on the head and tell you not to worry your pretty little self about such things and that s/he will take care of everything. If you want to actively direct the birth of your child, the former type of doctor is a much safer bet.

If you already have a doctor and s/he feels "natural childbirth" is a lot of foolishness, it would be well to seriously consider changing doctors. You will have enough to concentrate on during labor without feeling negativism on the part of your doctor. Talk to the doctor, find out where s/he really stands in regard to childbirth preparation. S/he will be the final authority on what procedures and medications may be administered during your childbirth. If you have a working relationship with the doctor, s/he will discuss recommendations with you and get your consent before action is taken. Aside from having utmost confidence in your doctor's professional abilities, you should be able to really talk with him/her. You should feel comfortable enough to discuss your concerns and wishes. Your goal is a rapport with the doctor, not dependence upon the doctor.

This feeling of rapport, pleasant in any doctor-patient relationship, is particularly important when a couple is planning a prepared birth. The laboring couple functions much more effectively in an environment of respect and encouragement. The communication set up during the prenatal care-giving can set the stage for such respect and encouragement from the doctor during labor and delivery.

Doctors differ in their opinions on father participation during childbirth. Some doctors absolutely won't allow the father in the delivery room; others will let the father actually deliver the baby (under careful supervision, of course). The number of doctors in the latter category is very small, but consumer demand and positive results are encouraging more and more doctors to re-examine their positions in birth and maternity care.

Most doctors fall somewhere between the two extremes. In the past it was difficult to find a doctor who would let a father accompany his partner into the delivery room. For a long time it was thought fathers would hamper the process by fainting, vomiting or just generally getting in the way. Fear of infection was also used to keep fathers out of delivery.

Today many, many doctors welcome the father and are firmly convinced that the father's presence is actually a helpful factor because of the calming effect his support has on the mother. Fathers very seldom faint or create a problem of any sort, particularly if they are trained. The trained father is aware of the common procedures and the normal chain of events in delivery. He knows what to expect and how to respond so he won't interfere with the hospital staff.

Usually the doctors who work regularly with prepared patients are the most liberal regarding father participation; however, don't take this Rule of Thumb for granted. Don't wait until your last prenatal checkup to ask for certain whether the father will be allowed in delivery. Ask early in your pregnancy. This one point accounts for many of the couples who switch doctors in the eighth or ninth month of pregnancy.

If the father of the baby won't be able to be with you during labor and delivery (or if he chooses not to be) some doctors and hospitals will allow a substitute coach. Ascertain ahead of time if your hospital will allow individuals other than the father in the sterile confines of the labor and delivery rooms. Some doctors and/or hospitals will not even allow the father into the delivery room if the parents are not legally married. Even though this seems to be an unnecessary value judgment on the part of the doctor and/or hospital, it is good to check this well in advance if your relationship is such that this could present a problem. Either change hospitals or doctors or work out some arrangement ahead of time that is satisfactory to everyone involved. But don't wait until you are in labor to do something about it.

Many doctors will agree to preliminary interviews with prospective patients at either no charge or a nominal fee. If this sort of arrangement can't be worked out, draw as much information from the receptionist as possible. She'll know what the doctor's basic attitudes are, even though she won't be able to answer specific, detailed questions.

Even though the doctor's attitude toward prepared childbirth will probably be the most influential factor in your choice of a doctor, several other factors are worth consideration.

Find out about the fee schedule. It is a fairly standard practice to charge one fee that covers all prenatal visits, the doctor's services at delivery, visits in the hospital while you are on postpartum, and a check-up six weeks after delivery. Sometimes a six-month checkup is included in the basic fee. **The physician's fee does not include the hospital costs such as room, medications, use of the delivery and labor rooms, nursery charges for the baby and other miscellaneous hospital charges.** These are completely separate matters.

The anesthesiologist's fee, too, is not included in the basic bill. The way it is handled varies from place to place and situation to situation. Some hospitals require the anesthesiologist to be present at every delivery, whether or not you plan to have an anesthetic administered. In these cases you will probably be charged a fee even if the anesthesiologist does nothing except stand in the delivery room. It is good to check local statutory requirements and hospital regulations regarding this so you will not be unpleasantly surprised with a rather stiff charge for possibly no services rendered! If there is an anesthesiologist's bill, it will probably be submitted separately from both the attending physician's bill and your hospital bill.

Find out early how much the doctor's fee is and what arrangements can be made for payment. Find out exactly what it covers and what extra charges there may be in case of complications at delivery. Some doctors include prenatal laboratory fees for blood work in the basic bill, some do not. In the latter case the lab usually submits a separate billing to you.

It is convenient if the doctor's office is reasonably close to your home, though not a necessity. During the last part of your pregnancy you will be making frequent visits to the office, and chances are good that you won't feel much like riding long distances every week or so when you are nine months pregnant. However, if it is a choice between a supportive doctor 50 miles away and a local doctor with whom you feel uncomfortable, go the 50 miles. Some women actually fly 1,200 to 1,500 miles for each of their prenatal check-ups and the delivery. That's stretching it a bit, but it does illustrate the importance of a supportive physician in a prepared birth.

Consider what hospitals s/he services. It, too, should be fairly close to your home if it is at all possible. Even if the hospital is an hour away, you will probably have no trouble at all getting there in plenty of time for the birth, but late labor is not the ideal time for a sightseeing tour. Labor room beds are much more comfortable than front seats of Volkswagens when you are in labor. Let your doctor know if you live a great distance from the hospital; you may have to be a little more conscientious about notifying your physician as soon as labor is established.

If a particular doctor delivers only at the most expensive hospital in the area and you simply cannot afford the most expensive hospital in the area, look hard for another doctor. If you can't find a doctor with whom you feel equally comfortable, decide whether you can be satisfied with a less pleasant doctor-patient relationship or whether you can come up with the extra money you'll need for the more expensive hospital.

Find out who will deliver the baby if your own doctor is unavailable when you go into labor. If your doctor does not have a partner, s/he probably alternates being "on call" with another doctor or group of doctors. Ask your doctor how the "alternates" feel about prepared childbirth and what support you can expect from each of them. If s/he does have a partner, or partners, someone else in the partnership will attend the delivery if your doctor is unavailable. You will probably see each of the doctors in a partnership during the pregnancy, so you will be able to ascertain for yourself what the varying attitudes about prepared childbirth are. Be aware that the views can vary greatly from doctor to doctor even in a partnership.

If your doctor practices alone and is out of town for a period of time during your pregnancy, s/he will arrange with another doctor to examine you while s/he's gone.

Many women feel much more at ease with a female doctor, particularly during pregnancy. Pregnant patients are often able to discuss their fears and concerns more fully and honestly with another female, especially if she has been through the childbirth experience herself. A female doctor who has had a baby can obviously empathize more readily and fully than can a male doctor who cannot possibly know how it really feels to be pregnant and give birth. Some male doctors tend to treat a pregnant woman's complaints and concerns as those of a neurotic woman.

The physical and emotional strains of pregnancy can be many. Some are obvious and some are vague, floating anxieties. A woman doctor who was in tune with herself during her own pregnancy is in a position to be most helpful and supportive of a pregnant woman. It's possible a woman doctor is more likely to be able to catch the faint, nameless distress signals you may be sending. On the other hand, some women doctors have undoubtedly gone through pregnancies that involved a very minimal amount of physical discomfort, and these doctors may tend to dismiss your complaints as not valid.

Two cautions if you are considering a woman doctor specifically: First, since there are comparatively few women physicians, some have quite a long waiting list of new patients. Start looking as soon as possible.

Second, just because she is a woman does not automatically mean she will be supportive of prepared childbirth nor that she will be particularly sympathetic to your individual problems. The fact that you're both women does not assure instant rapport. Choosing a female doctor is the same as choosing a male doctor; consider your own wishes, goals and prejudices. Use the same criteria you would in choosing a male doctor.

Happily, more and more women are entering the field of medicine as doctors. Their influence could easily cause some drastic changes to take place in maternal health care policies within the next few years.

Relationships between human beings are complex and affected by numerous underlying impressions. Beards, moustaches, size, age, sex and other physical features completely unrelated to professional competence can affect your attitudes toward an individual. These attitudes will, in turn, affect your relationship with that individual. For instance, even though most people don't actively consider the age of the doctor to be a crucial factor in the doctor-patient relationship, it can be. You may have conscious or subconscious preferences. Some women feel most comfortable with a young doctor, while others can't seem to develop trust in a young physician (particularly one who is younger than they themselves are). Some women like their doctor to be a parent figure type and tend to seek obviously older medical care-givers.

If you feel vaguely uncomfortable about a particular doctor, examine how that doctor affects you on a purely emotional nonobjective level. Don't silently scold yourself if you have what may be unreasonable prejudices, just admit to yourself that they exist and work from there. Either bow to the prejudices or overcome them, but don't accept a vaguely uncomfortable feeling without trying to identify the source of the discomfort. The right choice is whatever is right for you.

Another thing that is important to some people is whether the doctor will allow camera or taping equipment in the labor and delivery rooms. To some this won't make a bit of difference, but it is good to know ahead of time how your particular doctor feels about such equipment.

The question of photography invariably brings up the subject of modesty. The truth is that during childbirth, women usually have very little modesty. Most women find themselves more concerned with the event than with the perhaps revealing situation. The emphasis is on the baby, the excitement and the activity; it is not on the bare part of the woman's anatomy. Feelings of embarrassment can be lessened, too, by use of a more dignified delivery position than the normal lithotomy position.

Even if you don't want pictures of the actual birth, it is nice to have a picture of the seconds-old baby. S/he will never look quite like that again. Some hospitals keep a camera in the delivery room and routinely take a picture of every newborn with its parents. Ask ahead of time if this service is available.

Couples who are planning to use photography equipment in the delivery or labor rooms at all, will probably be required to sign a standard release form freeing the hospital of all responsibility if something should happen to either the mother or the baby as a result of the picture-taking. Good camera equipment and high speed film are necessary to get high quality pictures in the delivery room, because most hospitals allow only one flash picture to be taken in delivery.

Cassette tape recordings are easy to do, and are terrific for the baby book. However, it is difficult for the father to handle both a camera and a tape recorder, particularly during delivery. He will be quite busy with his coaching activities, especially if it is a first baby. And the expulsive phase of subsequent babies is often too quick to catch them on tape and film both. Don't attempt to do more than the father thinks he can comfortably handle, but do consider all of the options available.

Remember, though, that the father's prime function throughout the birth process is to give support. That duty should supersede all others. Pictures or recordings are frosting on the cake, not necessities.

> In our case, we didn't think about the possibility of photographing the birth when I was pregnant the first time, but early during my second pregnancy we decided we wanted birth photographs. Between the two pregnancies I started going to a marvelously empathetic, personable young obstetrician. When I became pregnant, I started asking him specific questions about his attitudes toward prepared childbirth. Everything was going along just fine until I told him we wanted to photograph the delivery. He said that that was certainly fine; we were welcome to take pictures of the baby in the delivery room as long as we didn't use flash photography.
>
> I wanted to make sure he understood that I meant we wanted to take pictures of the baby being born, not just the newborn baby. He looked at me with the oddest look on his face and told me we could take pictures of the mother, and we could take pictures of the baby. But, he said, we couldn't take pictures of my "bare bottom." He said the hospital lawyers had advised against allowing that sort of thing.
>
> I liked him very much, and it was a difficult thing to do, but I told him that I would just have to find another doctor. And I did. When Ami is 20 years old, I will probably not remember the first doctor's name, let alone what he looked like. But we will have the delivery pictures, and that was what was important to us.

MIDWIVES

One alternative to traditional maternity care patterns is the midwife. Midwife is an old, old word, but it hasn't been swept away by time. Even though the midwife is the primary source of maternity care throughout Europe and many other areas of the world, we in America tend to consider midwifery out-moded and not suitable for our highly technical, and extremely specialized, society. Our mainstream population labors under the misconception that midwifery is only for primitive, backward cultures.

One concern we have is that we don't know quite what a midwife is. Webster defines a midwife as "a woman who cares for women during childbirth." But that doesn't define her training and qualifications.

The midwife of yesterday, the so-called "granny" midwife, most often received her "training" by attending first the births of relatives and later the births of women throughout her community. She had little, if any, formal training and often was the only attendant at the birth. She developed proficiency at her craft through practice and necessity. These non-licensed midwives have delivered generations of babies throughout the world. In many societies these midwives are responsible for all of the maternity care provided, even today.

In America today there are basically two kinds of midwives: the midwife and the certified nurse-midwife. The governing body of nurse-midwifery in the United States, the American College of Nurse-Midwives (ACNM), defines a Certified Nurse-Midwife as "a Registered Nurse who by virtue of added knowledge and skill gained through an organized program of study and clinical experience recognized by the American College of Nurse-Midwives, has extended the limits of her practice into the area of management of care of mothers and babies throughout the maternity cycle so long as progress meets criteria accepted as normal." According to the ACNM, "nurse-midwifery is an extension of nursing practice into the area of management of care of mothers and babies throughout the maternity cycle so long as progress meets criteria accepted as normal."[1]

The ACNM is responsible for the certification of nurse-midwives; the establishment of qualifications, standards, and functions for the practice of nurse-midwifery; approval of nurse-midwifery educational programs; development of guidelines for nurse-midwifery services; and development of guidelines for continuing education of nurse-midwives.

Despite the ACNM certification programs for nurse-midwives, many midwives who are not nurses are also practicing in the United States today. The degree of training and experience these midwives have varies a great deal from woman to woman. Some of these midwives have been trained in very intensive midwifery programs abroad, but since they are not registered nurses, they do not qualify by ACNM standards to be certified nurse-midwives. Others of these midwives are self-trained and not very highly qualified. And a lot of the midwives fall somewhere between the two extremes in competence and experience. The midwives who are not nurse-midwives must usually operate outside of established health care systems in America because of the legal ramifications, and sometimes these women haven't the facilities available to handle the small percentage of births which demand emergency measures.

Midwifery as a whole is in a state of flux in the United States. Laws are changing by virtue of pressure from the public, pressure from the medical professions and tangible results. The extent to which the midwife and the nurse-midwife can legally function is governed by the legal jurisdiction in which she practices. According to the ACNM "in the U.S.A. a nurse-midwife always functions within the framework of a medically directed health service; she is not an independent practitioner."[2] Because one of the goals of this book is to direct couples toward finding medical care within established health care systems that are fully legal, the midwife who operates as an entity apart from a doctor and/or hospital is being largely ignored; the term "midwife," when used outside of this chapter, should be understood to mean nurse-midwife.

Midwifery is based in the belief that each family, regardless of culture, income level or background, deserves a safe and satisfying childbirth experience. The parents' right to self-determination and dignity can be accomplished only through comprehensive maternity care which includes emotional support as well as physical care throughout the birth cycle. The nurse-midwife is qualified and willing to offer such support.

The doctor/nurse-midwife team is one of the more innovative forms of maternity care available. In the team approach, the nurse-midwife completes most of the prenatal care. If she spots a potential problem developing, she alerts the doctor. As well as doing the routine prenatal exams, and counseling expectant parents, she will often teach childbirth education classes to groups of the doctor's patients.

The nurse-midwife often follows her patients through labor and delivery and is present at the hospital to help the laboring couple. Her personal knowledge of the parents enables her to offer the precise encouragement and coaching that will best meet their individual needs throughout the labor and delivery cycle. Her presence at the hospital can also offer the laboring couple a familiar mooring in a sea of the unfamiliar. In some cases, the nurse-midwife can also deliver the baby, usually under the doctor's supervision.

The nurse-midwife examines the infant at birth and may continue her association with the parents well into the postpartum period. She may help the new family adjust to the changed home situations and instruct the parents in baby care. This professional support during the postpartum period can help the family adjust more easily to the responsibilities and stresses of parenthood.

Many women are finding that the care given by the doctor/nurse-midwife team is the care that most completely meets their needs. The nurse-midwife's entire profession is involved with instructing, counseling and caring for expectant and recently-delivered parents. This almost total involvement gives her a special perspective and often intensifies her relationships with patients. Whereas patients often refrain from calling the doctor for seemingly unimportant questions because they feel s/he is too busy, the nurse-midwife makes a conscious effort to encourage patients to call for guidance and information at any time. The personal relationship that most patients develop with their midwife makes it easier for the expectant couples to express their concerns and doubts. Their questions can be handled in a relaxed, open manner when they feel someone has the time for them.

Increased use of midwives throughout American health care facilities can serve to very effectively reduce medical costs. Midwives care for the normal pregnancies, and free doctors to spend more time with the high-risk and problem pregnancies. It has been estimated that a nurse-midwife can see about three-quarters as many patients as can a doctor in the same time period. Serving fewer patients during a specified time span allows more time per patient. This tends to personalize service. The midwife's salary level is much less than that of the physician's.[3]

The American College of Nurse-Midwives has extensive information regarding the legal status and availability of Certified Nurse-Midwives throughout the United States.

Before my pregnancy, I had heard that my doctor was using a nurse-midwife in his practice. I hadn't known anyone who had used a nurse-midwife in delivery, and I was a little skeptical. But I had the utmost confidence in my doctor, and I wasn't about to consider finding another. On my first prenatal visit I was introduced to the nurse-midwife. She was a very friendly and outgoing person and I felt better already. We sat in her office and she thoroughly explained her background and the family-centered childbirth program that she and the doctor offered. She emphasized the belief that the childbirth experience is really an extension of the bedroom, and that the experience really involves only the father and the mother. She and the doctor, she said, were only there to do everything they could to make it a pleasant experience for us. The thought of being examined by a strange woman bothered me a little, but she was so friendly and reassuring that I felt quite positive about the whole

experience. My doctor uses a nurse-midwife because a doctor with a large practice cannot possibly get to know a patient on a very deep level over the course of nine months; so the nurse-midwife was there to make things a little more personal. The nurse-midwife handles only very routine, non-complicated pregnancies; thus freeing the doctor to become involved with the high risk pregnancies. I was told I could request to see either the doctor or nurse-midwife at any time. I came through the experience feeling totally convinced that I was very fortunate to have had such wonderfully personalized obstetrical care. The nurse-midwife and I had built up a very close relationship over the nine-month period, and I felt nothing but complete trust and respect for her.

CLINICS

The clinic is another option to the traditional care given by a private doctor. The clinic referred to in this section is the arrangement whereby a patient is examined by any of a number of staff personnel during her prenatal and postnatal visits. In many instances the clinic is located within the outpatient department of a hospital. The woman enters the hospital proper for delivery and is entitled to the same service as is a private patient at the hospital. **Clinics are lower-priced than private doctors, and many prenatal clinics provide excellent care for maternity patients.** Teaching hospitals quite often have good clinics; however, when searching for a hospital clinic, do consider the general merits of the hospital itself, rather than just the clinic, as related to the labor, delivery and postpartum experiences. Women who are clinic patients at a particular hospital usually receive the same quality of medical care and the same benefits as the women who deliver at the same hospital as patients of private physicians.

Clinics serve large numbers of people; therefore the hazards of group service prevail. Waiting in the clinic for an appointment can be very time-consuming. Clinics often function on a first-come, first-served basis and early arrival can ease the long waits. Sometimes clinic service tends to be impersonal. Depending upon the size of the clinic and the number of people served, it is possible a woman could go through an entire pregnancy without seeing the same doctor twice.

Clinics also offer the distinct disadvantage of never knowing who will deliver the baby. This is true to some extent even with a private doctor, but with a private doctor there are usually only two or three doctors "in the running." In a clinic situation, any one of a seeming multitude of doctors could be "on call" when a particular patient goes into labor. This necessarily somewhat impersonal and unknown atmosphere can frustrate a woman's attempts to control her own labor, but if she's a sporting type, she can consider the situation to be an extra challenge and handle it accordingly. In any case, be aware that the prepared couple is likely to have a bit harder time eliciting staff cooperation in a clinic situation. This of course differs from clinic to clinic; just be aware of the possibility if you are considering such prenatal care.

On the other hand, clinics offer some definite plusses in maternity care. **A growing number of clinics are using nurse-midwives for prenatal care.** The utilization of the nurse-midwife for prenatal check-ups as well as during labor and delivery can effectively reduce the clinic's impersonal atmosphere.

In addition to the physical aspects of care, clinics often have programs designed to deal with the emotional concerns of childbearing. Whereas private doctors are usually so busy with primary patient care that they cannot offer support or instruction in a systematic, organized program, clinics often have the personnel available to offer some sort of program aimed at educating clinic patients about childbirth. The private obstetrician's care for the patient is essentially completed with delivery. It is true that patients are visited during the postpartum stay in the hospital and are checked at six weeks and sometimes at six months postpartum, but the majority of the private doctor's job is done when the baby is born. Clinics frequently have programs aimed toward acquainting expectant mothers with baby care techniques, nutrition and related topics.

Prenatal information is given, too, but the breadth and depth of this educational effort is often severely restricted by time and staff limitations. The program is usually directed almost exclusively toward the mother, and is often held during daytime hours. Due to the lack of father participation in many clinic classes, it is best for the couple to attend other childbirth education classes together, in addition to the mother's participation in the clinic program. Often the prenatal education offered by the clinic does not give very extensive information about either breathing techniques or options in childbirth that differ from the standard hospital procedures of that clinic.

It could be difficult to exercise more than just very conservative alternatives in a clinic situation. If the choice is made to conduct a labor and delivery in an out-of-the-ordinary manner, the cooperation of the doctor is essential. It will take time and effort on the doctor's part to alert the appropriate staff as to the plans. The number of people served, as well as the uncertainty as to who will attend at an individual's delivery, makes personalized attention difficult to get.

Ultimately you must weigh the advantages of lower cost and the sometimes innovative care given (especially at the teaching clinics associated with medical schools) with the disadvantages suggested above and other disadvantages unique to specific clinics you may be considering.

POSTSCRIPTS ON CHOOSING HEALTH CARE

The goal of this section is not to give absolutes; it is to help you choose the medical care that you will be the most comfortable with. It is to help you choose what is right for you and your lifestyle. Once you've chosen a particular doctor or other health care system, try hard to function within the given parameters. Realize that each method and doctor has unique advantages and disadvantages.

Under any system, find out why the recommended procedures and routines are, indeed, recommended. The goal is not to become a problem patient, but to be an intelligent consumer of the medical care you are receiving. You'll get much more personalized service and consideration if you are a cooperative patient. However, cooperation does not necessarily mean being passive and instantly agreeable; it means a willingness to work with the doctor or other health care giver to solve medical problems and concerns in a way that both of you will be happy.

If you find out at any time during your pregnancy that you and your care-giver disagree violently about something that is important to you, weigh the situation. Realize that if it becomes a showdown situation when you are in labor, things will probably be done the doctor's way. If the doctor's views on medication, for instance, are drastically different than yours, realize that s/he is the one who orders medications when you are in the hospital. In a normal, non-emergency situation, it should be up to the patient to accept or reject medications. You should have confidence that the doctor will not recommend medications that are unnecessary for your particular situation. It can be physically and emotionally difficult to refuse medication during labor when a nurse tells you that "the doctor ordered it."

Remember at all times that you are the consumer. You are paying good money for the care-giver's services. **It is your baby and no one cares more about the health and well-being of that baby than you do.** If you consider your wishes to be reasonable and all attempts to reconcile the differences with your doctor are to no avail, change doctors. It is not unheard of for women to switch doctors during their eighth or ninth month when they discover, for example, that their present doctor does not allow fathers in the delivery room. **The probable added expense of changing doc-**

tors in midstream will be well worth it overall if you find a doctor who is more willing to consider your individual wishes.

> They wheeled me into delivery and the next five minutes was spent in adjusting the delivery table, fingerprinting, draping me and adjusting the mirror. I could hear the doctor scrubbing and I watched the nurses getting the birth certificate, bassinette and baby table ready. I felt, as I had in the labor room, as if I were on an assembly line—Pregnant Pelvis #X359 in final stages of processing. I shook the feeling off, thinking David and I would soon be together as a couple, watching our baby start, first slowly, then more rapidly, into the world. He pushed a stool to the end of the table, sat down and said to a nurse, "The father can come in now." While she went to the door, he grabbed two forceps blades and put in one side. David came in while he was inserting the other side. David sat down and not thirty seconds after David sat, the doctor pulled the head out until the nose was clear, glanced at the clock and said, "It's born at 6:20 exactly." He cleared the chin with one more pull of his hands, laid down the forceps, picked up a syringe, used it, then slipped the baby's body out. All through was total, dead silence. He said, "It's a boy" in a bored way, then nothing seemed to happen. I asked where the baby was and a nurse said, "Right here" and she picked him up off a table and showed him to us. They had been wiping him off so we wouldn't be "revolted." I said, "Oh honey, he looks like you" and they took him to a table behind me. The doctor said, "The father has to leave now" to the air and David left and started phoning while the doctor delivered the placenta. I felt empty and deflated emotionally—so disappointed. All that anticipation just to see my baby yanked out of my body the same way a doctor would pull a deep sliver from an anesthetized thumb with a pair of tweezers. The doctor got up, left without a word and they wheeled me into recovery. The entire delivery, including the stitching, took 10 minutes. I will choose my doctor very carefully, the next time.

done much to personalize childbirth; but unfortunately not all doctors and hospitals offer family-centered care.

Choosing a hospital for a prepared delivery is at least as important as choosing a supportive doctor or other prenatal health care system. No matter how carefully you have chosen your doctor, s/he will probably not be with you during the greater part of your labor. Unless you have a midwife who is committed to being with you during labor in the hospital, the majority of your time will be spent dealing directly with the hospital staff. A nursing staff that supports and understands prepared childbirth can make a great deal of difference. Some couples choose the hospital before they choose the doctor.

The location of the hospital should be considered. Most labors, particularly first labors, are long enough to get to the hospital with plenty of time to spare. Some women spend hours of their labor in the hospital labor room. Very seldom, in a precipitous birth situation, a women will not make it to the hospital before the baby is born. This is very rare, but if you are overly concerned about this possibility, choosing a hospital close to your home will lessen this worry.

Charges can vary a great deal from hospital to hospital, even within a given geographic area. Private rooms are more expensive than semi-private (two-person) rooms. And semi-private rooms are more expensive than ward beds. Hospitals charge for use of labor and delivery rooms. Hospitals charge for medications, anesthetics and nursery care. Hospitals charge for laboratory work. Some hospitals even charge for local telephone calls made from patient rooms. Contact the hospitals in your area and ask what the fees for various accommodations and services are. When you have a number of cost estimates, sit down and decide which hospitals you can best afford.

The hospital should definitely not be chosen entirely on the basis of cost; it should be chosen on the basis of services and alternatives offered. However, once you have figures you can decide whether you should request a private room or ward accommodations. You can decide whether you should discuss with your doctor the possibility of a shortened postpartum hospital stay. The cost of health care is incredible, but by careful comparison, you may be able to economize a little.

Whatever hospital you choose, do as much paperwork ahead of time as possible. Most hospitals offer a pre-registration to expectant parents. If the pre-registration is completed several weeks in advance of your due date, being admitted when you are in labor will be a much easier job. It is very easy to forget to pick up the necessary insurance forms and bank account numbers as you dash out of the house on your way to have a baby. While you are pre-registering, ask about financial arrangements. Find out what amounts of money will have to be paid when you are admitted, how much will be required upon discharge and what arrangements can be made for the balance. If you have no applicable insurance, or if you haven't built up a good credit rating, the amounts involved may be quite substantial.

By the way, the choice of private, semi-private or ward accommodations should be made on the basis of personal preference as much as on financial considerations. Some people find the solitude of a private room positively boring; others find the relative quiet to be very restful. Some find the company in a semi-private room or a ward to be pleasant; others find the lack of privacy extremely annoying. Some hospitals require the patient to have a private room if she wants rooming-in.

If the cost of the hospital stay is of major concern to you, some doctors will allow a mother to leave the hospital just a few hours after delivery, provided she is in excellent condition. Sometimes the baby will have to stay a little longer.

Some hospitals offer a tour schedule which may include films and orientation sessions. Orientation sessions are a must to attend, and many of your routine questions will be answered in the presentation. If you still have questions after the presentation, ask. No question is too trivial. It is easy for the hospital personnel conducting the orientation session to overlook something that seems quite obvious to the people who frequent the hospital almost daily. It is possible that your baby's birth will be the first time you've ever been a patient in a hospital. You don't know much about hospital routines, and you shouldn't be expected to know. Something that Aunt Martha, or Mrs. Johnson up the street, said about hospitals may be bothering you. Ask all the questions you can think of. If you're uncomfortable asking questions in a group of people you're unfamiliar with, buttonhole the discussion leader when the session is over. If you can manage, though, ask the questions in the group situation. The chances are good that someone else may be wondering about the same thing.

Some of the films that hospitals show are of prepared births; some are of Ostrich births. If you see a film of an Ostrich birth, be sure to counter the effects by seeing a film of a prepared birth. This is very important. Some of the films are of really negative experiences. Sometimes comparing the women's diverse experiences can give you a great deal of confidence in the wisdom of preparation.

A tour of the hospital facilities is very useful, and it can acquaint you with the services available. Seeing labor and delivery rooms before you are ready to use them can remove some of the fear of the unknown. Delivery rooms, especially, can be really frightening. They are filled with gleaming stainless steel and strange-looking instruments. An explanation ahead of time can ease tension considerably. If the hospital does not offer a regularly scheduled tour, request a personal tour. In the event you have taken a group tour of the hospital and still have unanswered questions, request a personal tour. If the hospital flatly refuses to let you inspect the labor and delivery area, the chances are that the hospital is not family-centered in its outlook. You must remember, however, that if labor and delivery rooms are in use, the hospital personnel will not allow anyone to go traipsing through them. If this is the case, the hospital will probably tell you that this particular time is a bad one, but you are welcome to come back another time.

In addition to the labor and delivery rooms, you should see the newborn nursery. Ask about any equipment you do not understand. And looking at the newborn babies can lend an air of reality to the pregnancy.

The hospital orientations, films and tours are most valuable when attended by both parents.

Staff support of prepared patients is very important. It is good if at least some of the labor room nurses have had training in prepared childbirth methods. In some hospitals, all prepared patients, regardless of the method of preparation they have learned, are called Lamaze patients. Knowing this can make it easier to question the staff. Nurses who don't understand the needs of the prepared couple have a difficult time dealing with the couple. Prepared childbirth demands concentration. Nurses who ask frequent questions, and expect immediate answers, during a patient's contractions can be extremely annoying. A supportive nurse will wait until between contractions to ask necessary questions and do the periodic examinations. Nurses who ask how the "pains" are, and those who offer medications every few minutes can sabotage the efforts of even the most confident couple. It is not important that the nurses know the specifics of each method of childbirth preparation; it is important that they are aware of ways to encourage and support prepared couples. Some staffs have unwritten agreements that if it is at all possible, only nurses who promote and understand childbirth preparation are assigned to care for prepared couples.

A labor coach is an essential part of a prepared childbirth experience. The father, or some other coach, should be welcomed in the labor room, not just tolerated. Some hospital personnel feel threatened by the presence of a coach. These people often misunderstand the role of the coach and tend to feel displaced by the coach. Staff people who have had experience with prepared couples realize this is not the case at all. The labor coach serves to complement the services allocated to the nursing staff, not curtail them. The labor coach has the signal responsibility of providing undivided attention to the laboring woman. Undivided attention by the nursing staff is practically impossible because of the work load. The labor coach is a buffer between the mother and the hospital staff. It is through the coach that the woman can communicate her feelings and wishes. The nurse is still in charge of medically monitoring the labor. She still takes blood pressures, operates fetal monitoring equipment, administers medications, and keeps the doctor notified of the mother's progress in labor.

The coach should also be welcomed in the delivery room. The birth is the culmination of nine months of pregnancy and a thousand dreams. Not allowing the coach to share in this emotional and exciting time is grossly unfair. The coaching is important to the mother in the delivery room as well as in the labor room. In most cases, the coach is required to sit or stand at the head of the delivery table during the birth. That's a fair request; the coach's responsibility is support and encouragement of the woman. These responsibilities can best be performed from a position near the mother's head. The medical personnel are moving about the room performing their individual functions; as with any team, the childbirth team functions most efficiently when all members have predetermined duties and assigned locations. That way everyone knows where everyone else is and what he is doing. The coach and the mother can watch the birth through a mirror attached to a wall or an overhead lamp. Sometimes a doctor will invite the coach to come around to the foot of the delivery table to watch, but don't count on it. Be certain well in advance of delivery that there is a mirror so you can watch.

Be sure you know your own hospital's requirements regarding prenatal classes. Some hospitals require that the labor coach has taken a childbirth preparation course in order to be admitted to the delivery room.

This requirement makes sense because the delivery room is a special, medical environment. The coach should know how to handle himself, and should know what procedures will take place. Some hospitals demand written proof of class attendance. Some even require that the coach has taken the specific prenatal class offered by that particular hospital.

Check rules regarding who is allowed in labor and delivery rooms. In most instances the father of the baby will be the labor coach, but sometimes a woman may choose to have someone else support her through labor. Some hospitals allow relatives, but not friends in labor and delivery. Some allow married fathers, but not unmarried fathers in labor and delivery. The legality of some of these discriminatory rulings could probably be tested, particularly those regarding married versus unmarried fathers, but if you plan to become a test case, do so well before your due date. If any of these considerations are important to you, choose a hospital that will allow you to choose your own labor coach.

Ask about the delivery table. Find out if it will adjust to a semi-sitting position. Many mothers find this position to be more comfortable, and to make pushing easier and more effective. If the table itself is not adjustable, a similar effect can be produced by putting pillows under the upper trunk of the mother, or by having the coach physically support the woman in this position during pushing. Even though such substitutions can be made if necessary, an adjustable delivery table is much preferred, particularly if the alternative is having the coach physically support her. The physical strain of supporting the woman in a semi-sitting position can reduce his effectiveness as a coach during this essential phase of labor.

Find out what labor room facilities are available. Are all labor rooms private? If they aren't private, what steps are taken to assure the most privacy possible? Prepared childbirth techniques demand concentration. Concentration is most easily achieved in an atmosphere of privacy and quiet. The hospital should make some sort of effort to keep prepared patients separated from Ostriches, for the comfort of both.

If it is essential to share a labor room with someone, she should be a prepared mother. Find out whether the hospital will allow your coach to stay with you even if you must share a labor room. Some hospitals assure couples that they will be able to remain together during labor and don't mention that this assurance does not apply unless you have the labor room to yourselves. Be sure the coach will be allowed to stay whether the other woman is prepared or not.

Some hospitals have special labor rooms set aside for prepared patients that are equipped for both labor and delivery. This arrangement avoids the necessity of moving during late labor; it also can make the delivery seem less pathological. The sterile, stainless steel of a regular delivery room tends to make the birth seem like a medical procedure. These special labor/delivery rooms are called birthing rooms.

It is good to know whether the hospital confines the laboring woman to bed. In most countries throughout the world, women in labor are encouraged to walk about until the membranes rupture. Conservative activity is considered to make labor easier by focusing the woman's attention away from her contractions as well as aiding in early engagement of the fetal head. In some hospitals, far too few, lounges are available for the prepared couple to use during the earlier stage of labor. The lounges, often equipped with televisions and adequate reading materials or game apparatus, can contribute significantly to the comfort of the woman laboring in the hospital. For safety and attendant legal reasons, the medicated mother is normally confined to bed. But the unmedicated mother deserves separate consideration, and the prepared mother is statistically more likely to be unmedicated than the Ostrich.

Some hospitals allow laboring women to use candy, honey or similar substances in the labor room to keep up energy. Many allow the use of ice chips to help the woman's mouth avoid dryness. The breathing techniques tend to dry out the mouth and the ice chips can be a great aid. Some hospitals allow the woman to continue to drink fluids throughout most of her labor. **The hospital policy regarding food and beverages should be checked out ahead of time.** It is also good to know whether the labor coach will be allowed to eat and drink in the labor room. It is inconvenient, and sometimes extremely disconcerting to the mother, if he must leave the room in order to eat.

Some hospitals require the coach to leave the labor room while the mother is being given vaginal exams; some don't. Many women feel the exams are the most uncomfortable part of labor, and the coach's presence can be comforting. Whether the coach can stay is often up to the discretion of the nurse or doctor who does the examination. In general, a supportive staff will allow the coach to stay if the mother wants him to, unless the hospital definitely rules against it.

Routine IV's are used in some hospitals. The intravenous feeding of glucose water sustains the mother's energy through labor; this may be helpful if she is not allowed to take other nourishment. IV's also provide a way for medications to be given almost instantaneously. Some people find the IV equipment—tubes connected to an IV bottle, and a needle inserted into the vein—to be upsetting. Once the IV is started, it is normally painless, but does hamper mobility.

Another fairly common piece of equipment in hospital labor rooms is the fetal heart rate monitor. These machines are used to monitor the fetal heart tones and the intensity of the uterine contractions. In some hospitals the fetal monitors are used on all patients if there is the time and equipment available; in some the monitors are used only on those patients who are considered high risk, those who develop a problem during labor, those who have been induced, or those who request the labor be mechanically monitored.

The two basic types of fetal monitors are internal and external. The external monitor is strapped across the laboring woman's abdomen. Two straps are used;

the upper strap holds a sort of pressure gauge to record the uterine contraction, and the lower strap is fitted with a device to pick up the fetal heart tones. The readings are indicated on either a scope or a printed read-out. Internal (or direct) monitors are more accurate and more complicated. The internal monitor has two small catheters which are inserted into the uterus through the cervix. One of the catheters is attached to the baby's presenting part, usually the head, with a small clip or screw electrode. This catheter measures the fetal heart rate. The other catheter is inserted farther up into the uterine cavity and it measures the intensity of the contractions. The measurements taken by both catheters are printed on a read-out. It is not uncommon for the mother's blood pressure to be monitored constantly along with the monitoring of the fetal heart tones and the strength of the contractions.

The machines cause loss of mobility, and can cause some problems with positioning in labor. The fetal heart tones cannot always be picked up, so the mother has to lie in one of the positions favorable for picking up her baby's heart tone; this can preclude even turning onto her side in some instances. Some women find the insertion of the internal monitor to be extremely uncomfortable and others don't find it painful at all.

These devices are definitely machines. They are sophisticated pieces of equipment and, as with all machinery, can appear quite impersonal to those unfamiliar with them. The whole area of routine fetal monitoring is an emotional and controversial one. The accuracy and interpretation of the readings has been questioned, particularly with the external devices. Undeniably, a reason that some doctors routinely use them is as protection from malpractice suits. However, it is also true that conscientious use of the fetal monitoring equipment can detect fetal distress very quickly. **If your hospital uses monitoring devices, it is good to have the equipment explained to you ahead of time.**

Another, much smaller, device is commonly used to

check the fetal heart tones during labor. This piece of equipment looks much like a small, portable tape recorder. The microphone is hand-held on the mother's abdomen and the fetal heart is amplified so that anyone nearby can hear it. This device is used periodically during the labor to screen for fetal distress. Some doctors have these machines available in their office, and women can listen to the fetal heart tones during prenatal visits. Be prepared for a very rapid heart beat; normally the fetal heart blips along at the rate of approximately 120-160 beats per minute. Because this device is used periodically instead of constantly, and it is small and portable, it does not hamper mobility nor cause discomfort of any sort.

If none of these devices is available, the nurse will check the fetal heart rate with a fetoscope, a sort of adapted stethoscope.

Find out whether the hospital allows photographic and recording equipment in labor and delivery rooms. Many hospitals will let cameras go into labor rooms, but not into delivery. If cameras are allowed, it is possible that flash photography is not. Necessary photography release forms can probably be signed when you pre-register. When you tour the hospital, pay special attention to lighting conditions in the various rooms if you are planning to take pictures. Be certain, far in advance of labor, that both the doctor and the hospital allow photography. Just because one does, does not necessarily mean that the other one does.

Ask what the hospital policy regarding the administration of anesthesia is. Most hospitals require an anesthesiologist to administer some of the drugs commonly used in childbirth. Some hospitals have an anesthesiologist on duty at all times. Some have one on duty during business hours and have somebody "on call" for the rest of the time. This could conceivably lead to a situation whereby a woman who wanted or needed a particular anesthetic could not have it if the anesthesiologist could not get to the hospital in time. Some hospitals that do not have an anesthesiologist on duty at all times require that the couple pay extra if they want the assurance of having an anesthesiologist at the hospital during off hours just in case anesthesia is desired. The fee is paid whether anesthesia is administered or not. Still other hospitals require an anesthesiologist to be in the delivery room whether or not anesthesia is requested or administered. Policies established by hospitals which do not have anesthesiologists on duty at all times can definitely cost the patients more money.

Find out what provisions will be made in the event that neither your own doctor, nor one of the back-ups, is able to reach the hospital before the birth. Will a nurse deliver the baby? Or a nurse-midwife? Is there a doctor at the hospital at all times for such situations? Nurses frequently deliver babies, and the only real problem is probably psychological. Some women want a doctor there, and it is good to know what procedures your hospital follows in this situation.

Liberal visiting hours, especially for the father, can make the hospital stay much more pleasant. During and after childbirth is a terrible time to separate a woman from her family and friends. A new mother certainly needs adequate rest, but the same number of people are likely to visit during a mother's postpartum stay whether the visiting hours are long or short; and several short visits spread out over several hours are much more restful and enjoyable than cramming 4 or 5 visitors in during an hour in the evening. Most women share different aspects of their childbirth experience with different people, and it is hard to do this when several people are visiting at once. Fathers should have special times to visit without the confusion and the distraction of other visitors. Childbirth is a very "together" experience and it takes some time alone with each other for new parents to fully comprehend what has happened. The hospital should also make some provision for a mother to visit with her other children. If the hospital regulations absolutely preclude visits by children to the mother's room, it is desirable if the mother can visit with her children in a lounge area. If the obstetric floor is on the ground level, children should be encouraged by the hospital to visit at the mother's window. Toddlers, especially, can be quite upset by maternal absence, so contact is important. Frequent contact with the mother during the postpartum hospital stay makes adjustment to the new family situation much easier for the older children. It is nice if the older children can see and touch the new baby during the hospital stay.

Some hospitals have sleeping rooms available so fathers don't have to leave. Other hospitals, a minute number, have apartment units available within the facility. A woman can check into the suite during early labor and stay there until her postpartum stay is completed. This is probably the ultimate in family-centered care. The woman can labor, deliver and care for her newborn in the relaxed, casual atmosphere of the apartment, yet have modern emergency facilities and professional medical attendants on the other side of the door. Medical assistance can be given at a moment's notice.

Some hospitals have policies that demand a woman must stay a specified number of hours in the hospital after she delivers. The length of a woman's stay should be based upon her medical condition, her home situation and her own wishes. As long as a woman is recoving well, and provisions have been made so that she won't overdo when she gets home, she should be released from the hospital as soon as she feels ready. If she enjoys the help with the baby and the rest she gets in the hospital, she should be able to stay; if she wants to go home, she should be allowed to, provided it is not medically contraindicated. On the whole, prepared women have shorter postpartum stays than Ostriches do.

Find out whether the hospital offers rooming-in. Rooming-in is an arrangement that allows the baby to stay with the mother rather than in a central nursery. There are four basic rooming-in plans and if the hospital offers rooming-in, it will probably be handled in one of the following ways.

The first is absolute rooming-in. Once rooming-in begins, the mother keeps the infant for 24 hours a day.

The baby cannot return to the central nursery at all under this plan. This means that the mother has full responsibility for the care of the baby. Many new mothers are very tired during the immediate postpartum period, and need more rest than this arrangement can afford. However, it is probably the rooming-in plan that offers the most realistic picture of life with a newborn, because the mother is charged with 24-hour care when she goes home. Some hospitals offer this plan in an attempt to discourage rooming-in. It is, of course, easier for the hospital if all babies remain in the central nursery and lie there like hamburgers waiting to be delivered to their mothers at 4-hour intervals. Since fathers are usually the only ones allowed to visit when the mother has the baby with her, mothers who have 24-hour rooming-in are not able to have other visitors.

Another basic plan is one which allows the mother to have the baby with her during the day, but not at night. The responsibility for the care of the baby rests with the mother during the day, and shifts to the nursing staff at night. This gives the mother the opportunity to care for the child during waking hours, and then allows her to get a full night's sleep. This plan doesn't offer the mother such a true picture of life with a little one, and some women are shocked into reality when they come home and no longer have a central nursery to care for the baby at night. Some hospitals allow the mother to return the baby to the nursery for periods of time during the day, too, if she wishes. With this arrangement, the mother can request the baby go to the central nursery during visiting hours, so she can receive visitors other than the father.

Under the third common plan, the mother is able to keep the baby with her as much or as little as she wishes. It's her choice whether she wants to keep the baby all night or return it to the nursery. This plan allows the mother to send the baby to the nursery any time she is feeling tired, or the baby is especially fussy. She can also arrange to have visitors other than the father.

The fourth plan is usually found only in new or newly-remodeled hospitals. The postpartum rooms are arranged around the outside of the central nursery or several rooms may surround mini-nurseries. The baby is kept in a "drawer" that can be opened from either the mother's side, or the nursery's side. When the baby drawer is pulled toward the mother's room, she is responsible for the care of the infant; when the drawer is pushed toward the nursery, the hospital staff is responsible. This situation is very convenient, because the mother can have the child immediately, whenever she wants him/her. It is not necessary to call the nurse and have her go retrieve the baby. If the baby is asleep, and the mother would like to go to sleep and be undisturbed, all she need do is push the drawer toward the nursery; this eliminates disturbing the infant during the transfer to the central nursery. Some women find the close proximity of the infant, even during the times the hospital staff is responsible for the care-taking, to be comforting. In a traditional setting the nursery can be quite a distance from the mother's room. With the nursery so far away, a woman can hear a baby's cry and have no way of knowing whether it is her baby or not.

Many women find it comforting to have rooming-in because they learn to care for the baby under supervision. It's nice to have an "expert" readily available if you have questions. Newborn babies are very tiny and very helpless. And they can be extremely demanding. When most people think "baby," their internalized picture is of a baby 5 or 6 months old. It can be shocking to realize just how small a newborn is. It's hard to understand how a newborn can possibly have all the working parts in such a small package. It is not uncommon for new parents to feel a sort of panic when they realize that they, and they alone, are responsible for the day-to-day care of this helpless human. Certainly these thoughts go through the heads of expectant couples, and often they are even verbalized during the pregnancy. However, the thoughts become very real and very concrete as they leave the hospital with the infant. Parents who have started to care for their baby during the postpartum stay are much more confident upon leaving the hospital. The nurse can assure the parents that a particular infant behavior is normal; she can help the parents with problems as well-defined as getting diapers to fit, and as open-ended as comfort mechanisms to try when the baby is fed, dry and still fussy. Many different opinions exist regarding every area of baby care. Ask questions, get answers, and then make up your own minds. It's helpful to view the hospital staff as resource people. Caring for the baby under supervision during rooming-in can clear up many questions and build confidence in your capabilities.

If a hospital does not have rooming-in, or if the parents opt against it, the father will probably not be able to touch the baby during the hospital stay. As close as he may be allowed to get is pressing his nose against the thick glass of the nursery window. This "hands off" policy can make an early father-child relationship more difficult to establish. Hospitals, especially the ones which have no rooming-in arrangements, maintain that the father-child separation reduces infection among the newborns throughout the nursery. However, research has consistently shown that the nursery and the nursery staff are the greatest sources of infection in the infants.[1,2]

Ask whether the father is allowed to hold the baby in the delivery room. Some fathers are upset by not being able to touch the infant at this point. This will quite possibly be up to the doctor in attendance, but it's good to check normal hospital procedure.

Find out how soon after delivery mothers usually get to see their babies. Some hospitals require even the healthy mother and baby to wait 12-16 hours to be together. Most hospitals let the mothers have the baby about 4-6 hours after birth. The baby is usually kept in a warming unit for the first hours after birth to stabilize the infant's temperature. Temperature stabilization is, of course, important, but experience in hospitals where it's been tried indicates that the baby whose mother is relatively unmedicated during labor and delivery will not suffer an abnormal temperature drop if s/he is quickly dried and wrapped in a warm blanket and then given to the mother to hold.[3]

The importance of frequent maternal-child contact during the early postpartum period is being recognized. Research has been done that seems to indicate that early maternal-child separation can affect later maternal behavior. According to the research, maternal-child separation during the 24 hours postpartum tends to interfere with normal maternal responses to the infant.[4] The research indicates that this early period can be crucial to establishing normal maternal-infant bonds. It has even been suggested that there may be a biochemical mechanism involved during the immediate postpartum period that produces an increased sensitivity toward the newborn.[5] Early establishment of rooming-in can help the bonding process.

How much mother-infant contact the new mother wants during the postpartum stay is largely a function of her physical condition and her perception of what Mothers should be like. A woman who has had a long and difficult labor, or who has had a Cesarean birth obviously has a greater physical need for rest during the hospital stay than the woman who has had a fairly short, relatively easy labor and delivery.

Some women feel an overwhelming need to be with the baby constantly from the moment of birth. Other women, no matter how easy the delivery was, prefer to use the time in the hospital resting and letting others care for the baby. These women may view the responsibilities of motherhood as beginning when the hospital stay ends, or they may need as much rest as they can get because of heavy family responsibilities when they return home. In any case, the choice of having or not having rooming-in should be yours. As with any aspect of the childbirth experience, what is right for you is very individual. You should choose what is right for you; not what was right for your next-door neighbor. Feeling comfortable with your choice is important.

Check to see whether the father may accompany the mother to the recovery room. In most instances, the mother will spend some time in the recovery room after she leaves the delivery room. A close check is kept on her blood pressure, involuting uterus and general condition. The length of time spent in the recovery room can range from a few minutes to several hours depending upon the mother's condition and the availability of rooms on the postpartum floor. A prepared mother is often on such a high following delivery that she finds it impossible to sleep. If the time spent in the recovery room can be shared with the father, it can be a very special time. Being completely alone in the recovery room, or sharing it with an Ostrich who has just had a "horrible" experience can be a real bummer.

In deference to the importance of the immediate postpartum period in maternal-child bonding, some hospitals are establishing mother-infant recovery rooms. This service allows hospital staff to keep a close check on both the mother and the baby during the critical postpartum period, and it allows the mother and child to become acquainted with each other. The time spent in the recovery room can be extremely lonely for the new mother, especially if she's too excited to sleep; being separated from her new little person and the father is the prime cause of the loneliness.

If you're plannng to breastfeed, find out whether you can breastfeed the infant on the delivery table. Some hospitals have absolute rules against this. The major argument against the practice is that some babies have too much mucus, or are too tired, to actually suck; doctors are concerned that if the baby refuses to suck, the mother may feel rejected. And some pediatricians and other health care practitioners feel it is important to give the infant a test feeding of glucose water before s/he goes to breast. The test feeding is done to help determine whether the baby is hooked up and working properly top to bottom, and to clean out mucus from the baby's system. However, many family-centered hospitals and doctors are allowing the mother to feed the infant on the delivery table with no ill effects at all.

In some hospitals, it is the practice to bring the baby to the mother while she is in the recovery room. **In the recovery room the mother can devote her full attention to the infant; in the delivery room there is much going on that can interfere with the relaxed atmosphere that is recommended for nursing.** Many doctors and mothers prefer that the first nursing take place in the recovery room, just a few minutes after delivery, rather than on the delivery table.

Colostrum, the substance in the breasts that precedes the milk, provides antibodies to the newborn. The earlier the infant can ingest the colostrum, the earlier the antibodies can start to be built up by the child. If the mother does not feel well enough to attempt the first nursing shortly after delivery, it should definitely be delayed; however, it is nice to have the option available. Early and frequent nursing, such as that afforded by rooming-in, helps to establish the mother's milk supply.

When you visit the hospital nursery before the baby is born, check the tags attached to the babies' beds. The tags indicate the baby's last name, sex, birthdate, birth weight, length and feeding method. If the nursery has a large number of breastfed babies, the staff is probably fairly supportive of breastfeeding and has had experience working with breastfeeding mothers. This, of course, is not always the case, but it's a good indicator.

It is true that the most common cause of failure in breastfeeding is lack of support for the breastfeeding mother. A supportive nursing staff can help the mother with many early questions about breastfeeding and can give important encouragement to the new mother. An unsupportive or antagonistic staff can do much toward sabotaging breastfeeding efforts.

Some hospitals will bring the baby to the mother on a demand basis; when the baby appears hungry, s/he is taken to the mother to be nursed. Other hospitals hold to rigid schedules and will only take the baby to the mother at predetermined times. If the baby seems to be hungry between the times s/he is scheduled to be with the mother, some nurseries feed formula or glucose water to the child, often without the mother's knowledge or consent. In some instances, hospital nursery personnel routinely supplement breastfeeding babies "just to be sure the baby is getting enough to eat."

For the proper establishment of breastfeeding, it is important not to supplement breastfeeding with formula or water unless it is absolutely necessary. If the infant is fed in the nursery shortly before s/he is taken to the mother, s/he won't nurse properly. S/he simply won't be hungry. If s/he doesn't stimulate the breast by sucking, the breast won't produce milk. Breastfeeding is an example of supply and demand in its simplest terms. The more the baby sucks (demand), the more milk will be produced (supply). The best way to establish an adequate milk supply and build a good nursing relationship between the mother and the baby is demand feeding, especially during the early days of life.

This section has been an attempt to acquaint you with some of the differences in hospital care. Too often it is assumed that all hospitals offer the same services and quality of patient care. Not all of the points mentioned in the chapter will be important to you; and those that are of importance will not all be of equal importance. Choose the factors that are most important for you and choose the hospital on the basis of its performance on those points. Before you start your search for a suitable hospital, it is helpful to realize that it is likely that no hospital will serve your needs perfectly. Choose the hospital by considering the things that are the most important to you.

Many things that are not routine hospital policy can be achieved with the help of your obstetrician and pediatrician, or your general practitioner. These health care-givers, if family-centered in their approach to maternity care, are often willing to "bend" hospital rules a little if couples make reasonable requests. If a hospital does not offer a particular service you would like, request it. When you do the requesting, remember the old adage that you can catch more flies with honey than with vinegar. Request, don't demand. Have reasons thought out ahead of time for your requests. For instance, if the hospital does not allow fathers in the delivery room, you're not going to get the father of your baby there by asserting that it is your baby and you are going to do whatever you feel like doing. You have a much better chance of getting him there by expressing a desire to share your birth experience; point out that the baby is a tangible result of your love for each other and that it is really important to you to have the father's physical presence at the moment of birth. These reasons may look a little schmaltzy printed out in black and white, but if you analyze your feelings, you will probably come up with about the same reasons for wanting to be together at the birth.

Anyway, do remember that the hospital administrators are people, just like you. They love and hate and laugh and cry the same as you do. They also feel threatened when they are put on the defensive. When you request something that the hospital does not routinely offer, you are in effect questioning the authority of the hospital. Even when you are making a perfectly logical request, you must realize that this is the initial reaction that the hospital personnel will have. If you are belligerent in your approach, the administrators will react accordingly with a determined effort not to bend to your wishes.

Even if the hospital still does not allow something that you think is important, your mentioning the request is not in vain. Hospital rules change slowly and under the pressure of consumer demand-requests. If enough consumers demand a particular service and the hospital (money-oriented as it probably is) is losing patients because of a program that is not family-centered, eventually the hospital will probably change its policies.

If the hospital does allow you something that is not often offered, do not abuse the privilege afforded you. And do write a note of thanks after the baby is born. Positive results mean that the next couple who requests the same or similar services will have an easier time getting the hospital to agree.

Many geographic locations do not offer a choice of hospitals. Often it is these hospitals, the ones that have a monopoly on patients in a given area, that are the slowest to change. The patient can't say she'll go to the hospital down the street—there isn't one. Make requests particularly carefully in this case. You shouldn't let lack of a service, or refusal of a request ruin your birth experience. All you can do is accept the situation and make it the best you can. And, in a charitable vein, you can hope that the request you've made, and the way you've conducted yourself as a prepared couple, will pave the way for future couples to enjoy family-centered maternity care at the same hospital.

It's helpful to talk to couples who have recently delivered at the hospital you are considering. It's much better if the couples you talk to were prepared couples because you are more intensely interested in a full range of things than the Ostrich couple is. Discuss what about the hospital both partners liked and disliked. Ask what sorts of problems, specifically, came up during the hospital experience. Find out how they handled problems and whether they could suggest ways to prevent the same problems from happening during your experience. Ask whether they have, since the birth, thought of more effective ways particular problems could have been handled. See whether there are any services they would have liked to have had that they hadn't thought of before the birth, and were not allowed to have because prior arrangements hadn't been made. When dealing with the hospital, remember that it is best to request a service, for instance rooming-in, even if you aren't sure you will want to have it when the time comes. In most cases if it is written on your chart, you will have the choice of accepting or rejecting the service when the time comes. If it is not written on your chart, you may not be offered the service at all, nor will you be allowed to have it if you request it while you are in the hospital. It goes without saying that if you don't care either way about something, you shouldn't hassle the hospital to give you special privileges and then change your mind after permission has been granted and paperwork has been completed.

Recently-delivered couples can be very helpful in offering practical suggestions for dealing with the hospital staff. Fathers, particularly, can be extremely helpful regarding the labor part of the hospital stay. He has a little more time to take notice of all the things that are happening than does the mother; she's busy resting between contractions as labor progresses. It's best to talk to both parents because each has a unique perspective on the birth experience and each may remember a particular incident in a different light. Recently-delivered couples can also instill lots of confidence in expectant parents regarding the effectiveness of prepared methods and the necessity of having a labor coach. Don't feel as if you are imposing on these people. Most couples, particularly prepared ones, really enjoy discussing their experience with most anyone who will listen!

If you don't know anyone who has delivered at the hospitals you are considering, perhaps a childbirth education teacher can direct you to several suitable couples. Your doctor or midwife may be able to help you find couples, too. If there's no other way to find someone, you can always check the "Birth" listings in the vital statistics section of the newspaper.

The family-centered maternity care movement makes progress every time a prepared couple has a satisfying birth experience.

Choosing a Pediatrician

Some individuals who provide prenatal and delivery care also provide for fairly long-term care of the newborn. When the mother's doctor is a general practitioner, a "family doctor," s/he will assume responsibility for the newborn as soon as s/he's born. A nurse-midwife is trained to give comprehensive care to the mother and the infant after delivery, but she operates in a support role, and her care continues only as long as the newborn's progress meets criteria accepted as normal. Some nurse-midwives continue to supply actual care to the newborn past the immediate care given at birth; others provide only counsel and support after the birth examination. Mother-infant clinics provide care to the newborn and for months, sometimes years, after birth.

However, in most cases the doctor who cares for the baby on a permanent basis is not the doctor who is involved directly with the pregnancy and birth. It is the parents' responsibility to engage a doctor to care for the baby. Usually this doctor is a pediatrician, a doctor who specializes in caring for children.

The mother tells her prenatal doctor what pediatrician she has chosen, the doctor indicates such on the chart, and the hospital staff automatically notifies the pediatrician when the baby is born. An initial exam is given by the personnel attending at the birth and the pediatrician conducts a thorough exam sometime within the 24 hours following birth. Unless there is some reason to expect a problem, the pediatrician is usually not present at the birth. When the pediatrician is notified of the birth, s/he is given pertinent information regarding the baby's condition, the length of the labor and what medications and anesthetics the mother was given during labor. This information helps the pediatrician determine whether s/he should cancel the next appointment to examine the infant immediately, or whether s/he can wait until a little later to do the examination. Realize that this is a separate service, and will not be included in the hospital billing. The pediatrician will submit a separate bill, and you will pay him/her directly.

If you have not chosen a pediatrician prior to the birth, the hospital will probably have one of the staff pediatricians examine the baby. Be sure what arrangement will be made if you don't have your own pediatrician.

A pediatrician should be chosen just as carefully as the prenatal health care is. Your association with the pediatrician can conceivably last through several years and several children. Having a pediatrician whose judgement and advice you can depend upon can ease you through many childhood tragedies and minitragedies.

When choosing a pediatrician, it is helpful to interview doctors during the pregnancy period. This is something that can be done well ahead of the time the pediatrician's services will be needed. Some doctors will talk with prospective consumers for no charge and others will not. Even if a charge is made for the doctor's time, it is money well-spent if you find a suitable doctor. The interview method can be very effective for choosing a pediatrician that the family feels comfortable with. Some of the things that parents need answers to are tangible things such as location of the office and cost for office calls; some of the things are intangible and can be judged only by personal interview. The doctor's expectations of the family, attitudes and general manner are some of the intangible points that will interest prospective patients.

The pediatrician's competency is, of course, extremely important. Ask about the doctor's education. Find out whether s/he is certified by the American Academy of Pediatrics.

The office location can be important. Some parents must depend upon public transportation, and riding a long way can become a burden. Regular check-ups are important, and the more trouble it is to keep appointments, the more likely it is that appointments will be broken or not scheduled to begin with. It is particularly easy to allow check-ups to slide when the child appears to be perfectly healthy. In case of emergency, it is good to have the pediatrician close at hand.

Find out whether the pediatrician is on staff at the hospital you have chosen for delivery. If s/he is not, or if s/he cannot conduct the newborn exam for some other reason, s/he should offer to arrange for a colleague to do the examination. It is preferable if the pediatrician is on the staff of the closest children's hospital. A hospitalized child deserves all the familiar faces it is possible to provide. Hospitals are scary places, particularly to small children, and a child shouldn't have to develop confidence and trust in a new doctor at such a stressful time.

If the pediatrician is a member of a group practice, will the child have a personal doctor, or will s/he see a different doctor each time s/he visits the office? Children really do seem to like stability, especially in unfamiliar surroundings. It can also be easier for you to build a trusting relationship if you deal primarily with one doctor.

What emergency and weekend services are available? If the physician operates within a group, it is likely that the doctors in the group will take turns being "on call." If s/he has no group, nor partner, the doctor should have a well-defined and stable plan for handling emergencies when s/he is not available. Doctors who practice alone often will exchange services with other doctors who practice alone. It is, of course, impossible for any doctor to be available at all times, but qualified medical care should be easily accessible in the doctor's absence.

Find out how large the pediatrician's practice is. If the practice is too large for the number of doctors involved, appointments will be difficult to obtain, and the doctors may view the patients as charts rather than as little people. You shouldn't have to call too far in advance to get an appointment for a check-up, and you should always be able to schedule your child very quickly in the instance of serious illness or emergency. Many offices allot a certain amount of time each day, often in the afternoon, for the benefit of children who need immediate care. In a group practice one doctor may take all of these children on a given day. In this case, it would be possible that you could be dealing with a doctor other than your own, but at least your child's primary doctor would be near if his/her presence became necessary.

Obtain a fee schedule. It is always good to know in advance approximately how much the medical care will cost. Ask how much the fee for the newborn examination is. Remember that the pediatrician's fee for this exam is not included in the hospital bill.

The pediatrician's opinion and approval of breastfeeding is very important, particularly to a new mother. The doctor remains the expert, and his/her approval and support can be crucial to the mother's success in the venture. A pediatrician who "solves" every breastfeeding problem by suggesting that the mother supplement breastfeeding with formula, does not support nor understand breastfeeding as a whole-body phenomenon. It is most desirable to have a pediatrician who advocates breastfeeding if you are planning to feed your baby that way. Remember that support, not mere tolerance, of breastfeeding is necessary. Pediatricians who recommend the early introduction of solids to breastfed and bottle-fed babies alike are not actively supportive of breastfeeding.

Find out how family concerns about the baby's health are handled. Ask whether the doctor is willing to talk frequently with the parents when they have questions. Many parents have many questions, especially during the early weeks. It's good if the pediatrician is willing to answer the very basic questions over the telephone. Of course, if there is a problem that goes beyond routine questions, the baby should be examined.

Ask how s/he feels about mothers working outside of the home. If you are planning to work outside of the home after the baby is born, whether by choice or through necessity, it is good to have your pediatrician's support in this. If s/he feels your working will have an adverse effect on the child's physical or emotional development, you will probably feel guilty. It may seem silly, but subtle or overt indications of disapproval can undermine your confidence in your own parenting abilities. The pediatrician who does not disapprove of working mothers can probably offer some very helpful suggestions about how to make the most of the working mother's "family" time.

Talk with the pediatrician about schedules and timetables. This will give you some sort of an indication whether s/he issues edicts or offers guidelines to parents. Baby care can be handled in any number of ways. Some parents feel most comfortable with simple guidelines to follow; other parents feel the need for more structured, precise instructions. Choose the approach that is right for you, and be sure that the pediatrician can adjust his/her attitude to fit your needs. Most doctors fall somewhere between the two extremes, but some pediatricians want all instructions followed to the letter and others simply refuse to give detailed instructions for general baby care.

Every person possesses special, personal life rhythms. Development is individual and can only be predicted by referring to "averages." The individuality of the person involved must be considered. Parents who are capable of viewing their infant as a separate person can accept the baby's individuality for what it is and do not try to force the child into some predetermined schedule of development. For instance some babies cut teeth at 3 months, and some cut teeth at 12 months. If you expect your child to crawl at 6 months, and s/he doesn't crawl until s/he is 9 months old, it is possible to worry yourself into an absolute tizzy. Trying to make your baby conform to a structured pattern of growth and development is an extremely frustrating experience for everyone concerned. **It is good if the pediatrician's philosophy of child development and care is openly appreciative of the individuality of each child.**

Certainly, one of the doctor's important functions is to diagnose when a child's behavior and/or development is grossly abnormal, but a wide variety of behavior and development fall within the range of normal.

By the same token, babies simply can't tell time. They can only respond to the messages they receive from their systems. Parents who attempt to rigidly schedule their baby's eating and sleeping often end up feeling frustrated and thwarted. And a demand feeding schedule makes breastfeeding much easier to establish and maintain. If the pediatrician advocates precise schedules and the parents prefer a demand arrangement, or vice versa, it can cause problems.

It can also create problems if the family and the pediatrician hold vastly differing opinions about what size a family "should" be. Even though family size is a very personal decision, the doctor can indicate disapproval in many subtle ways, often unintentionally, when the family deviates a great deal from the pediatrician's idea of perfect family size. The woman who has decided to have only one child shouldn't feel pressured by the pediatrician to have more. Nor should the woman who is in the middle of her fifth or sixth pregnancy be made to feel guilty about it. Many factors influence family size; personal preference, family economics, ecological concerns, and religion, as well as an element of chance, all count.

The religious bearing of the pediatrician is important to some families. If you think compatibility of belief could affect your relationship with the doctor and your confidence in his/her suggestions, find out about what religious views s/he holds.

Talk with the doctor about circumcision. Circumcision is an emotional and controversial topic. Usually the pediatrician is not the one who performs the circumcision, but s/he is the one who cares for the growing infant and child, so s/he can point out some positive and negative aspects of circumcision. If you have strong feelings one way or the other about it, it is good if your doctor's opinion is middle-of-the-road or agrees with yours.

Consider the age of the pediatrician. Some parents prefer young doctors because they feel comfortable with a doctor near their own age, and feel s/he will treat them as equals more than will an older doctor. Some parents would rather have an older doctor because s/he is more experienced than a young doctor, and because they feel good about the doctor's being a parent figure (or grandparent figure) for their child. Some parents prefer one or the other for different reasons. Some parents really don't care at all how old the doctor is. If you think the age factor will affect your relationship with the doctor, interview doctors with that bias in mind.

Some parents feel best when their children are cared for by a woman. If you would prefer having a woman pediatrician, by all means make a determined effort to seek one out. If you don't have any strong feelings one way or the other, be sure to interview at least a couple of women doctors, as well as a couple of men doctors, before you choose your baby's pediatrician.

Ask whether the physician employs a pediatric nurse-practitioner. The nurse-practitioner can be compared to a nurse-midwife. The nurse-midwife cares for the pregnant and delivering woman as long as everything is going along as it should be. The nurse-practitioner does the same thing for the child. She does the well-child exams and gives general instructions to the parents. When the child is ill, or when the nurse-practitioner discovers something questionable during an exam, she notifies the doctor. The nurse-practitioner is a registered nurse who has received additional special training in pediatrics. Usually, but not always, a nurse-practitioner is a woman. Many families find the doctor/nurse-practitioner combination suits their needs perfectly.

During the interview, watch for signs that the pediatrician has a sense of humor and really seems to like children. A child is often apprehensive about going to the doctor, even if s/he adores the pediatrician, simply because it is a new experience and the doctor is always poking, prodding and listening to the child's body. A child is often sick when s/he sees the doctor, and may come to automatically associate the doctor with unpleasant feelings. In addition to the strange sensations and the unfamiliar environment, if the child senses animosity on the part of the doctor, it can set a pattern of intense fear and distrust of medical personnel that can last for many years. **Watch closely for the indications that the doctor likes children; a child knows when someone truly likes him/her and when someone is only pretending.** It's some sort of sixth sense that children have.

After the interview, take some time to think about how you felt about the doctor and the interview. Did you feel comfortable? Did you feel s/he was entirely honest with you, or that s/he tailored the answers to what s/he thought you wanted to hear? Did the doctor treat you as a peer; as a partner in the job of keeping your child happy and healthy? Did the doctor seem to think the interview was a waste of time, or did s/he seem to appreciate your taking the time and effort to choose your child's doctor with such care? Did you feel that this was the person to whom you want to entrust your child's health care? Did you feel "right" about the doctor and the interview?

After you've interviewed several doctors, and selected the pediatrician you feel will best serve your needs, contact those doctors you did not choose. It is not necessary to talk personally with the doctors, nor to indicate what doctor you have chosen, but it is much more thoughtful to let the doctors know of your decision than to leave them up in the air, particularly if they didn't charge you for the interview time.

Talk again with the pediatrician you have selected. The pediatrician writes orders for the care of your baby while s/he is in the hospital. If you are requesting things that are not routine in your hospital, it is essential you make arrangements with your pediatrician for the requests that directly affect your baby. If you want to nurse your infant on the delivery table, for instance, your pediatrician will have to file orders to that effect before the baby is born. If the hospital does not routinely allow a particular practice, it's much more likely you'll be allowed to go ahead if you have the support of the pediatrician. If the requests pertaining directly to the baby are made through the pediatrician, it is usually more effective than direct requests, and you have a greater chance of positive reaction on the part of the hospital.

If you do plan to nurse on the delivery table, your pediatrician will have to write an order that it is okay for the baby to nurse before the test feeding is given. Do remember, however, that just because the pediatrician approves nursing on the delivery table, it does not necessarily mean that you will be allowed to do so. It will take the cooperation and approval of the physician attending the delivery as well.

A concerned, caring pediatrician may be able to help you get permission to keep the infant with you during the recovery period if you feel well enough to do so. Some hospitals absolutely do not allow this practice, but the only way changes are made is through consumer request. And consumer request is even more effective when it comes through medical channels and carries medical sanction. Through appropriate orders, the pediatrician may also be able to help you initiate early father-child contact if the hospital does not routinely allow it.

The pediatrician's support of a rooming-in request is often helpful, particularly in hospitals that do not encourage rooming-in. It's easier to convince the hospital personnel that breastfeeding is easier to establish with rooming-in than with carefully-spaced four-hour feedings when such a claim comes from the pediatrician. If the hospital absolutely won't allow rooming-in, the pediatrician can leave orders that the baby be fed on a demand schedule.

If you wish your baby to be entirely breastfed, and that is best for the smooth establishment of breastfeeding, the pediatrician can leave orders with the nursery staff that the baby be given no formula or glucose water. If you feel very strongly about this, you and your pediatrician can jointly order that the baby be given no artificial nipples; this order precludes the chance that any formula or glucose water is given to the baby as a part of routine feedings in the nursery.

It is a good idea to discuss with your doctor how s/he feels about the various medications and anesthetics used during labor and delivery. Pediatricians have usually had contact with many newborns whose mothers have received varying doses and combinations of drugs. Because of this extensive experience and observation, s/he may have recommendations about which drugs s/he feels affect the babies the least. Some of the drugs affect the baby in ways that are still not fully understood, and the use of every drug carries with it some degree of risk. The goal is not neces-

Pregnancy

Pregnancy is undoubtedly one of the most exciting times of a couple's life together. It is a roller coaster ride of hopes, dreams, love and emotional adjustments from the time the pregnancy is established until the baby is born. After the birth, the postpartum roller coaster takes over!

During pregnancy, much attention is focused on the "due date." Despite all the attention, **fewer than 5 per cent of all babies born are born on their official due date.** The doctor calculates the due date (or EDC —estimated date of confinement) by counting back three calendar months from the first day of the woman's last menstrual period and adding seven days to that date. This is only an estimation since a pregnancy can last anywhere between 240 and 300 days and still be normal. The average duration of pregnancy is 38 weeks (266 days) from the probable date of conception; or 40 weeks (280 days) from the first day of the woman's last menstrual period.[1]

The importance of early and constant prenatal care cannot be overemphasized. Even though a pregnant woman is not sick, she should be regularly checked in order to spot potential problems early and thus avoid complications which could be dangerous to both herself and her baby. From about the third month of pregnancy until around the seventh month, doctors usually see normal prenatal patients once a month. During the seventh and eighth months the mother is usually seen every two weeks, and during the ninth month she is seen weekly. These frequent appointments can become very boring, and seem quite pointless when the pregnancy is going along as it should be; however, keep making the appointments and continue to keep them faithfully. The old adage that an ounce of prevention is worth a pound of cure is especially applicable in this instance.

The first prenatal visit is often made to confirm pregnancy. After the pregnancy is confirmed, a complete physical is performed on the expectant mother. The entire body is involved and affected by pregnancy. The health care provider will find out as much as possible about the woman's past illnesses and medical problems by taking a complete medical history. This history, together with laboratory tests which will be ordered, will help determine whether the woman is likely to experience any particular problems during the childbearing cycle.

The prenatal physical consists of several tests and measurements. It differs from place to place exactly which are routinely done on all pregnant women, but the following are very frequently a part of the initial prenatal examination done after pregnancy is confirmed.

The woman's weight is recorded at the first and every subsequent visit. A rapid weight gain or loss can indicate there is a problem of some sort developing. For years physicians restricted women of normal prepregnant weight to a weight gain of no more than 20 pounds over the course of the pregnancy. Women who were overweight were limited much more drastically and sometimes even encouraged to lose weight during the pregnancy. Women who were underweight were allowed to gain as much as 30 pounds. However, gathering evidence seems to suggest that weight gain should not be strictly limited; low birth weight babies seem to be directly related to minimal weight gain in the mother. It is becoming more and more evident that the rate and cause of weight gain is more important than total weight gain. If the weight is gained from eating nutritious foods, and if it is gained at a steady rate rather than jumps of 8 to 10 pounds in a two-week period, it is usually no problem. It is true that gains of 45 to 50 pounds are excess in most cases, but a gain of 25 to 35 pounds is not unreasonable for most women. Doctors are starting to treat women as individuals regarding weight gain, and looking at their particular dietary patterns and weight gains as something that should be judged individually. In any instance, the food consumed during pregnancy should be nutritious. A direct and proven relationship exists between poor maternal nutrition and spontaneous premature labors, toxemia, low birth weight babies and other problems.[2]

A woman's blood pressure is watched very carefully throughout the childbearing cycle. Blood pressure is taken by wrapping a blood pressure cuff around the upper arm of the woman and then pumping the cuff up in order to apply pressure to the blood vessels. As the pressure is released, two measurements are taken. A typical blood pressure might read 110/70. The top number, the 110, is the systolic pressure and it indicates how much lateral pressure the blood exerts on the walls of the blood vessels while the heart is contracting. The bottom number, the 70, is the diastolic pressure and indicates how much pressure the blood exerts while the heart is at rest. A substantial increase in blood pressure can indicate toxemia, a serious complication of pregnancy.

Urine analysis will be done throughout the pregnancy. In many cases the doctor will give the patient a little bottle to take home with her and ask her to bring an early morning urine specimen to her next prenatal appointment. This same course of action will be followed during the entire pregnancy. The urine is tested for both sugar and albumin. The specimen should be collected before the woman has eaten anything because sugar is more likely to appear in a specimen taken after a meal. Even the normal pregnant woman can have a decreased kidney threshold for glucose, so it may spill into her urine; this is more likely to happen after a meal. If albumin is present in the urine, it is another indication that toxemia might be developing. Urine analysis also provides a simple means of detecting some infections in the pregnant woman.

During the prenatal physical, the doctor will perform a pelvic examination to check internal measurements to determine whether the pelvic measurements and motility of the coccyx appear to be adequate to allow a normal-sized baby to pass. This preliminary examination gives the doctor some idea of what the chances are of a normal, vaginal delivery. Later in the pregnancy, if the fetus appears to be larger than normal, or if the mother's measurements are smaller than average, the doctor may do an x-ray pelvimetry. This subjects the fetus to some of the radioactive material, so should be avoided unless a problem is suspected. In cases of **cephalo-pelvic disproportion (when the baby's head is too large to pass through the mother's pelvis)** a Cesarean delivery will have to be performed. If the baby is in a position other than head down, and the mother's measurements are small or just average, the doctor may advise x-ray pelvimetry to ascertain the exact size of the fetus and the mother's pelvis. During the pelvic exam, the doctor will also check the vagina for any abnormalities which might affect the delivery process.

The doctor also measures the fundal height. The fundus is the upper, rounded end of the uterus; the fundal height is the distance from the pubic bone to the fundus. Growth of both the uterus and fetus in relation to gestational age can be determined by fundal height measurement because the fundal height growth is somewhat uniform from individual to individual. The doctor makes the measurement with either a tape measure, or, more commonly, a set of calipers. The measurement is taken in centimeters.

Some of the superficial cervical cells and fluid may be taken for a Papanicolaou (Pap) smear. This is a test done to detect cancer of the cervix at its earliest stages. The cervical smear is examined under the microscope and classified as a Class 1, 2, 3, 4 or 5 smear. Class 1 and Class 2 smears have a complete absence of possibly cancerous cells and are considered normal. The Class 3, 4, and 5 smears contain cells that are either actually malignant or give indications of possible malignancy. A second cervical smear may be used for a Gonococcus (GC) test; this test detects gonorrhea in the pregnant woman.

Several blood tests may be taken. A Complete Blood Count (CBC) is done to identify how many of each type of cell is in the blood. A Venereal Disease Reference Laboratory (VDRL) test is used to screen for syphilis. A Rubella titre may be done to determine whether or not the pregnant woman has had, or been exposed to, rubella (German Measles). A pregnant woman's blood is typed (A, B, AB or O) and tested for the presence or absence of an antigen known as the Rh antigen.

An antigen is a protein substance which causes production of other specific substances called antibodies. Antibodies usually react against antigens foreign to one's body, but not against one's own antigens. **Blood which has the Rh antigen is classified as Rh + blood; blood which doesn't have the Rh antigen is classified as Rh − blood.** Therefore, the Rh + and Rh − designation indicates the presence or absence of the Rh antigen. It is extremely important to determine the pregnant woman's Rh factor. In the case where the mother is Rh − and the father is Rh +, it is possible that the baby will inherit the Rh factor and be Rh +. During pregnancy small amounts of fetal blood may cross the placenta and enter the mother's blood stream.

An Rh − mother carrying an Rh + fetus will produce antibodies to destroy the foreign Rh + antigens in her blood stream. This is a protective device called sensitization. The first Rh + fetus is usually not affected because the sensitization takes place gradually. However, at delivery there may be a more extensive exchange of blood. This causes the mother to manufacture more antibodies. In future pregnancies, these antibodies may cross the placenta and destroy the fetal blood if it is Rh +. Within the last decade or so an anti-Rh immune globulin called RhoGAM has been developed. **Administration of RhoGAM within 72 hours of termination of an Rh + pregnancy, whether by birth, abortion or miscarriage, prevents the mother from forming the antibodies and therefore protects the next Rh + fetus.** The RhoGAM must be administered after every Rh + pregnancy to be effective. Rh incompatibility has caused countless fetal and neonatal deaths over the centuries, and the development of the RhoGAM globulin is a great advancement in maternity care. If the doctor feels it advisable, s/he may order an Rh titre done several times throughout an Rh − woman's pregnancy in order to determine the amount of antibodies the mother's blood has produced to react against the Rh + antigens. Something less than 15 per cent of the total population is Rh −. No chance of an Rh problem exists if the mother is Rh + and the father is Rh +, or if the mother is Rh + and the father is Rh −, or if both are Rh −. The only time the possibility of a problem exists is when the mother is Rh − and the father is Rh +. And if the result of the union is an Rh − fetus, no Rh problem exists.

Another blood incompatibility, the ABO incompatibility, is more common, but less serious, than Rh incompatibility. The ABO mechanism is much like the Rh mechanism, except the ABO incompatibility usually affects the first-born baby, too.

Blood incompatibility is not something that a pregnant woman should be overly concerned about since the development of RhoGAM and other protective and screening devices. The important thing is that the health care practitioners be aware of all pertinent details. Blood incompatibilities can lead to death of the fetus or baby in the most severe cases, but that is very uncommon today. Sometimes an exchange transfusion is necessary for the newborn, but most commonly the affected child will merely be jaundiced for the first few days. The jaundice is caused because red blood cells are being destroyed faster than the liver can excrete them. As the red blood cell is broken down, a yellow substance called bilirubin is produced. Presence of this bilirubin in the child's system causes the skin to take on a yellowish cast. When the bilirubin concentration is dangerously high, the baby may be placed under bright lights ("bililites") to help destroy the bilirubin. More frequently, as the baby's liver matures, it starts handling the bilirubin and the jaundice disappears by itself after the first week or so.

The whole subject of transmission of blood groups and blood incompatibilities in very complex and beyond the scope of this book; the information given here is very basic. If you have further questions, be sure to ask your doctor.

The doctor may check the woman's breasts for conditions, such as inverted nipples, which may require special preparation during the pregnancy period in order that breastfeeding may be easier.

The doctor may suggest that the woman visit her dentist because total health care is so important to producing the most comfortable pregnancy and the healthiest child possible. X-rays should be avoided, if possible, during pregnancy. If the mother has dental x-rays done, she should wear a lead apron to minimize the chance of any radiation reaching the developing baby.

Certain things will be done at each prenatal exam, but the rest of the prenatal exams will not be nearly so complete, or so lengthy, as the one during which the complete physical is done. **Weight, blood pressure and fundal height will always be recorded.** A urinalysis will be done at each visit, preferably with an early-morning specimen. The doctor will listen for fetal heart tones, and will palpate the abdomen to determine the size and position of the fetus and uterus. Until the last weeks, the position of the fetus is unimportant because until then it has enough room in the uterus to turn complete somersaults, and s/he frequently does. As the fetus grows, there is no longer room for such antics and during the last weeks the fetus usually settles into the position it will have when labor begins. The position at this time is important because it determines the presenting part of the fetal body. The presenting part is that part of the fetus which is nearest to the os, the opening of the cervix. This is the part that will emerge first from the mother's body at birth.

In approximately 96 per cent of all term births, the head is the presenting part of the fetus.[3] The head is the largest and heaviest single part of the fetal body, and it usually settles down into the mother's pelvic cavity. The head presentation is called a cephalic presentation. The second most common presentation is the breech presentation in which the buttocks, a foot or a knee proceed from the uterus first. In some very rare cases the shoulders or back may be the presenting part. Presentations are more fully discussed in the chapter dealing with special labors and births.

During late pregnancy the doctor may do a vaginal or rectal examination in order to determine whether any ripening, effacement or dilatation of the cervix has taken place.

The prenatal visits should be viewed as an opportunity for the woman to assure herself that the pregnancy is progressing normally, as well as a time to ask questions about anything regarding the childbearing cycle that she may be wondering about. Many people become tongue-tied at about the time the doctor says, "How do you feel?" or "Do you have any questions?" Most people suddenly feel fine and have no questions at all—until they walk out of the door. It is important to regard the doctor as an individual willing and prepared to answer questions. In most cases the doctor is being well paid for medical services and it is reasonable for the patient to expect just that. If the doctor never seems to have time to answer questions, or to explain things adequately, complain. Let your caretakers know what you expect of them in the way of service, advice and answers. Because of the Tongue-tie syndrome and the Sudden Loss of Memory syndrome, it is usually helpful to jot down questions as they occur to you between visits. Keeping a slip of paper in your purse, or the pocket of your favorite coat, might be a good idea. Every time you think of a question or a concern, or if you have some physical sensation you want to ask the doctor about at your next visit, you can write it down on your piece of paper and be ready the next time s/he asks whether you have any questions.

Doctors usually give their patients a list of danger signals to be reported. Some should be reported as soon as they happen, even if it is in the middle of the night; some should be reported as soon as the doctor's office or clinic next opens. Presence of one or more of these conditions may or may not be indicative of a serious complication, but that is for the medical personnel, not the expectant mother, to decide.

The doctor should be notified immediately of any:

1. **Vaginal bleeding. Bleeding is never normal in pregnancy.**
2. **Sharp abdominal pain or severe cramping.**
3. **Dizziness.**

If any of the following occur, the doctor should be notified as soon as the office or clinic opens, sooner if the symptoms persist during a long period when the office or clinic is not open, for instance over the weekend.

1. Disturbances in vision such as dimness, blurring, flashes of light or dots before the eyes.
2. Persistent nausea or vomiting.
3. Puffiness or swelling of hands, face and feet; a woman often notices this upon arising in the morning and finds her rings are tight.
4. Severe, continuous headache.

5. Painful or burning urination.
6. Irritating vaginal discharge.
7. Chills and fever; or oral temperature of more than 100°.
8. Sudden escape of fluid from vagina.
9. Marked decrease in urine output.

FETAL DEVELOPMENT

The development of the baby from the union of an egg from the mother's body and a sperm from the father's body can only be classified as a miracle. The ovum measures about 1/25 of an inch across. It is fertilized, usually in the upper portion of the fallopian tube, by the male sperm. The sperm is much, much smaller than the ovum, and the father usually provides some 20 million to 500 million sperm cells per ejaculation. The fertilized egg continues on down the fallopian tube and implants somewhere in the uterine lining that has built up since the preceding menstrual period. This lining nourishes the zygote, as the fertilized egg is called. From the third to the fifth week of gestation, the developing baby is called an embryo, and after the fifth week, it is called a fetus. During the early weeks, the egg is nourished by the uterine lining and the yolk sac of the egg.

By the end of the third month of gestation the placenta has taken over the function of providing the fetus with food, oxygen and water. The placenta is the organ that serves as a go-between for the mother and the fetus. The fetus and the placenta are connected by the umbilical cord; one end of the cord is attached to the center of the placenta and the other end is attached to what will be the baby's bellybutton. At term the umbilical cord is some two feet long and about three-quarters of an inch in diameter. The cord contains two arteries and one vein twisted together and protected by a substance called Wharton's jelly. The vein supplies substances to the fetus and the arteries remove waste products. When the baby is born, the placenta weighs approximately one pound and is eight inches in diameter and one inch thick. For a long time it was thought that the placenta filtered out all "bad" things and that the baby received only the good and pure things. It is now known that almost everything that the mother ingests, including alcohol, most drugs and nicotine from cigarettes, crosses the placenta and enters the fetal blood system. The mother provides the fetus with its needs through the porous blood vessels of the umbilical cord; the mother's blood doesn't actually enter the cord.

Because the normal menstrual cycle is 28 days (4 weeks), doctors often refer to periods of lunar months, or four-week periods of time, in describing fetal development. Conception, usually about 14 days after the start of the woman's last menstrual period, begins the first lunar month. **At the end of the first lunar month the embryo is approximately ¼ of an inch long and has a tail.** Even by this time organs have started to become differentiated, blood is pulsating through tiny, tiny arteries and the arms and legs have just begun to form. The backbone has formed, and the beginnings of the digestive system are visible.

At the end of the second lunar month the fetus is about 1 inch long and weighs just about one thirtieth of an ounce. During this month the embryo became a fetus and began to resemble the human form. The head is very large because of brain development. The fetus has arms, legs, fingers, toes, elbows and knees by the end of the month. The tail has reached its greatest development; from now on it becomes less and less prominent. The external genitalia have appeared, but sex is not visually distinguishable.

By the end of the third lunar month the fetus is more than 3 inches long and weighs approximately one ounce. Specialization is occurring; the fingers and toes have become shaped and even the early teeth buds are present. The external sex organs are developing. At this time the fetus is moving about in the uterus, but the movements are too weak for the mother to feel. **During the fourth lunar month the fetus grows to a length of 6½ inches and to a weight of 4 ounces.** By this time the placenta and the umbilical cord are well-formed. Movements are more vigorous, but few women feel them yet.

At the end of the fifth lunar month the fetus is about 10 inches tall and weighs 8 ounces or so. It is during this month that the doctor will probably be able to first hear the fetal heart through the fetoscope. This is also an exciting time because most mothers feel the fetus moving for the first time. This is called quickening. Lanugo (fine downy hair) appears all over the body of the fetus. Most of the lanugo disappears by the time a term baby is born.

During the sixth lunar month the fetus grows to about 12 inches and 1½ pounds. The skin is red and wrinkled, but the fetus does look just like a miniature baby now. During the next few months the fetus develops subcutaneous fat. About now the vernix caseosa, the substance which protects the fetal skin from the liquid environment, starts to develop. The head is still large in proportion to the body; eye brows and eye lashes are formed.

At the end of the seventh lunar month the fetus is about 15 inches tall and weighs approximately 2½ pounds. A baby born now has a fair chance for survival if s/he's given expert medical care. **By the end of the eighth lunar month the fetus is approximately 16½ inches long and weighs about 4 pounds. During the next month the fetus grows some 2½ inches and just about 2 pounds.** Between the middle and the end of the tenth lunar month the fetus is at full term and will probably be born. At birth the baby is usually between 7 and 8 pounds and between 19 and 22 inches long. Boy babies are usually slightly bigger than girl babies.

The fetus and the amniotic fluid are contained in the amniotic sac (or bag of waters) during life in utero. The amniotic fluid serves to protect the fetus from outside stimuli; this protection is why the fetus is seldom damaged, even if the mother takes a very bad fall. The amniotic sac protects the fetus from infection and provides it with a constant temperature.

The fetus can move about easily in the liquid environment and can exercise in utero. The production and removal of amniotic fluid is still not fully understood, but we do know that approximately one third of the volume of the fluid is replaced every hour. At that rate approximately six gallons of amniotic fluid is exchanged daily during a good portion of the pregnancy. By around the fifth month the amniotic sac contains approximately one quart of fluid. At about the seventh month the amount of fluid is automatically adjusted to approximately one pint. This reduction in the amount of fluid gives the growing fetus more room to move.

The sex of the baby is determined by the sperm from the male at the moment of conception. Each normal body cell, except the sperm and the ovum, contains 23 pairs of chromosomes. These chromosomes determine the person's hair color, eye color, height, bone structure and the other characteristics that humans have. When the sperm and the ovum unite to form the eventual baby, the fertilized egg has 46 chromosomes (23 pairs); 23 chromosomes from the mother and 23 chromosomes from the father. Normal male cells, except the sperm cells, carry both an X and a Y sex chromosome. The female cells carry only X sex chromosomes. If the sperm cell (which contains only 23 chromosomes, instead of the 23 pairs of chromosomes that other body cells contain) is carrying an X sex chromosome, the baby will be a girl because the mother only has an X chromosome to offer. If the sperm cell is carrying a Y sex chromosome, the baby will be a boy because the fertilized egg will have both an X and a Y sex chromosome.

The sex of the unborn baby can be determined by examining the amniotic fluid. However, the process of amniocentesis, the withdrawal and subsequent study of amniotic fluid through the pregnant woman's abdomen, is only performed when some genetic disease in the fetus is suspected or when the baby has gone long past the woman's EDC. It is a relatively safe procedure, but an expensive one that should be avoided unless medically indicated. Using amniocentesis to determine the sex of the fetus merely out of curiosity would be foolhardy.

NUTRITION

Nutrition is a big and complex subject. Many women don't know much more about nutrition than what they heard in their high school home ec classes. Pregnancy is an excellent time to supplement (or replace, if high school home ec was very long ago) that knowledge and learn a bit about the subject. Many good books are available dealing with both general nutrition and with nutrition as it relates specifically to pregnancy. Suffice it to say here that the growing fetus has many nutrition requirements and s/he gets only what the mother ingests. If the mother ingests only ice cream, french fries, popcorn and Pepsi, that's all the fetus will get. If she ingests a nutritionally sound diet, that's what the baby will get. Considering that research has shown that good nutrition in the mother is directly related to her baby's brain development,[4] most mothers would probably rather their baby got the nutritionally sound diet rather than the popcorn diet. Iron is particularly necessary for the mother and fetus during pregnancy. During pregnancy, the fetus is storing up iron to use for as long as six months after birth. This depletes the mother's iron supply drastically, and physicians often prescribe an iron preparation for the expectant mother to take. Adequate amounts of protein are also very important.

BODILY CHANGES

Many changes, some slight and some extremely obvious, take place in the woman's body during the childbearing cycle. It's very apparent that the most noticeable change is in the size and the shape of her abdomen. In its prepregnant state the uterus weighs approximately 3 ounces and measures roughly 3 inches by 2 inches by 1; when it contains a term baby the uterus weighs approximately 3 pounds and measures somewhere in the area of 12 inches by 9 inches by 8 inches. Some women carry their babies right out front and others carry them farther inside their bodies. Some women carry their babies very high and some women carry their babies very low. A woman is not necessarily consistent from one pregnancy to the next; she may carry one baby high and outside and the other low and inside. It is impossible to predict how a particular woman will carry her baby and how "big" she'll get during the pregnancy. How the baby is carried has absolutely nothing to do with the sex of the baby. Normally the pregnant woman will start to "show" her expanding uterus around the fourth or fifth month.

As the abdominal wall stretches to accommodate the growing uterus, pink or reddish striations may occur in the skin of the abdomen and thighs. These marks are known as striae gravidarum, but are frequently called simply stretch marks. These marks occur when the deep connective tissue is stretched and ruptured. The striae gravidarum never completely disappear, but they look like whitish scars instead of pink marks after delivery. A dark line between the umbilicus and the bottom of the abdomen may develop. This is called the linea nigra. The external genitalia may darken, and chloasma, the so-called mask of pregnancy, may develop on the woman's face. Chloasma is characterized by dark blotches of pigmentation; the spots usually disappear after delivery. Vascular spiders are small, bright red spots which may appear on the body. These marks will disappear upon delivery of the child.

The umbilicus (bellybutton) is also involved in the abdominal changes. At about the seventh month of pregnancy the umbilicus is no longer a depression; it is just a darkened area on the abdomen. During the last weeks of pregnancy, the umbilicus may be pushed out further and actually protrude.

The cervix, the neck at the opening of the uterus, becomes shorter, more vascular and produces increased secretions during pregnancy. The vagina, the birth canal, experiences an increase in the muscular layer and develops a blue coloration. Whitish vaginal discharge is very common during pregnancy.

Some obvious changes occur in the pregnant woman's breasts. During the third month the breasts begin to enlarge and become firmer. Often the breasts will be very tender, and a woman may experience some tingling or throbbing in the nipple area. The area which surrounds the nipple, the areola, darkens near the end of the third month. Sometimes, usually about a month later, brownish spots may appear on the skin surrounding the areola. This is called the secondary areola. Blood supply to the breasts is increased and the veins may become very apparent through the skin. Many A and B cup women are pleased with the increase in the size of their breasts. Many C and D cup women are equally displeased. If a woman has large breasts, it is particularly important that her breasts are adequately supported during pregnancy. Many claim that poor breast support during pregnancy, rather than breastfeeding, is what causes sagging breasts.

A normal woman who doesn't overeat during her pregnancy gains between 20 and 30 pounds on the average. The weight gain is usually distributed as follows:[5]

Fetus	7.5 to 8.5 pounds
Placenta	1.0 - 1.5 pounds
Amniotic Fluid	1.5 - 2.0 pounds
Uterus and Breasts	5.0 - 5.5 pounds
Blood and Fluid	4.0 - 7.0 pounds
Muscle and Fat	1.0 - 6.0 pounds
	20.0 to 30.5 pounds

The blood volume and fluid content of the body increases by about 30 per cent approximately 4 pints, during pregnancy. This increase means the heart has more blood to pump and the pulse rate increases by 10-12 beats per minute by about the 36th week of pregnancy.

The pregnant woman's diaphragm may be displaced as much as an inch by the upward expansion of the uterus. To compensate for this, the thoracic cage widens, producing a lateral expansion of the chest. The pregnant woman's respiration is deeper, and she takes in more air than the nonpregnant woman, but her respiration rate does not increase. The expectant mother is oxygenating the baby's blood as well as her own. Taking three or four deep breaths before rising from a sitting or lying position can help relieve possible dizziness or breathlessness.

COMMON DISCOMFORTS

Many of the common discomforts can be directly related to the physical changes in the body that are a direct result of the pregnancy. **Nausea, particularly in the morning upon arising, is the most common complaint during the first trimester (three-month period) of pregnancy.** Somewhere around 50 per cent of all pregnant women suffer from nausea during the first months of pregnancy; some of these vomit. Some people feel that "morning sickness" is entirely due to emotional causes and the power of suggestion, but there is growing evidence that disturbances in the metabolism of glucose and changes in the hormonal balance may be responsible for the feeling of nausea. Some women find it helpful to eat a light sweet snack, such as milk and toast with jelly, before going to bed at night. Others find that eating a couple of dry soda crackers or some dry toast about a half hour before getting up in the morning helps to control the nausea. Some women have found that adding an egg to their diet helps; others have found that a diet high in protein is helpful. Trial and error is about the only way to find out what is most helpful to a particular individual. Some women are bothered less by nausea if they eat several small meals during the day instead of three larger meals. The period of nausea is usually confined to between the end of the fourth week of gestation to about the twelfth week. If nausea and vomiting are particularly severe, the doctor can prescribe medication.

Another frequent complaint is constipation. It is probably caused by pressure from the expanding uterus, and can usually be helped a great deal by appropriate diet. Adequate fluid intake and roughage in the diet help; roughage is provided by fruits, vegetables, coarse foods and whole grain breads. Prune juice, figs and raisins may help the problem. A regular pattern of moving the bowels each day, for instance after breakfast, is recommended to help establish regularity. Some women find it easier to move their bowels if they elevate their legs on a footstool (or a child's potty chair) while sitting on the toilet. This leg elevation places the body in a semi-squatting position that is physiologically more correct for moving the bowels than the familiar sitting position. A pregnant woman should not take any medication, sold over-the-counter or by prescription, unless it is recommended by her physician. This includes laxatives and enemas.

Regular evacuation of the bowels, coupled with some minor dietary restrictions, can also help prevent flatulence. The gas is usually caused by bacterial action in the intestines, and some foods, such as beans, parsnips, corn, sweet desserts, fried foods and candy, are particularly prone to the production of gas.

Many women develop varicose veins during pregnancy. A varicose vein is one which is enlarged due to stretching, and consequent thinning, of the vein wall. Progesterone, one of the hormones associated with pregnancy, causes muscles to relax and may be responsible, at least in part, for the lack of tone in the walls of the veins. Pressure exerted in the pelvis by the uterus and the increased flow of blood from the uterus act to impede return of the blood from the legs. Articles of clothing that bind tightly around the legs should be avoided, as should long periods of standing. Support hose and, in more extreme cases, elastic bandages may provide relief. Frequent elevation of the legs helps relieve the aching connected with varicose veins.

In some cases a pregnant woman may be instructed to lie on her bed with her legs and feet elevated at a ninety degree angle to her body; this is accomplished by placing her buttocks against the wall and resting her heels against the wall.

Hemorrhoids are varicose veins of the rectum. Avoidance of constipation is the best way to avoid hemorrhoids, because they are usually caused and worsened by straining to move the bowels. The doctor can prescribe hemorrhoidal preparations that will afford relief.

Leg cramps are frequent complaints, particularly during the latter months of pregnancy. These muscle contractions are due to the pressure the growing uterus is applying to the nerves which go to the legs. Cramps are usually sudden and painful. The cramp can be relieved by forcing the toes back toward the face; this is usually best accomplished while in a sitting or reclining position. It is often necessary to apply pressure on the foot with the hand, and it is helpful to push down on the knee at the same time in order to straighten the leg. The legs are much more prone to cramping when the woman is tired or cold. Leg elevation can help in avoidance of cramps.

Swelling (edema) of the lower extremities is common during pregnancy; if severe it may be a sign of toxemia. Toxemia is more suspect if swelling of the hands and face is also present. In most cases the swelling is of no consequence, but it may be uncomfortable. Regular rest periods throughout the waking hours can help alleviate the problem. Swelling of the vaginal area can be relieved by applying a cold compress to the perineal area. A very cold bottle or can of juice wrapped in a thick towel can be utilized quite nicely for this purpose.

Backache is also common. A woman's center of balance changes as her abdomen is distended by the growing uterus and fetus. In compensation for this, she tends to sway her back and push her shoulders back. As in the nonpregnant condition, good posture can do much to alleviate backache. Low-heeled shoes help assure proper posture. Relief from backache can be provided by doing pelvic rocks. Fatigue, improper bending, and improper lifting intensify the problem and should be avoided. Backache should be relieved by physical rather than chemical means if at all possible. The pregnant woman should not take anything, even anything as reputedly innocuous as aspirin, without the consent of her doctor. Too little is known about the effects of drugs on the unborn baby. Aspirin, for instance, slows clotting time and may be associated with hemorrhage in the newborn if taken in large enough quantities during late pregnancy.

Despite the fact that pregnant women actually breathe in more air than nonpregnant women, a feeling of a shortness of breath is common. Again, the expanding uterus is a cause. It is applying pressure on the diaphragm in this case, and the problem is particularly prevalent during the last weeks when the uterus is at its largest. Sleeping in a semi-sitting position, propped up by pillows may help the woman who has so much difficulty in breathing that she finds it hard to sleep.

The burning sensation known as heartburn may occur at any time during the pregnancy, but is particularly common during the last 12 weeks. Apparently, progesterone causes relaxation of the cardiac sphincter of the stomach; relaxation of this muscle allows some of the contents of the stomach to re-enter the esophagus. This causes the burning that is felt behind the lower part of the sternum. Heartburn has absolutely nothing to do with the heart. Greasy and spicy foods should be avoided, and large amounts of food should not be eaten at one time. Baking soda, a common remedy for heartburn, should not be taken because of its sodium content. The sodium frequently causes excess fluid retention. Your doctor can recommend low-sodium antacids that may help. Some women find that eating celery relieves heartburn. Sitting tall and breathing deeply can also help relieve the discomfort caused by heartburn.

Bleeding of the gums and nose is a frequent complaint of pregnant women. It may be caused by a vitamin C deficiency, and eating citrus fruits and other sources of this vitamin may help relieve this minor problem.[6] It may be caused by the pregnant woman's increased blood volume putting additional pressure on capillaries.

During the first trimester many women experience fatigue and drowsiness. This overall feeling of tiredness usually subsides after the first weeks of pregnancy and does not reoccur until the strains caused by the enlarging uterus become more and more prominent near term. Sleeplessness is very common during late pregnancy because many women, especially those with particularly large abdomens, find it almost impossible to get comfortable. This, coupled with awaking two or three times during the night to go to the bathroom, contributes to a generally fatigued condition. It is important to the mother, as well as to the baby, to get an adequate amount of rest throughout pregnancy. This is particularly important as labor approaches, because the well-rested woman is much better able to cope with the strains and pressures of labor than is the fatigued woman. If sleeping is difficult due to the where-to-put-the-stomach problem, experimenting with pillow props will probably help. Practicing relaxation techniques taught in childbirth education classes can help women make the most of even short periods of rest during the day. It is extremely important to learn to interpret body signals and follow them. If the body says that rest is needed, it is. And it should be taken as soon as possible.

A frequent desire to urinate is almost universal among pregnant women. During the early weeks, before the uterus has risen out of the pelvis, this is caused by the enlarging uterus stretching the base of the bladder. This stretching causes a sensation just like that felt when the bladder is distended with urine. As the uterus rises out of the pelvic cavity, the pressure on the bladder is lessened and the frequent desire to urinate is lessened. Toward the end of the pregnancy, the uterus may apply renewed pressure on the bladder and produce again the frequent desire to urinate. The only way to cope with this symptom of pregnancy is to accept it with an element of humor. Nothing anyone can do will change it. Fluid intake should not be restricted in an attempt to lessen the problem; fluids are very important at any time, and particularly so during pregnancy when the body must work for more than one.

Due to increased vaginal secretion, increased vaginal discharge is normal during pregnancy. This should be considered of no consequence unless it is particularly abundant, is yellow or greenish in color, is odorous, is irritating or is accompanied by burning during urination or causes itching. If these symptoms occur, or if the presence of discharge is upsetting, the doctor should be consulted. Douching and feminine hygiene sprays are both medications of sorts and should not be used unless the doctor specifically recommends such.

Dizziness and fainting are relatively common in pregnancy and may be caused by the pressure the enlarged uterus applies to major blood vessels and the consequent drop in blood pressure. The frequency and persistence of this problem depends to some degree on the size and the position of the fetus. Another cause of dizziness and light-headedness may be pooling of blood in the legs allowed by relaxation of the blood vessels. This is caused by hormonal changes. Rapid position changes by the expectant mother, standing for extended periods, fatigue, excitement and nervousness can all bring on the dizziness. The problem can be minimized by moving slowly to avoid causing blood pressure changes, and by sitting instead of standing as often as possible. Dizziness should definitely not be ignored; it should be reported to the doctor. S/he'll be able to decide whether the cause is serious or not.

Many women experience dizziness, caused by hyperventilation, while practicing prepared childbirth breathing techniques. The breathing techniques are designed partially to supply the laboring woman with the extra oxygen she needs to cope with the stresses of labor. As the oxygen level increases, there is an abnormal loss of carbon dioxide from the blood. This causes first a tingling sensation in the extremities and face, and then a feeling of dizziness and restlessness. Hyperventilation can be helped by rebreathing one's own air for several breaths. This can be accomplished by breathing into cupped hands or a paper sack. This serves to rebalance the oxygen-carbon dioxide level in the blood. Hyperventilation is less of a problem during labor than during practice because oxygen requirements are increased during labor.

Itchy skin may be experienced during pregnancy. Sometimes the itching is localized on the stretching abdomen and breasts and sometimes it is generalized over the entire body. Cold cream, hand lotions, calamine lotion, baby powder or other soothing salves may be helpful in controlling the itching.

Due to total body adjustments, many small, temporary changes may take place during the childbearing cycle. Increased or decreased appetite, increased or decreased hair growth, voice changes and more rapid temperature changes can all be associated with pregnancy.

Good posture and body mechanics can do much toward relieving the minor discomforts of pregnancy. Backache, particularly, can be minimized by proper posture. Carrying the uterus back and inside the body instead of unnecessarily pushing it forward reduces the strain on the back muscles. The legs, rather than the back, should absorb the effort during stooping, lifting and carrying movements. Low-heeled shoes can aid in attaining good posture.

Varicose veins, leg cramps and swelling are all directly related to poor circulation. As often as possible, the pregnant woman should make herself really comfortable, remove sharp angles from her limbs and elevate her legs; all of these things contribute to improved circulation. Binding, tight clothing should be avoided. Frequent rest periods are essential, particularly during the last trimester of pregnancy.

EMOTIONS

Most women exhibit less emotional stability during the childbearing cycle than during other, less stressful periods of their lives. This generally means that emotions, good or bad, are felt more intensely during pregnancy and the postpartum period than they normally are. Therefore, a woman who is usually very even-tempered and stable may exhibit some signs of becoming more emotional; a woman who is normally quite emotional may become even more so. In some cases, a woman who is normally very emotional may become more calm and even-tempered during the childbearing cycle, but this is the exception rather than the rule.

Pregnancy is, without a doubt, a very stressful time. Long before anyone else becomes aware of the pregnancy, the expectant mother knows she is growing a baby inside of her body. Some women identify the growing fetus as a person from the very early stages of pregnancy, and others view the fetus as an object, but not necessarily as a person. Pregnancy brings with it an entirely new state of consciousness. Many women feel as though their defenses against outside stimuli are lowered. This brings a feeling of not being able to cope. The pregnant woman can't even control what is happening inside her own body; the growth and movement of the fetus is simply not directly controllable by the woman—so she often feels that she certainly can't cope with, nor control, outside stimuli.

Mother-child conflicts that have been buried for years can emerge during pregnancy. The woman is moving from being the Child to being the Mother. She must suddenly reconstruct her perception of what is "right." She is to be the mother now; she must view the world now from the perspective of a mother rather than that of a child. It's very common for a pregnant woman to feel a need to re-examine her relationship with her own mother.

Sensitivity, dependence, passivity and introspection are all very common during pregnancy. Moods frequently swing from a high high to a low low. Lots of pregnant women are very irritable. Fears and feelings of stress often result in increased dreaming and easier and more total recall of dreams. It is not at all uncommon for a pregnant woman to have explicit dreams about giving birth to a deformed, dead or premature baby, giving birth to several babies, or giving birth to kittens. Talking out these dreams with a caring person can help immeasurably. Realization that these dreams are only manifestations of free-floating anxieties and fears involved with the entire childbearing cycle can put the dreams in their proper perspective. The dreams are not omens of awful things to come.

Pregnant women, without even trying, seem to think of numerous things to be afraid of. Unless the fears become obsessions, they can be healthy. Really thinking something through can result in many creative solutions to a particular problem should it actually come up.

Some of the most common fears during pregnancy relate to the health and well-being of the mother and the baby. The fear of miscarriage, often prevalent during the early months of pregnancy, gives way to a fear of starting labor prematurely. Fears of giving birth to a defective or retarded infant are very frequent. Before pregnancy, a woman usually feels that her future baby couldn't possibly be the one in 10,000 who has a rare disease; during pregnancy the same woman often feels that somebody has to be the one in 10,000 and it is probably her baby. Seeing a retarded child, in person or on television, seems to be particularly effective in triggering this it-must-be-me response. Fear of ugly birthmarks is common. In days past, it was believed that if a mother were frightened by something during the pregnancy, a bear for example, the baby would be born with a birthmark in the shape of a bear. The myth has persisted because babies are often born with temporary splotches on their skin. People with imagination can make the splotches resemble anything they please. It's kind of like finding animals or ice cream cones in the clouds.

Fear of great physical discomfort, particularly during the labor and birth cycle, is promoted by the stories of "knowing" women. Childbirth education can lessen these fears to a great extent. Some women are intensely afraid of the physical mechanics of the birth; they are afraid the baby won't come out and that the baby and/or mother will die. Fear of the necessity of a Cesarean delivery is common. Again, childbirth education can reduce these concerns a great deal.

Other fears are related to less concrete, less well-defined issues. Many women, especially those who have spent very little time around children, are concerned about their own ability to parent. Lots of women have never even changed a diaper until they meet their own infant's wet bottom. Parenting includes a wide variety of behaviors, and expectant parents often are afraid life as they knew it will completely dissolve after the baby is born. The fear of being tied down to the house and the baby is something that most women must deal with. Happily, sharing of parental responsibility is becoming more and more popular, but in the final analysis, primary responsibility for the care of the baby rests with the mother in most cases. A woman is almost forced into re-evaluation of what she thinks a "good" mother is. Mothers on television and down the street seem to be so unharried and unselfishly giving in their relationships with their children. These feelings, and appropriate resolution, are really more involved with the postpartum period, but mothers usually begin dealing with this concept of "mother" during the pregnancy.

A woman is frequently afraid of losing her figure. This is entwined with dismay at the appearance of her own pregnant body. This feeling is accentuated a great deal if the male partner shows displeasure with the changes in her body during pregnancy. Perception and appearance of the woman's body deals directly with the sensitive area of sexual responsiveness and communication. Pregnancy often alters a woman's sexual response; sometimes her desire for sexual activity increases and sometimes it decreases. Sexual relationships are particularly complex because they involve attitudes toward the pregnancy, toward the appearance of the pregnant body, toward parenthood, and the sexual relationship the couple had before the pregnancy. Many, many factors influence sex, and it must be realized that the degree of sexual responsiveness during pregnancy is not necessarily the degree of responsiveness that will exist after the baby is born. Communication between the partners is the best way to adjust to any changes in sexual appetite or responsiveness. As the pregnancy progresses, experimentation with position and technique can help solve the problem of the interfering tummy. If intercourse is physically uncomfortable for the woman, other forms of sexual stimulation and gratification can be utilized.

Concerns about possible marital problems, especially related to sexual and economic problems, are very common. These problems are all involved with the couple's changing perception of their relationship, their responsibilities and their having a baby to care for very shortly. It is important to remember that many of the fears that the mother must deal with must also be dealt with by the father. Sometimes the father's position is given much less attention; this is probably due to the traditional Ostrich Approach to childbirth. In the Ostrich Approach, the father is supposed to get her pregnant and pay the bills. The father who wants to share parental responsibility and who wants to help his lady through the labor and delivery experience becomes much more involved in the pregnancy from the beginning. Much fuss is made over the pregnant woman; about all the man gets from his peer group is a knowing leer. A line of open communication, hopefully developed before the pregnancy, is important to the relationship throughout the childbearing experience. Both man and woman should be able to express concerns about all aspects of the experience in an open and caring atmosphere. Communication can make the difference between remembering the pregnancy and postpartum period as one of happiness or remembering it as one long period of negative feelings. That is not to say that communication will necessarily remove all fears and make all problems go away; it is to say that communication can help a couple stay on top of things and live with fewer we-should-haves later.

All women have both positive and negative attitudes about the pregnancy and the growing fetus. It doesn't matter whether the baby is a wanted, planned-for baby, or whether s/he is a surprise baby. At some period in the pregnancy, both parents are likely to feel that this is a very poor time to have a baby. Either the car needs fixing, or the furnace breaks, or the father loses his job, or wants to change jobs, or the mother is offered a terrific job at a terrific salary, or any one of a hundred other things makes this a very inopportune time to be pregnant. During bouts of morning sickness or during times when every woman in the world has a 22" waist and she is eight months pregnant, or when she has to take a maternity leave from the job she absolutely loves, the expectant mother may resent the coming baby. It's very common to feel resentment toward both the baby and the father when the expectant mother awakens for the second or third time during the night to go to the bathroom. These feelings of resentment are normal, and should not produce feelings of guilt.

Emotions and emotional response to situations can be affected by hormonal changes within the body, by poor nutrition, by fatigue and by particularly stressful life situations during pregnancy. Proper nutrition, especially inclusion of adequate sources of B-complex vitamins, coupled with plenty of rest can provide a base for an emotionally happy pregnancy. Couples should be aware that the emotional aspects of pregnancy are particularly prevalent during the third trimester.

LATE PREGNANCY

Several things happen during late pregnancy that signify that labor will be starting soon. Braxton Hicks contractions are the uterine contractions that precede true labor contractions. The Braxton Hicks contractions start during the early weeks of gestation and occur regularly throughout the pregnancy. These contractions exercise the uterine muscles and allow the uterus to enlarge to accommodate the fetus as it grows. During late pregnancy, when the uterus is expanded almost as far as it will expand, the surface area of the uterus is larger and the woman often becomes aware of these contractions. Sometimes these contractions can be very strong and often they are mistaken for true labor, particularly by women who know very little about the childbearing cycle.

Two to four weeks before a woman delivers her first baby, "lightening" may occur. The baby "drops," and the presenting part of the fetus settles into the pelvic cavity. In most cases, lightening will not occur until labor actually begins if the mother has previously borne children. Sometimes a first-time baby does not drop until labor begins. The settling of the presenting part of the fetus into the pelvic cavity is technically called engagement; the presenting part is said to be engaged.

Once engagement has occurred, the resultant pressure on the bladder will cause the mother to feel a frequent desire to urinate. This, coupled with other minor discomforts of late pregnancy, can make it very difficult to get sleep during this period. Engagement can produce pressure on the sciatic nerves; this may cause shooting pains down the legs. During the end of the pregnancy, the baby is often less active; s/he must rest in anticipation of the big day, and, too, there is not much room left in the uterus.

Increased vaginal discharge, a heaviness in the lower abdomen, menstruation-like feelings and backache with lower back pressure are frequently experienced shortly before labor begins.

As the end of the pregnancy approaches, sleep becomes more and more difficult to get. A special effort must be made to get adequate amounts of rest and to avoid fatigue and exhaustion if the woman plans to play an active part in her labor and delivery. The childbirth experience is much easier to handle, both physically and emotionally if the woman enters it well-rested. This is particularly true if her labor is long. It must be remembered that labor is very physical, and good body condition can help a great deal.

Changes in appetite, either an increase or a decrease may occur shortly before labor. During the several days prior to delivery, the woman may experience a weight loss of 2 or 3 pounds. Most women welcome this weight loss after gaining for nine months! Diarrhea is common during the last few days before delivery; this appears to be nature's way of cleaning out the woman's system in preparation for labor and delivery.

A great spurt of energy is frequently experienced shortly before labor begins. This is known as the nesting urge, and the expectant mother tackles jobs such as cleaning closets, waxing all of the hardwood floors or washing all of the windows. It's probably a good idea to do the large jobs over several days and to maintain fairly short working periods. No one, not a doctor, a nurse, a midwife, a next-door neighbor or a childbirth education teacher, can predict exactly when a woman will go into labor. Going into labor after four or five hours of very physical housework is not the ideal situation. Chances are good that the urge to get all sorts of big jobs done at once, before the baby comes, is due to a subconscious fear that after the baby comes there won't be time to do anything except care for the baby for months to come. On the other hand, some women experience a sudden decrease in energy just preceding labor.

During the last weeks of pregnancy, the doctor may do vaginal examinations to determine how much the cervix has ripened and if any dilatation or effacement has occurred. Dilatation and effacement are more sure signs of impending labor than are the other probable signs of labor.

True labor starts in one of three ways:

1. Loss of the mucus plug
2. Rupture of the membranes
3. Regular, rhythmic uterine contractions

Labor: First Stage [Dilatation and Effacement]

Labor is defined, rather unromantically, as the process by which the products of conception are expelled from the mother's body. Depending upon the parents' outlook, expectations, understanding and preparation, labor can be an unequaled adventure and time of closeness, or it can be a terribly frightening and painful experience.

During labor the neck of the uterus must open, and the baby and placental materials must be pushed out. To accomplish this, the cervix must efface and dilate. The cervix is the bottom, neck-like part of the upside-down pear-shaped uterus; this projection normally extends about 2 inches into the vagina. Effacement is the softening and thinning of this neck until it is a part of the lower uterine segment. Dilatation is the opening of the cervix to allow the baby to pass through.

DILATATION AND EFFACEMENT OF CERVIX

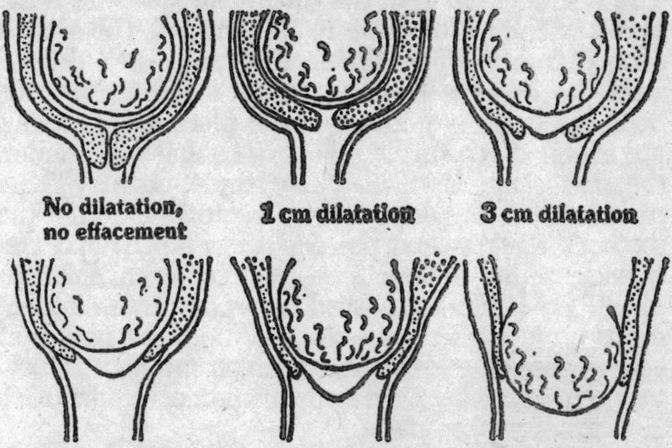

No dilatation, no effacement
1 cm dilatation
3 cm dilatation
5 cm dilatation, 100% (full) effacement
8 cm dilatation
10 cm (full) dilatation

During labor the uterus is divided into two distinct segments. The upper segment contracts and pulls up the lower part of the uterus, thus causing effacement and dilatation. The contractions also push against the baby and force it down into the pelvic basin. The presenting part of the baby pushing against the cervix helps dilatation.

The cervix starts to efface (thin) before it starts to dilate. As effacement continues, dilatation begins. Dilatation continues after effacement is complete. In other words, effacement starts first and dilatation ends last, but for a period of time both are taking place at same time.

Effacement is measured in percentages, and dilatation is measured in centimeters; the cervix is completely opened at 10 centimeters. Zero effacement and zero dilatation means that the cervix still extends the full distance into the birth canal and is still closed. Fifty per cent effacement and 2 centimeters dilatation indicates that the cervix only extends into the vagina about one inch and that the cervical opening is 2 centimeters in diameter.

The process of labor is divided into three stages. The first stage is from the time labor starts until the cervix is fully dilated at 10 centimeters. The second stage is from the time the cervix is completely dilated until the baby is born. The third stage is from the time the baby is born until the placental materials are expelled. To further simplify talking about labor, the first stage is divided into three phases. These phases blend into one another in actual labor, but the mother's feelings and the character, length and frequency of her contractions do differ from phase to phase. Pre-labor, established labor, and transition are terms often used to differentiate the three phases of active first stage labor. It's common for some effacement, and possibly even some dilatation, to take place before active labor starts.

Presence of one or more of the following signs indicates active labor is imminent:

1. The membranes rupture
2. Pink (or bloody) show appears (loss of the mucus plug)
3. Regular, rhythmic contractions begin

Ruptured Membranes

The membranes (or bag of waters) is the term used to refer to the thin, semi-transparent sac which contains the baby and the amniotic fluid. During the pregnancy, the sac and the amniotic fluid prevent anything from reaching the fetus; this precludes infection of the fetus through the vagina. The fluid also keeps the baby's body temperature even, gives the fetus a buoyant environment and cushions the fetus from bumps and falls the mother's tummy may take.

It doesn't hurt when the membranes rupture, and usually the only way a woman can tell it has happened is fluid loss from the vagina. Sometimes there may be an audible indication, a pop like a balloon breaking or a soft squeak like the sound of a finger rubbing against a rubber inner-tube. The fluid may gush out and seem like gallons, or it may just dribble out. Sometimes a woman doesn't realize her water has broken, and she thinks she is leaking small amounts of urine. However, unlike urine flow, a woman usually has absolutely no control over the flow of the amniotic fluid. If the baby's presenting part is pressing down hard on the cervix, and thereby acting like a plug, it's possible that no fluid can escape when the woman is in sitting or standing positions; in prone positions the fluid is able to escape because gravity is no longer pushing the baby against the cervix as hard as it was in the upright positions. For mattress protection, it's a good idea to have a plastic sheet or a very thick mattress pad on the bed during the last weeks of pregnancy. Several thicknesses of toweling work quite well.

The membranes may rupture before labor starts or at any time throughout labor. If contractions haven't started before the membranes rupture, they usually do within the next day; however, it could take as long as two weeks for contractions to begin spontaneously.

In some cases, albeit very rare, the membranes are still intact when the baby is born. The physician in attendance usually ruptures the membranes artificially during the advanced phase of first stage labor if they have not spontaneously ruptured beforehand. Sometimes the membranes are artificially ruptured during the earlier part of first stage labor in an attempt to increase the intensity and frequency of contractions.

Most doctors want to be notified immediately if a woman thinks her membranes have ruptured. Because of the risk of infection to the fetus, many doctors will induce labor if it has not started spontaneously within 24 hours after the water has broken. As a precaution, intercourse is not advised once the membranes have ruptured. If the woman is told to remain at home until contractions start (in the assumption that they will start soon), it's best to keep activity to a minimum because labor will more than likely start within several hours. It's also a good precaution to take a temperature reading every four hours; if the temperature goes over 100° the doctor should be notified. Most doctors allow their patients to take showers after the membranes have ruptured, but advise against taking baths.

There's no such thing as a "dry birth." Even if the membranes rupture early, a dry birth is impossible because the placenta produces fluid after the water breaks; in addition to this fluid lubrication, the baby is covered with vernix caseosa, the white, oily, cheesy substance that covers the baby's body to protect the baby's skin in utero.

Pink Show

Another sign that may shortly precede active labor is pink (or bloody) show.

It is very common for a woman to have increased vaginal discharge the day or so before active labor begins. During pregnancy a mucus plug blocks the cervix and acts as an additional protection against foreign substances entering the uterus. This gelatinous plug is about the size of a pencil lead and is attached to the cervix with tiny blood capillaries. When the plug breaks loose, the capillaries break, so there may be some blood mixed into the mucus discharge. The mucus may be blood-tinged, or lightly streaked with blood, but it is not bloody per se. Any real bleeding should be reported to the doctor immediately. Again, as with ruptured membranes, pink show is an indication that active labor may start soon; it is not proof absolute. Loss of the mucus plug is painless.

Contractions

The third, and most conclusive, indication that active labor is beginning is the presence of regular, rhythmic contractions. Normally, but not always, contractions get progressively stronger and progressively closer together. This allows both the mother and the fetus to adapt to the increasing strength of the uterine contractions. It is common for false labor contractions, or Braxton Hicks contractions, to precede true labor contractions.

Sometimes the false contractions can be quite strong and seem quite regular, so the character, strength and regularity of the contractions must be examined in order to determine whether the contractions are true or false labor. True labor contractions usually occur at fairly regular, gradually shortening intervals. Even if the contractions do not come exactly every 15 minutes (for instance), they will probably develop some regular pattern. False contractions occur at very irregular intervals and do not get closer together. The intensity of true labor contractions gradually increases, while the intensity of the false contractions remains the same. For most women the true labor contraction seems to start around the back and to radiate toward the front, hold for a few seconds in the front and then reverse its course. The false contraction is usually centered mostly in the abdomen. True contractions are intensified by walking and false contractions are either not affected or are relieved by walking. False contractions may sometimes be stopped altogether by walking.

Changing your activity is a good way to determine whether the contractions are true or false. A change of activity will usually cause no change in the frequency or intensity of the true contractions, or will cause them to get harder. However, false contractions often go away or become less intense when activity is changed. If the membranes haven't ruptured, a warm bath is a good test; true contractions will go right on, but false contractions are usually relieved a great deal. It's a good idea to have someone help you in and out of the bathtub so you don't injure yourself.

True contractions cause effacement and dilatation; false contractions do not (or do so to a much lesser degree). Only medical examination can determine whether effacement and dilatation are taking place. Even if the false contractions do not produce noticeable progress, they do exercise the uterus and the cervix and prepare them for the upcoming labor.

Describing a uterine contraction is very difficult. No two labors are exactly alike, and no two people perceive a contraction in exactly the same way. Some women have compared contractions to gas pains or menstrual cramps. Some women experience a mild ache in the back, some feel even true contractions only in the front. Many women think early labor contractions are indigestion.

As labor progresses, the contractions get longer, harder and closer together. The interval between contractions is timed from the beginning of one contraction to the beginning of the next contraction. The length of the contraction is timed from the start of the contraction to the end of the same contraction. It is most common for a contraction to start gradually and build to a peak and then recede. They've been compared to ocean waves. During the last part of labor, particularly, it is common for contractions to have two or even three peaks.

The uterus is an involuntary muscle, like the heart, and it is impossible to stop it from contracting. When people speak of controlling a contraction, or handling one, they are speaking of retaining the ability to relax the rest of the body during the contraction, thereby allowing the uterus to work most efficiently. If the entire body is allowed to tighten along with the uterus, the muscle tension can spread and intensify any discomfort that the uterine muscles may be producing. Left to its own devices, without interference from surrounding muscles, the uterus can accomplish its job in the most efficient way possible.

Throughout labor, the interval between contractions should be used to relax totally and prepare for the next contraction. Contractions are much easier to handle if the couple is ready for each one; otherwise the peak can be overwhelming. Good oxygenation and circulation of the blood is important during labor because the uterine muscles use a great deal of oxygen during the contractions. If the muscles do not receive an adequate supply of oxygen, the lactic acid is not removed and muscle cramps and pain may result.

LABOR CHART

First Stage (Dilatation and Effacement)		
Pre-Labor	Established Labor	Transition
0-4 centimeters	4-7 centimeters	7-10 centimeters

Second Stage (Expulsion)	Third Stage
Birth of Baby	Delivery of Placenta

STAGE 1 LABOR—PRE-LABOR PHASE

This phase is defined as the time that the cervix dilates from 0 to 4 centimeters. Actually the cervix starts out at a little more than 0 dilatation because of the mucus plug, but for ease in explaining the phases of first stage labor, pre-labor is usually defined as being from 0 to 4 centimeters. Remember that sometimes the cervix is dilated to 2 or 3 centimeters before contractions are felt.

During the pre-labor phase the uterus is pulling up the cervix, and the body of the uterus is becoming shorter and thicker. Both dilatation and effacement are taking place.

Pre-labor contractions can be between 15 and 45 seconds long and they are usually 10 to 30 minutes apart. From the time the first contractions are felt until the cervix is dilated to 4 centimeters is normally between 5 and 8 hours for first-time mothers; however, it can be less than an hour or go on longer than a day. Subsequent labors usually go faster than first labors.

A very common feeling when contractions first start (after waiting nine months or more) is one of excitement. Another frequent feeling is that there's so much that's still not done. There's a real tendency to want to scurry around and wash the dishes, put a load of clothes in the washer and scrub the kitchen floor. It's important to squelch the desire to do any of these things. A woman shouldn't do anything that is physically strenuous during early labor; rest and relaxation are important at this time because the advanced parts of labor require a great deal of energy. If contractions start during a time when you normally sleep, you should try to sleep or rest quietly for as long as you can.

It's a good idea to keep a written record of the length and frequency of contractions. This information will help the doctor or midwife determine how your labor is progressing. For energy, small amounts of easily digestible food should be eaten frequently during this phase of labor unless you feel nauseous. Light foods, high in carbohydrates and proteins, are recommended. Fruit juices, toast with honey, and gelatin desserts are all good. Dairy products should be avoided because they do not digest quickly or easily. Small feedings every 2 to 4 hours during early labor will help sustain energy.

A warm bath or shower, if the doctor or midwife doesn't object, can be very relaxing and refreshing at this point. After the bath or shower is a good time to apply fresh make-up (if you normally wear any) so you'll look your best going into labor. It can really help the morale if a woman knows her hair and make-up look good.

It's good to practice the breathing techniques during these early contractions, but not with every contraction. The use of breathing techniques at this point is for practice and building confidence only, not for distraction. The longer you wait to use a particular breathing technique for real, the longer it will be useful. The longer each technique works, the less chance there is of "running out" of techniques before the baby is born.

Most first-time mothers go to the hospital sometime during this phase of labor.

STAGE 1 LABOR—ESTABLISHED LABOR PHASE

During this phase, the cervix dilates from about 4 centimeters to approximately 7 centimeters. Effacement may have finished during the pre-labor phase, or it may complete during this phase. When effacement is complete, dilatation usually progresses more rapidly.

Contractions during established labor are usually between 40 and 60 seconds long and are often less than 5 minutes apart. By the end of this phase the contractions normally occur every 2 or 3 minutes. Average length for this phase of labor is somewhere between 1 and 4 hours.

The mother may feel like walking during this stage, and this activity probably helps to promote engagement of the fetal head. However, most hospitals confine the laboring woman to bed, so be prepared for this possibility. Almost without exception, American hospitals confine laboring women to bed after the membranes have ruptured, whether or not they have received any sort of medication. If the membranes did not rupture during pre-labor, they may during established labor. Dilatation often speeds up after the membranes have ruptured.

Physical and mental relaxation remain important, because the hardest part of labor is still ahead. Reading, doing needlework or playing cards are all activities that many women find to be enjoyable, and somewhat distracting, during this phase. Sleeping is fine as long as you can stay asleep both between and during contractions. Once the contractions are strong enough to require use of breathing techniques, or strong enough that you can no longer walk or talk during the contractions, you shouldn't sleep between the contractions. Sleeping between the contractions will cause each contraction to catch you unaware and unprepared; awaking at the peak of the contraction makes it very difficult to "catch up" with the contraction and control it.

It is common during this phase for dilatation to slow down or seem to stop. This is called reaching a plateau, and it is very discouraging. When regular, strong contractions continue for an hour or two and no progress in dilatation is being made, a lot of women have the thought that if labor is "This bad now, what will it be like later?" One good thing to know about a plateau is that once things start happening again, dilatation is often quite rapid.

Toward the end of the established labor phase, dependence upon the labor coach and the medical staff increases. Even women who are usually very independent seem to need someone to lean on emotionally during the latter parts of labor. Attention may wander as dilatation progresses and it is important to keep using the focal point and breathing techniques through each contraction. Communication with the coach becomes critical as this phase ends and the next phase of first stage labor begins. Let the coach know what s/he can do to help you.

Backache during this phase is common because of the way the baby may be pressing on the spine. A back rub or counter-pressure applied to the lower back during contractions may help. Ice chips, if the hospital will allow them, can help to keep the mouth from becoming too dry. A lip balm brought from home, or petroleum jelly available from the nursing staff, can keep the lips from chapping. Some hospitals will allow the use of hard candy, preferably lollipops, during labor. The sugar in the candy helps to maintain energy, and the candy keeps the mouth moist. Candy on a stick is best because the coach can remove the candy from the mother's mouth as the contraction starts. It's possible to choke on the small round candies because it's hard to remove them during contractions. The sour flavors are better than the sweet flavors because the sweetness sometimes causes nausea. A little squirt of honey also provides quick energy.

It is important to check with the doctor or midwife, and with the hospital, to see whether they all allow the candy or the honey. Some hospitals generally restrict the use of candy or honey, but will allow such things on the doctor's request. Some hospitals strictly prohibit the woman's taking anything at all by mouth because the possibility always exists that general anesthesia may be necessary for the birth; for instance in the case of an emergency Cesarean delivery. It is important that the patient's stomach be empty when general anesthesia is administered because it is possible that the patient may vomit, then aspirate the vomitus.

Women who have had children before often show up at the hospital during this phase of labor.

STAGE 1 LABOR—TRANSITION PHASE

During transition the cervix completes dilatation and stretches over the baby's head. When transition is completed, it is time to start pushing the baby out into the world.

Contractions during transition are the longest and most intense of labor. They can be from 50 to 90 seconds long and sometimes are as long as 2 minutes. The contractions can come every 2 or 3 minutes, and there is very little time for rest between them. This phase of labor is definitely the hardest, and the most uncomfortable, but it is also the shortest phase of stage 1 labor. Transition averages somewhere between 30 and 60 minutes, but it can be as short as one contraction or as long as 2 hours or so.

Transition is usually easily recognizable, even when a woman doesn't know how far her cervix is dilated. It is good for the coach to be thoroughly acquainted with the signs of transition, because often the woman is too involved with the intensity and frequency of the contractions to realize she is in transition. The coach's ability to recognize the signs of transition is particularly important if the woman has been on a plateau at 5 or 6 centimeters, for example, for quite a while. She may begin to dilate very rapidly, and go into the transition phase before the hospital staff expects her to. Observation by the coach can be extremely helpful.

Following is a list of things that many women feel during the transition phase of labor. These are called signs of transition. Some women have several of the signs, and some experience none of them. Having three or four of these signs is average. Rest assured that nobody experiences all of them.

1. A feeling of panic
2. A trapped feeling and the desire to escape
3. The desire to go home—it's common to want to come back later to finish all of this
4. Confusion and disorientation—this may be disconcerting to the coach
5. Extreme discouragement, the feeling that labor is never going to end
6. Great anxiety about the safety of both self and baby
7. Extreme excitement
8. Extreme irritability—the back rub that felt so good five minutes ago may now be extremely irritating. If the coach has been stroking the hair back off the face, a typical reaction in transition is telling the coach to quit messing up her hair
9. Sensitivity to attitudes, words and noises
10. Need for understanding from those surrounding her
11. Need for companionship—most women don't want to be left alone at all at any time during labor, and especially during transition
12. Extreme dependence on coach and staff—more dependence on coach than on staff if rapport has not been established with staff during earlier labor
13. Restlessness, an inability to get comfortable for more than a few seconds
14. Extreme drowsiness between contractions, extreme desire to go to sleep—feel very little rest between contractions
15. Trembling and uncontrollable shaking of limbs or total body
16. Nausea—may vomit
17. Heavy show, often streaked with blood
18. Dizziness; a whirlpool sensation
19. Prickly feeling in skin, often in fingers
20. Extreme sensitivity to touch—may want to be touched a great deal; or may not want anything or anybody to touch her

21. Red splotches on the face—called a "face mask"
22. Numbness in buttocks
23. Muscle cramps in calf, thigh, buttocks
24. Pain or ache in thighs
25. Severe backache or back pressure
26. Chills
27. Extreme warmness
28. Rectal pressure or the desire to "push"
29. Cold feet—due to decreased circulation; long, warm socks help relieve this discomfort

The membranes will probably rupture during transition if they haven't already. If they do not spontaneously rupture, the doctor will probably prick them at this time.

Transition is, without a doubt, the most difficult phase of labor. Transition is what all childbirth preparation is really directed toward. Strong and caring coaching is very important to the laboring woman. Relaxation is important during transition, but many women find it difficult to achieve during this part of labor. Practice during pregnancy and good communication between mother and coach can make transition easier to handle. Good communication with the coach can lead to good communication with the hospital staff because the coach can alert the medical personnel to any needs the mother may have. Any changes in physical or emotional attitudes should be reported to the staff.

During transition, more than at any other time during labor, it is important to remain alert and be ready for each contraction. When contractions come very close together and peak possibly 2 or 3 times, they are hard to handle anyway; if the couple is not ready for the contraction, it is practically impossible. Complete concentration on each contraction, as it is happening, is essential. It's a waste of time to worry about the previous contraction that may have been handled poorly, and it's a waste of time to worry about the next contraction (which may not be anyway!).

Realize during transition that the contractions are

not going to get any harder. Keep in mind that this is the shortest phase of labor and may only be 20 or 30 contractions long. Ask to be checked frequently to determine dilatation; rapid progress seems to make it all easier. Counter-pressure on the lower back during contractions can be a big help during transition. The coach can apply this pressure, or the woman can lie on her own fists or on tennis balls or something of a similar shape. It's no use to suffer through discomforts that can be relieved. Let the coach know if you want socks put on, or pressure applied to your back, or your abdomen rubbed.

Transition is the time when women lament over getting pregnant and when some vow to "never let him get near me again."

The intention here is not to frighten people, it is to explain labor as many women see and feel it. Transition is by no means uncontrollable; neither is it a game. Diligent practice and good communication between the coach and the laboring woman are the keys to making this stressful time into a tolerable phase of labor. Remember that it usually lasts no more than 30 to 60 minutes.

Sometime during the end of transition, the woman will probably get the "urge to push." It is important to control this urge; it is important to avoid pushing until dilatation is complete. Premature pushing can cause the cervix to swell or lacerate. Some women never have this urge, but most do. It is an unmistakable feeling, and very difficult to control if it is a strong urge. Techniques are taught in childbirth education classes that help women control this urge; unfortunately a lot of the couples don't think this is an important part of the training and tend to disregard this information. Trying to explain how difficult this urge is to control is difficult in itself. Maybe an example would help.

Picture yourself in a crowded theater sitting in the middle of a row. Suddenly you feel as if you have to vomit. The tendency is to try really hard to contain yourself until you are out of the auditorium section and at least into the lobby, if not in the restroom.

When someone feels really ill, it is hard to control the urge to vomit. When a woman in labor feels the urge to push the baby out, it is hard to control that urge. To clarify: in no way does this mean that a woman feels like vomiting when she feels like pushing; this was only used as an example because the urge to push and the urge to vomit are both nearly uncontrollable bodily functions.

Sometimes the woman interprets the urge to push as an urge to evacuate her bowels. This is because the baby's head presses on the rectum and tailbone as it descends into the pelvis.

It is extremely important for the coach to notify the medical personnel as soon as the woman indicates a desire to push. In some cases she may be able to verbalize the desire to the coach, and in other cases she may be caught entirely by surprise in the middle of a contraction and just start grunting or pushing involuntarily. The coach should be alert to these indications and help her to use the techniques taught in class to avoid pushing. The importance of the coach's job during this part of labor cannot be overstressed.

When the cervix is completely dilated, the medical staff will give the mother the go-ahead to start pushing along with the contractions. The urge to push occurs with the contractions; it does not remain between the contractions. This is the beginning of the second stage of labor and contractions from here on out are much different from those experienced during first stage labor. The job is not yet completed, but the passive part is; during the second stage of labor (the expulsion of the baby) the mother is able to work actively with each contraction.

MORE ON FIRST STAGE LABOR

It's a good idea for the mother to notify her labor coach as soon as she is fairly certain that she is in labor. This is especially important, of course, if the coach's job is such that s/he can't be contacted directly, or such that s/he must make arrangements with a supervisor or other employees before s/he can leave.

It is not an imposition, nor an interruption, to contact the coach at work. Remember that the coach is probably almost as excited about the baby's birth as you are, and is very anxious to know when labor starts. It's even a good idea during late pregnancy to be with the coach as much as possible. That doesn't mean that the mother and coach must go everywhere together, but it's good for the coach to be fairly close and for the mother always to know how to reach the coach on very short notice.

Early labor is the time for both the mother and the coach to eat. As mentioned before, the mother should eat small amounts of high protein, high carbohydrate foods. She should avoid dairy products. Digestion is slowed during labor and the stomach should be empty by the end of labor in case general anesthesia is necessary. It doesn't matter what the coach eats, but if the sight or smell of a particular food nauseates the mother, it should be avoided.

Someone should pack a lunch for the coach to eat at the hospital. Coaching can be a strenuous job, and if the coach doesn't take a lunch to the hospital s/he may have to leave the mother during labor to get something to eat. This can be very distressing to the woman in labor. Even if the coach is not allowed to eat the lunch in the labor room, it is much quicker to sneak down the hall to the Fathers' Waiting Room for a few minutes to down a sandwich than it is to go to the hospital cafeteria and order a meal. Whatever the coach chooses to take in the lunch should have a thoroughly non-offensive odor because the sense of smell is heightened during labor. The smell of tuna fish, for example, may be very strong and very unpleasant to the laboring woman. The coach should not approach the delivery room on an empty stomach; it's an exciting environment and it's easy to become light-headed.

A woman shouldn't exert herself with unnecessary physical activity during early labor. She should relax in preparation for late labor and delivery. Sometimes this is easier to do if the situation is put in the proper perspective. It's almost a certainty that she will wash those same dishes hundreds of times; she will only have this baby once. It makes sense to do everything possible to assure it will be the best experience possible.

Either the coach or the mother should record the frequency and duration of the contractions in order to be able to report accurately to the doctor or midwife. Doctors and midwives usually give their patients specific instructions regarding when they want to be contacted. Some want to be notified when the contractions are 10 minutes apart (usually for multiparas); some when the contractions are 5 minutes (or less) apart; some when the contractions are becoming progressively stronger; some when the contractions are between 45 and 60 seconds in length; and some when the contractions become so strong that the mother can no longer walk or talk during the contraction. The intensity is important because most medical personnel judge progress in labor more by the intensity than by the length and frequency of the contractions. The doctor or midwife will alert the hospital, so they'll be ready for you.

Showering or bathing, washing hair and just generally getting ready for the trip to the hospital are good things to do during early labor as long as the activities don't take too much energy. Early labor is a good time to get the giggles and excitement out, because it's hard work between then and the time the baby is born. Labor is called labor because it is the hardest work most people will ever do.

Pelvic rocks are good for relief of backache during early labor, and it's good to do them at home because it's possible that the nursing staff won't allow you to assume a hands and knees position once you've checked into the hospital.

Deciding just when to go to the hospital depends upon what your doctor or midwife tells you as well as how you feel about hospitals. If you feel comfortable with your doctor or midwife, and feel that s/he will level with you and treat you fairly throughout labor; and if you think that the hospital personnel will be receptive and supportive, go ahead and enter the hospital early in labor. But if you aren't sure about your doctor's real feelings about prepared childbirth, and you aren't sure about the reaction of the hospital staff to prepared parents, it might be a good idea to wait until later in labor to go to the hospital. It's difficult to judge progress by the frequency of contractions. Some women's contractions start out 5 minutes apart; other women are dilated to 5 centimeters when their contractions are still 15 minutes apart. The length and intensity of the contractions are more important in judging progress. It is a rule of thumb that when contractions are between 55 and 65 seconds long, and when the first level of breathing is no longer adequate, the cervix is probably between 4 and 6 centimeters dilated. This is usually a good time to go to the hospital because you'll be there early enough to check in and have all of the preliminary procedures completed with plenty of time to spare before the birth, but you won't be there so early that you will spend hours and hours in the hospital labor room when you would have been much more comfortable in your own living room.

If you live a great distance from the hospital, or if you have a particular fear of not making it to the hospital in time for the birth, by all means go to the hospital early. Some women can't really relax until they are in the hospital labor room, and that's just fine; a woman should spend the early part of her labor in whatever environment allows her to be the most comfortable both physically and emotionally.

Naturally, if the doctor has indicated that there may be some sort of problem during labor, for example, a disparity between the size of the baby's head and the size of your pelvis (cephalo-pelvic disproportion), you should be in the hospital early. If the doctor has indicated that your labor might progress particularly rapidly, it's a good idea to plan to go to the hospital as soon as you have any signs of labor. The doctor can predict a rapid labor if your cervix has dilated to 2 or 3 centimeters during the latter part of pregnancy, or if you have had rather quick labors in the past. The prediction is only a prediction, not a promise, but it is based on hard facts that pertain directly to you.

If you have company when you go into labor, don't feel impolite if you ask them to leave. If you want them to stay for a little while longer, that's fine, too, but your wishes are paramount. It is your baby, your labor and your show. Do whatever will make it easiest for you. It's nice if the coach can be the one to ask people to leave, then you don't have to deal with "guilt" feelings yourself—and most people feel a certain degree of guilt when they ask company to leave.

Both a suitcase and another, smaller, bag should be packed and ready about a month before the baby is due. The suitcase should be filled with things you'll need during your stay after the baby is born. The other bag, often called the "goody" bag in childbirth classes, should have things in it that you will be using during labor. You must have two separate containers because the suitcase is usually whisked off and put in a locker for safekeeping as soon as you check into the labor room. It takes up too much space to be left in the labor room, and there would be no way to keep an eye on it while you and the coach are in the delivery room having the baby. Obviously, some of the things you will need in your suitcase, such as your toothbrush, will have to be put in at the last minute. It's a good idea to tape a list of these last minute items and where each is kept if the item itself does not dictate its location, so the coach can gather them up as you're leaving for the hospital. The list taped on the outside of the suitcase can save harried searches for elusive items and trips back to the house for forgotten items.

The following is a list of the things to pack in your suitcase. Some hospitals provide a few of the articles, but it's a good idea to take everything on the list just to make sure you have all of the things that you need.

To Use in the Hospital

Nightgowns: should be washable, and should be designed so that it is easy to put the baby to breast if you are planning to breastfeed. Either short gowns that can be lifted up, or gowns that fasten down the front are appropriate. The number of gowns you will need naturally depends upon how long you plan to stay in the hospital, but it is a good idea to have at least one for each day you plan to stay, plus an extra.

Slippers: hospitals simply will not let patients pad around their halls with bare feet, so even if you never wear slippers at home, take a pair to the hospital.

Robe: this, too, should be washable. Taking a robe is essential, because you'll probably be down the hall several times a day to check on the baby, especially if your hospital doesn't have rooming-in, or if you do not choose to have it. Even if you do have rooming-in, you should have a robe because it's nice to visit with other new mothers and to look your best for visitors.

Nursing bras: bring at least two. The nursing bras should be at least one cup size larger than your normal nonpregnant size. If the nursing bras are purchased during the last month or so of pregnancy, they should fit or be slightly larger. For the best support, nursing bras should have fairly wide straps and good cup support. If you're not planning to nurse, the hospital may provide a binder for you to wear at first. After the binder is removed, you will need a bra with good support.

Sanitary pad belt: the hospital will probably provide a sanitary pad belt, but it's a good idea to have one of whatever style you like best because the hospital is sure to have a different style.

Sanitary pads: the hospital will provide these, but sometimes charge the patient per pad. At some hospitals each new mother receives a "gift pack" filled with products of all kinds that relate to babies and the postpartum experience. The gift packs are provided by advertisers and sometimes contain boxes of sanitary pads. Even if you don't take any to the hospital with you, be sure to have some at home waiting for you.

Going-home outfit: your nightgown, robe and slippers is a perfectly acceptable (and very comfortable) outfit for the trip home. If you take clothes, be sure that they are not tight. Chances are very slim that you will be back to your pre-pregnant size. Something that you wore when you were 4 or 5 months pregnant is suitable. The baby usually gets hungry on the way home, so the clothes you wear should be two-piece or fasten down the front.

Personal toiletry items: comb, brush, shampoo, shower cap, rollers, bobby pins, hair styler/dryer, toothpaste, toothbrush, deodorant, powder, perfume, cold cream, hand lotion, lanolin for nipples, hand mirror, nail file, razor, and make-up. If you're not sure whether you will use a particular item or not, take it. It's better to have it if you want it.

Watch or clock: otherwise you may never know what time it is.

Small change: some hospitals have telephones in each room; some don't. It's handy to have a little money to buy newspapers and small items at the hospital gift shop in case you forget something at home.

Camera: if you're planning to take pictures in the delivery room, the camera should be in the "goody" bag. Be sure to have plenty of film and flash bulbs. Mothers who have rooming-in have plenty of opportunities for good pictures during the hospital stay. Nurses are usually happy to take a picture if they aren't too busy.

Reading materials: it's good to have some entertaining, light reading materials. Interruptions come constantly, so serious reading is often difficult to really get into. If you're planning to breastfeed, it's a good idea to take a book or two about breastfeeding. This information will give you courage and a sense of purpose. This is particularly important if the hospital staff is less than supportive of breastfeeding.

Writing materials: the postpartum hospital stay is an ideal time to write some long-overdue letters; it will probably be several weeks before you can find the time again. Pens, pencils, stationery, address book and stamps are good to take. If you plan to use birth announcements whose design does not focus on the sex of the baby, you can address the envelopes sometime during the last couple weeks of your pregnancy and just fill in the vital information in the hospital. Take the forms necessary to write up your birth report for the childbirth education instructor. Details of the labor and birth are so easily forgotten if you wait too long to write the report.

Projects: needlework, knitting, crocheting are all appropriate and relaxing to do in the hospital.

Book or pamphlet of postpartum exercises: ask your doctor when you can start doing exercises to get your abdomen and legs back into condition. For the first few days you will necessarily take it pretty easy, but you can usually begin doing isometric types of exercises as soon as you want to. Kegel exercises should be done on the delivery table and frequently during the first few days.

Prenatal vitamins: if your doctor prescribed prenatal vitamins during your pregnancy, s/he will probably want you to continue taking them while you are nursing.

For Going Home

Diapers and pins: take a couple of diapers and diaper pins. Many of the disposable diapers have tapes, and thus eliminate the need for pins.

Plastic pants: if you use cloth diapers, you should have plastic pants or a waterproof pad for under the baby.

Undershirt: these certainly aren't essential, but many parents use them for newborns. Some baby undershirts snap down the front and some pull over the head like an adult undershirt. The ones that open down the front are usually easier for inexperienced parents to put on the baby.

Nightgown or stretch suit: bring something cute, but not the best, most expensive thing you have. It's very likely that no one but you two will see the baby on the way home. And the outfit will probably be dirty by the time anyone comes to your house to see the new little one. Save the fancy things until the baby is seeing other people.

Receiving blanket: square receiving blankets are much more logical than the rectangular ones. There usually seems to be a foot or bottom sticking out of the rectangular kind. Make certain that all of the baby's clothes have been washed before s/he wears them. It is particularly important that the receiving blanket is clean because if the baby is born on the way to the hospital s/he should be wrapped in the receiving blanket and taken to the hospital immediately.

Heavier blanket or bunting: if the weather is chilly, it will be necessary to wrap the heavier blanket or bunting, as well as the receiving blanket, around the baby. But do be careful not to overbundle the little one. If the car is comfortable for you in regular clothes, it is comfortable for the baby in a receiving blanket.

Goody Bag

The following items may be of use during labor and should be taken in the "goody" bag. Few people use all of the things, but again, it is better to have them along and not use them than want them and not have them.

Watch with second hand: some people use regular wrist-watches, and others use stop watches; one of the two is essential for proper timing of contractions.

Pencil or pen and small notebook: this is for the coach's use in recording contractions, comments and progress. This record of labor will be a really nice addition to the baby book. However, it is important that the coach does not get so involved in note-taking that s/he is not able to coach effectively. The notebook will be helpful when you are writing your labor report for your childbirth education instructor.

Lollipops and/or honey: to keep the mouth moist and supply energy. The lollipops should be the sour kind. Some couples go through dozens of lollipops at home before labor ever starts, so be sure to have a large supply.

Photographs, drawings and masking tape: choose drawings or photographs that you find interesting or particularly meaningful. Tape one to the hospital wall and use it for a focal point. When you tire of one, have your coach put up another. Some women prefer pictures of babies, others especially like geometric designs. Whatever the focal point is, it should be interesting enough or personally meaningful enough to hold your attention during what could be a long labor.

Washcloths or sponges: it's a good idea to have at least two of whichever you choose. Damp sponges or washcloths can be used to cool your brow and face. One can be soaking in a sink of cool water while you are using the other one. In hospitals that do not allow ice chips or candy, you can suck on a wet washcloth to moisten your mouth and tongue. This substitution also comes in handy during transition because most hospitals withhold even ice chips at this late stage in labor. The mouth becomes particularly dry when the techniques designed to control the urge to push are used. Most hospitals will supply you and your coach with the washcloths, but again, it's better to bring your own and not have to use them than to not have access to any at all. Be sure the sponge is real; plastic sponges taste funny.

Lip balm or petroleum jelly: this is to prevent chapped lips. The hospital may be able to provide you with glycerine lemon swabs, too.

Talcum powder and body lotion: to use in both effleurage and back rubs; the powder or cream will decrease friction and prevent skin irritation.

Tennis balls: applying effective counter-pressure for a long period of time is very tiring for the coach. If your coach runs out of energy, you can put the tennis balls between you and the bed at the point of greatest discomfort; this if often quite effective. Some childbirth instructors suggest taking a very cold can of soda; it can be used in the same way and it has the added advantage of being cool and refreshing. And when you get tired of using it to apply counter-pressure, your coach can drink it! Other instructors suggest taking a brand new, unused paint roller to help the coach give back rubs that are not so tiring. Of course, the tennis balls or paint roller should be clean and unused; the nurses probably won't let you use them if they're not.

Heavy socks: in case your feet get cold during labor, particularly during transition. A rather large pair is a good idea because they will be easier for you or your coach to put on your feet, and because they won't feel tight. Woman in labor tend to be sensitive to tight clothing.

Snacks for the coach: in addition to the lunch, it's a good idea to have a candy bar or some other source of quick energy for the coach. Avoid taking your particular favorite, because you won't be able to have any. Chances are that you wouldn't want any late in labor, but one can't be sure.

Playing cards, board games or books: in case you are in the labor room for a long time, it's nice to have one of these things along to while away the time. Again, the activity shouldn't be strenuous, but you will know when you no longer feel you can comfortably keep your mind on a game or book.

Labor guide, student manual: bring written material that both of you (particularly the coach) can use to review techniques during labor. Charts showing dilatation and the stages and phases of labor are useful in helping you to visualize progress. A student manual from your childbirth education class, notes or this book can help you remember just what you were supposed to be doing with those tennis balls and washcloths.

Class certificate: if your childbirth education instructor does not routinely hand out class "diplomas" be sure to ask for something that verifies your attendance at the classes. Some hospitals require proof that the coach has attended childbirth education classes before they will let him/her into the delivery room. Don't rely just on what you've heard that the hospital requires or doesn't require. There have been cases where a certificate is not required by the hospital, but an unsupportive staff member (or physician) has asked to see a coach's certificate and then refused the coach admittance if s/he cannot produce one. This is obviously extremely unfair, but it's best to avoid the possibility because by the time you've hassled it out with the hospital staff and/or administration, the baby will probably have been born and the coach will have missed the birth.

Insurance forms, hospital forms, and identification: if you haven't yet returned the pre-admission forms to the hospital, you'll have to take them with you when you enter the hospital. Some insurance forms may be required when you check into the hospital; find out ahead of time exactly what you'll need. If you are covered by some sort of government-supported or private employer/employee plan, it will be necessary to take your identification card. Women entering a civilian hospital under the military CHAMPUS program are required to have their government identification cards no matter how much paperwork has been filled out in advance.

List of phone numbers and phone change: it's most likely that both of you will be very anxious to let the world know about the arrival of the baby. The coach should have a pocketful of change and a list of all the people s/he's supposed to call. Minutes after the birth is no time to have to call directory assistance for phone numbers. A list also eliminates the possibility that someone will be overlooked by mistake.

Paper bag: should be lunch-size. You can breathe into this sack in case you hyperventilate during labor. Breathing into the sack, or into cupped hands, can cause the symptoms of hyperventilation (tingling sensations in the extremities, face or lips; possible numbness in hands and feet; general restlessness) to subside. Hyperventilation is caused by an imbalance of oxygen and carbon dioxide in the blood.

Rebreathing one's own air, through use of a paper bag or cupped hands, brings the carbon dioxide level back up to where it should be.

Transistor radio: can be used for distraction during labor, and can be used for enjoyment during the postpartum hospital stay.

Cassette tape recorder and tapes: can be used to record the labor and delivery experience, or for distraction during labor. This, too, can obviously be used during the postpartum stay. If you plan to record either in the labor room or the delivery room, you will have to check with your doctor to ascertain whether s/he and the hospital allow taping. If the hospital does not routinely allow taping equipment, perhaps your doctor can write special orders suggesting that you be allowed to do so. This approach may or may not be successful.

Camera and film: most hospitals allow only one flash photo to be taken in the delivery room, so a 35 millimeter camera with fast film is the best bet. An Instamatic may work, but the chances of getting really good pictures is much better with a 35 mm. If you are planning to shoot color, be certain the photographer (usually the coach) sees the delivery room ahead of time in order to choose the appropriate film. It's a good idea to take a test roll ahead of time if you can talk the labor/delivery room nurses into letting you enter (or stand at the door) of their sterile room. If there is no way you can examine the delivery room ahead of time, do ask the doctor about the light source. The hospital Public Information office may be able to help you, too. Space in the delivery room is usually very limited, so tripods and large equipment are not allowed most places; a hand-held camera will have to suffice. You must have the support and permission of your doctor to take pictures in delivery. Remember that even if you do not want pictures taken of the actual delivery, it is nice to have pictures of the minutes-old infant as s/he's being cleaned up and handed to the mother.

Since no one knows exactly when the baby is going to decide to be born, it is important to be prepared for the birth to take place at any time during the last month or so. Having a full, or near-full, tank of gas in the car at all times during the last few weeks is advisable; particularly if the country is in the throes of a real or imagined fuel shortage. Know how to get to the hospital and how long it takes to get there. Know an alternate route, in case of traffic jams, construction or road blocks; know how long the alternate route takes. In choosing routes to the hospital, it is good if the road is as smooth as possible. A woman in labor can notice ruts, dips and patches in the road that she has never noticed before. Know what hospital entrance to use at night, and what entrance to use in the daytime. Be sure you know.

Having a clean blanket and a couple of clean towels in the car can be helpful in case your membranes rupture or the baby is born on the way to the hospital. Whatever you wrap the baby in must be clean, not semi-clean.

As much paperwork as possible should be completed and returned to the hospital prior to labor. This makes the admitting procedure much shorter and much more pleasant when you arrive in labor.

If you have other children, have at least three or four places ready to take them at a moment's notice. If you aren't having someone come to your home to care for them, have suitcases packed with their belongings ready and waiting ahead of time.

The drive to the hospital should be quick and efficient, but not reckless. Unless you have a police escort, traffic laws and common courtesy to other cars should be strictly obeyed. Getting in an accident on the way to the hospital is very inconvenient.

If you feel an urge to push (or "bear down") on the way to the hospital, use whatever breathing techniques you've been taught in order to avoid pushing. Let your coach know what you are feeling. Remain calm. Unless you are very near the hospital, the coach should pull the car out of traffic and stop as soon as possible. In a situation like this, the urge to push will probably be too strong to control for more than several contractions. After the car is stopped, assess the situation and determine whether or not you think you can make it to the hospital before the birth. If you decide that it is probable that you can, proceed carefully, using the techniques you've learned in order to control the desire to push.

If you decide that it is not possible to reach the hospital, stay where you are. Remove your undergarments and prepare to greet your baby. Do not, under any circumstances, have the coach hold your legs together to delay the birth. This was a fairly common practice in days gone by; nurses used this technique to delay the birth until the physican arrived. It's true that the baby didn't arrive until the doctor did, but the baby whose mother was treated in this manner was often brain-damaged.

The baby that is coming this fast usually doesn't need much pushing help from the mother. Allow the baby to ease out with the contractions. If you push with great force as the baby is coming out, there is a much greater chance of perineal lacerations. Before the baby is born, put the clean towels under yourself. Support the baby's head as it is born; remember that the head naturally turns to one side as it is born to allow for rotation of the shoulders. Do not pull on the baby. Be sure to support the baby's whole body as it emerges.

When the baby is born, dry him/her thoroughly, wrap in the clean receiving blanket and support him/her in a position that allows the mucus to drain. A position whereby the infant's head is lower than its feet is adequate; you don't have to stand it on its head. If the baby does not cry or start breathing spontaneously as soon as it's born, massage its body gently to stimulate breathing. Put it to breast if the umbilical cord is long enough to do so without pulling it taut. Being held close to the mother's body will comfort the infant and keep it warm even if s/he doesn't feel like sucking.

Ideally, by this time, a police car will have stopped to see what is happening and will be ready to escort you on to the hospital. Even if that hasn't happened, continue to the hospital and go directly to the emergency entrance. If you have a police escort, the police officer will have radioed ahead and the hospital staff will be waiting for the three of you.

It is just as well if the placenta is not born until you arrive at the hospital. Do not cut the cord; just leave it attached to the baby. If the placenta is born before you arrive at the hospital, wrap it up with the baby; it will provide the infant with extra warmth. Remember, even if the placenta is born, do not cut the cord.

Assuming the baby isn't born on the way, the following is a general idea of what will happen when you arrive at the hospital.

Thanks to advance pre-admitting paperwork, the admitting procedures in most hospitals are not too difficult. Usually the mother's signature will be required at least once at the time she enters the hospital. In some hospitals all mothers are met at the admitting area with either a wheelchair or a stretcher; in others the mothers are allowed to walk to the labor room. After the mother signs the necessary papers, she is usually escorted to the labor room while the father completes the rest of the paperwork. If contractions are especially strong, or she feels a definite need for coaching, the paperwork can be completed later. **It is not legally necessary to have registration completed before birth.**

The nurses in the labor room area will be waiting for you. They should have a complete history on you that your doctor, midwife, or clinic provided during the last month or so of the pregnancy. Your prenatal history, name, age, occupation, number of previous pregnancies, number of miscarriages, religion, due date, address and other pertinent data will be on the forms that the doctor gives the hospital. In addition to this information, the labor room nurses will need information relating to the progress of this labor. They will ask when the contractions started, how strong and frequent the contractions are, whether you've had any discharge or bloody show, if and when your membranes ruptured, whether you feel nauseous at all, what and when you last ate, and whether you have any known allergies to medications. Some hospitals may ask a couple of questions more or less, but all focus on gathering this information. Be sure to tell the nurse that you are a prepared mother; tell her that whether she asks or not. If the nurse asks questions and expects answers in the middle of contractions, just ignore her until the contraction is over. Then explain very politely that you will be happy to answer any number of questions between contractions, but that during the contractions you must do your breathing and relaxation techniques in order to control the contractions. If she does not seem to understand, or does not seem to accept your position, be insistent. Just refuse to answer anything during a contraction.

Some hospitals require the mother to weigh before she is admitted to the labor/delivery area.

The perineal area (the area around the opening to the vagina) is washed to disinfect the area in preparation for the birth. A clean perineum lessens the chance of contamination through the birth canal. The pubic hair may be clipped or shaved in order to further insure a perfectly clean perineum. Some doctors order a "full prep," but most order a "mini-prep." When a full prep is given, all of the pubic hair, including that in the front, is shaved off; when a mini-prep is given, just the hair between the legs, the hair around the birth canal opening, is shaved off. A few doctors don't order their patients shaved at all, but most do; being free of hair facilitates episiotomy repair as well as promoting cleanliness. If you have a real aversion to being shaved, discuss it with your doctor prior to entering the hospital.

Many hospitals collect a urine specimen if you're not too far along in labor. Some hospitals catheterize you in order to collect a sterile specimen. Catheterization consists of inserting a small rubber tube into the bladder; this is a fairly painless procedure if you are relaxed.

Most hospitals give an enema in order to clean out the lower bowel. One of the reasons advanced for giving an enema is so the mother will not push anything else out when she is pushing the baby out. Actually, there is not usually very much in the lower bowel of most laboring women because of the natural diarrhea which is often present during the last couple of days preceding labor. Having a lot of material in the lower bowel can interfere with the progress of labor. Enemas are sometimes given expressly to stimulate labor; they may be repeated during labor if the labor is going very slowly or if a plateau is reached. If you wish, you may be able to give yourself an enema at home before you go to the hospital, but do so only with permission from your doctor or midwife.

Soon after you arrive in the labor/delivery area, you will be checked to determine how far labor has progressed. An internal exam, either vaginal or rectal, will be done to determine cervical effacement and dilatation. While she is doing the examination, the nurse will also feel the baby's presenting part to estimate its position and station. The nurse will feel your abdomen both during and between contractions to establish the strength and character of the contractions and to judge the position of the fetal body. After the examination, the nurse will report the pertinent data to your doctor or midwife.

The station of the baby refers to how far down the presenting part is. The baby is at a minus (−) station when the presenting part is above the ischial spines (two bony projections of the pelvis); it is at zero station when the presenting part is even with the ischial spines; and it is at a plus (+) station when the presenting part is below the ischial spines. The presenting part is out into the world at about a +4 or +5 station. Each "station" is equal to approximately one centimeter.

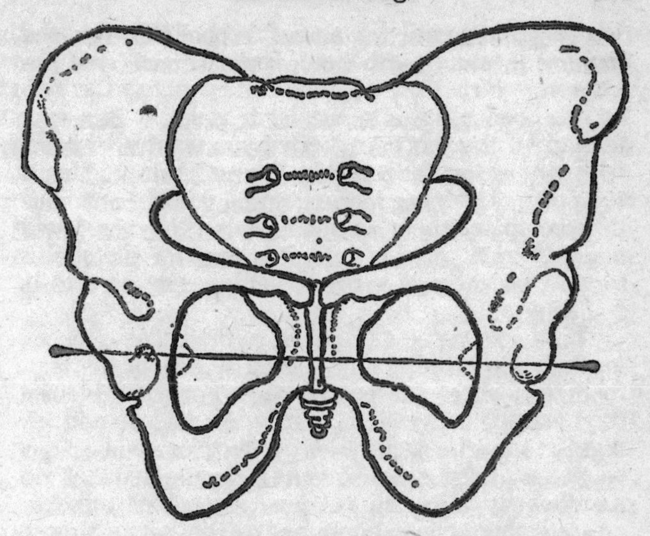

It is possible that the nursing staff could determine that you are not in active labor and send you home again, but that's okay. Next time you go to the hospital you will know exactly what will happen to you!

The nurses also take your blood pressure, temperature, pulse, and respiration rate. The fetal heart tones are recorded, too. The rate of the baby's heart beat can help the medical personnel determine whether the baby is in any trouble. It's fun to listen to the fetal heart beat if the hospital uses one of the machines that amplifies the heart beat.

A few hospitals give baths or showers as patients are admitted, but not very many do.

All of these procedures really don't take too long, but it will probably seem like an unusually long time to the coach who is waiting to come in and begin coaching. If labor is extremely far along, or if a particular nurse is especially supportive of prepared childbirth, the coach may be allowed to rejoin the mother as soon as the admission papers are finished, but normal procedure is for the coach to wait in the Fathers'

Waiting Room until the mother is completely prepped, examined, and questioned. Even if the staff has assured you that the coach will be contacted as soon as s/he can come into the labor room, it is a good idea to let the nurse know that you want your coach with you as soon as possible. Remember that many of the patients they see in the hospital don't have anyone to accompany them through labor. They deal with many Ostrich patients, and it is easy for the staff to forget that there is a coach waiting out there to be contacted.

The whole process of riding to the hospital, checking into the hospital and getting settled in the labor room can affect the contractions. For some women, the contractions get temporarily less intense and less regular; sometimes they even go away for a while. Some women experience more intense and more frequent contractions for a period of time. Sometimes these increased contractions continue, so the whole process acted like a stimulant to labor. Other women experience no definite change as they enter the hospital; the contractions just continue gradually getting stronger and closer together.

It's common for a woman to have more difficulty in handling the contractions when her coach is not with her. The farther along labor is, the more prevalent this is. Usually the problem resolves itself when the coach is able to join her in the labor room.

Temperature, pulse, respiration, blood pressure and fetal heart tones are recorded at intervals throughout labor. Periodically either a vaginal or rectal examination will be done to determine how cervical dilatation is progressing. Many nurses request that the coach step out into the hall when they're doing this exam, but there is certainly no medical reason to have the coach leave.

Some nurses make the request in order to save the mother embarrassment and others do it because they themselves are uncomfortable when the coach is there (particularly a male coach) while they are examining the patient. If you wish to have your coach remain, ask. It is not effective for the coach to say, "I want to stay." You must say, "I'd like to have him stay. I like to have him here, and the contractions are much easier to handle when he's here." It is possible that these exams could be quite painful, and proper breathing and relaxation are very important; some women find this very difficult to achieve when the coach is wandering around out in the hall. The early exams are usually the most difficult because as the labor progresses, the baby gets closer to the outside world and can be felt more easily by the nurse.

Another difficulty with examinations is that medical personnel often have the mother lie on her back for the exam. Most women find a side-lying, or partially-sitting position to be the most comfortable for labor, and some are extremely uncomfortable in a flat-on-the-back position. In fact, lying flat on the back is not recommended during the latter parts of pregnancy, nor during labor because such a position restricts blood circulation to the fetus. Some staff people will examine you while you are on your side; if the back-lying position is particularly uncomfortable, ask whether the exam can be done while you are lying on your side.

If the nurses do not automatically tell you about your progress after each examination, be sure to ask. Ask about your effacement, dilatation and the station of the baby. Most medical personnel measure and report in terms of centimeters, but some use the term "fingers." In this case, one finger is equal to approximately 2 centimeters. Some people have slipped into the incorrect habit of using the terms "finger" and "centimeter" as indicating the same measurement; however, this is not the proper use of the words. **If you are the slightest bit confused about what is meant, ask for the progress in terms of centimeters.** It is possible that two different people may check your progress at almost the same time and come up with different figures. This is because estimation of size may differ from individual to individual. This is usually not a problem if the people have worked together for a period of time; they will have made adjustments and know how to make the numbers agree.

If you want to be examined more frequently, or if you feel that the contractions are getting a lot stronger and you haven't been checked for a while, ask for an exam. It is certainly your right to know how your labor is progressing. This is particularly important if you are attempting to determine your need for medication.

At this point, an explanation may ease your mind. The people who are examining you do not insert 3 or 4 fingers; they insert two and determine the distance between fingers when one is on each side of the dilating cervix.

In many countries, a woman is allowed to labor in a lounge reserved for women in early labor. She is accompanied into the lounge by a family member or friend and allowed to remain there until her membranes rupture or until she feels the need to enter the labor and delivery rooms. In this situation, she returns to the labor and delivery area periodically to be examined. A few hospitals in America offer the laboring woman this option, but in the United States it is almost a universal practice to confine the laboring woman to her labor room bed from the time she enters the hospital until she is taken to the delivery room. Be prepared for this when you enter the hospital.

The use of routine medications in many American hospitals causes hospitals as a whole to limit the movement of laboring women as a precautionary measure. This is becoming more and more important as malpractice lawsuits are becoming more and more prevalent.

Communication with the hospital staff throughout labor and delivery is extremely important. Every time you come in contact with a new staff member, point out that you are a prepared mother. They deal with many, many Ostriches who don't know anything about what is going on; it is easy for them to forget that some women enter childbirth with a positive attitude and want to know all about how things are going.

Undeniably, some nurses are supportive of prepared childbirth and others definitely are not. Almost every hospital has some of each kind. Sometimes a doctor can assign a supportive nurse to his/her prepared patients, but usually there's absolutely nothing you can do to insure that your particular labor room nurse will be supportive. However, by choosing a hospital that is family-centered in its approach, the chances of having a supportive staff is greatly improved. If you find yourself in the position of having a nurse who doesn't seem to understand what you are trying to do, try communicating with her. Explain that you must be allowed to concentrate fully on each contraction as it happens and that you will be happy to change position for examinations, answer questions, etc., between contractions, but that you simply can't breathe and relax properly if you attempt to do these things during contractions. If she still doesn't seem to respond to your wishes after you've explained your position a couple of times, consider having the coach explain the problem to another staff member and see whether a staffing adjustment can be made. It can be embarrassing to ask for a different nurse, but remember that it is your body, your baby and your childbirth experience.

Let the nurse know how you feel and what you would like. The nursing staff is in the hospital solely to care for you, the patient. The coach can act as a buffer between the mother and the nurse.

Communication with the coach is also important. It is virtually impossible for the coach to know exactly what you want at each point during labor. A comfort measure, such as a particular method of back massage, may be very effective during early labor, but lose its impact in late labor. The only way the coach will know its effect has changed is to tell him/her. If the labor room is too warm or too cold, tell the coach. If you need pillows re-arranged or the blanket adjusted, tell the coach. The coach is the one person that is there to offer you undivided attention and support. The nurses have other patients to care for, phones to answer, doctors to communicate with and even breaks to take. The coach is there for you. The only way for the coach to know exactly what you want is to communicate with him/her.

It is particularly important to communicate effectively about medication. Prepared childbirth is based on the premise that each couple should be allowed to make choices regarding their own childbirth experience. It is not important whether a couple chooses to use medication; what is important is that the couple be allowed to make the choice. Medication is an area of great conflict and source of much disappointment if expectations are too high, or if medical people are too forceful in "offering" it.

Some doctors order routine medications for all of their patients; the nurses can sometimes make it seem as though the woman has no choice but to accept the medication. Actually, a woman has the legal right to refuse all medication. The decision to accept medication or not should be the parents'. They should certainly use judgment based on information, and on their individual situation and expectations; but the decision should be theirs. Communication among all of the parties involved can make everyone happier.

The mother should urinate about once an hour during labor. If the bladder becomes distended with urine, the progress of labor will be hindered and she may have to be catheterized in order to remove the urine. It's easy for the mother to be unaware that she has a full bladder during labor; she is busy concentrating on contractions. If the bladder is full enough, it could be causing the contractions to be more painful than they otherwise would be. Before the membranes rupture, you'll probably be allowed to get up and walk to the bathroom. After the membranes rupture, you may have to use a bedpan.

To improve circulation, it is important that the mother change position at least once an hour. It's easiest to remember to do this if you just change position every time you urinate.

The fetal heart tones will be monitored in one way or another throughout labor. Some hospitals use fetoscopes (adapted stethoscopes), some use devices that amplify the heart tone so that anyone in the room can hear it, some use external fetal heart monitors and some use internal fetal heart monitors. The various methods of monitoring the fetal heart tones are explained briefly in the Choosing a Hospital chapter. **The fetal heart rate is normally between 120 and 160 beats per minute. Any prolonged rate outside of this range can indicate some sort of fetal distress.**

When dealing with either the external fetal heart monitor or the internal fetal heart monitor it must be remembered that this kind of monitoring is constant. It does not happen just when the nurse decides it is time to listen; the equipment it attached and stays there throughout labor. The presence of the machine can be intimidating. If the position of the machine causes the coach to be separated from the mother, all efforts must be made to adjust the position of either the mother's bed, the machine or the coach. Use of a fetal heart monitor is no reason to separate the couple. **If the staff is not sensitive to the spatial problem that the machine may be creating, it is up to the coach and the mother to alert the appropriate people.**

Another common problem with the monitors, particularly those that have a print-out on paper, is that some nurses tend to ignore the mother and pay attention only to the information that the machine is spitting out. Certainly the machine is telling the nurse how often the contractions are coming, how strong they are, the fetal heart rate and sometimes even the mother's blood pressure. But it does not tell her if the mother would like to have the window closed, or if the mother is feeling a great deal of discomfort. If you have a fetal monitor and feel as if the staff is paying more attention to the machine than to you, let them know how you feel.

If you do not understand what the machine is doing, ask for an explanation. It is your right to know what this thing is that is recording your body's involuntary movements and your baby's heart beat. The fetal heart monitors are a source of great controversy among opposing factions in the medical profession. Realize that they can be of great value in detecting fetal distress; realize, too, that they are just machines. Some women find the monitors to be extremely uncomfortable, especially the insertion of the internal monitor, but most don't seem to experience any special discomfort. If you are hooked up to one of the monitors that produces a read-out on a strip of paper, the nurse may give you a section of the paper for your baby book if you ask. Ask while you are in labor, because it may not be available the next day.

Some hospitals require that the bed rails be put up as a safety precaution. This is a practice directed mainly toward medicated mothers, but a hospital may require it for unmedicated mothers as well. Don't let the rails bother you. Sometimes the nurses will let the coach lower the rails on the side of the bed next to the coach so that s/he can coach more effectively. If this is not allowed, it is not too difficult to adjust the coaching to meet the situation. The rails do not have to be a barrier between the coach and the mother.

Ideally, each woman is provided with a private labor room. Unfortunately, this doesn't always work out. Most hospitals try to assign one patient per labor room until they run out of space. Even when labor rooms must be shared, most staffs attempt to keep prepared women together. This makes it a lot easier on a prepared couple; the breathing and relaxation techniques take concentration and a distraught Ostrich in the next bed can be very distracting. Some hospitals allow the labor coach to stay only if the mother is in a labor room by herself; if the other bed is occupied, the coach has to leave. Check this out a long time before the baby is due. If the hospital won't assure you that you can be together during labor even if you do not have a labor room by yourself, change hospitals if it is at all possible. One of the basic principles of prepared childbirth methods is the use of a labor coach.

If it becomes necessary for you to share the labor room, ask to have a prepared mother. If that is impossible, and you must share the room with an Ostrich, labor may be a bit more of a challenge for you. It's very difficult to concentrate if the woman in the other bed is thrashing around or crying out with each contraction. And it can be disturbing to hear her refer constantly to the contractions as "labor pains." Several things can be done to make the situation more tolerable. First, try to tune her out; try doubly hard to concentrate on each contraction totally. Try playing a cassette recorder or a transistor radio very quietly if the nurse will let you. Talk with your coach. Put cotton in your ears if nothing else seems to work.

Ask the nurse if there is anywhere you can be moved. It is possible that a labor room has opened up since you were admitted. If there is no empty labor room, ask if it's possible to be moved in with someone who is prepared, or someone who is quieter. Don't ask to have the other woman moved; she is uncomfortable enough already.

If there is absolutely no other way to cope with the situation, your coach may want to offer to teach her some of the breathing techniques. Of course this approach should be taken only if the woman seems receptive. However, most laboring women are willing to try anything that might eliminate the discomfort. There's no time to go into complicated explanations, and it's unreasonable to expect her to catch on immediately to each method, but unprepared women are often helped immensely by using just the beginning techniques. It's better than nothing. It's also important to remember that the coach is there to coach you, not the other woman. If you feel s/he is taking too much time with the Ostrich, let her/him know.

The importance of proper rest and complete relaxation during and between contractions throughout the first stage of labor cannot be overstressed. The first stage is a passive time; the goal is to let the body function most efficiently on its own. The second stage of labor, the expulsion stage, is completely different. It takes a lot of energy and a lot of effort. Most women are pleased when the cervix is completely dilated and they can do something physically active in the birth process.

When the doctor, nurse, or midwife tells you that your cervix is completely dilated, the opening will measure approximately 10 centimeters (about 4 inches) in diameter. Then it's time to push the baby out into the world.

I was worried that I wouldn't be able to recognize the signs of labor, such as when contractions begin, when transition begins, etc., but it seemed to come naturally.

Two weeks before my due date I began losing my mucus plug. It took three weeks in all. I'd never heard of that before.

But each time I didn't concentrate on breathing and focal points and realized how much worse it was that way, I was able to gain control again with the next contraction. I really noticed the difference that using all of the techniques made.

I kept saying I was hungry and thirsty, but I wasn't allowed my sucker or even any water. I thought I would starve before it was over.

When I gave birth to our daughter 2½ years ago, I hadn't been to any Lamaze classes. I wasn't aware of what was happening and fell asleep on the delivery table after the saddle block. Being so alert and experiencing the birth of this baby was such a rewarding, unforgettable moment for both of us. I've never seen Tim so moved. He had to go home and take four Excedrin tablets . . . I felt terrific!

FETUS IN UTERUS

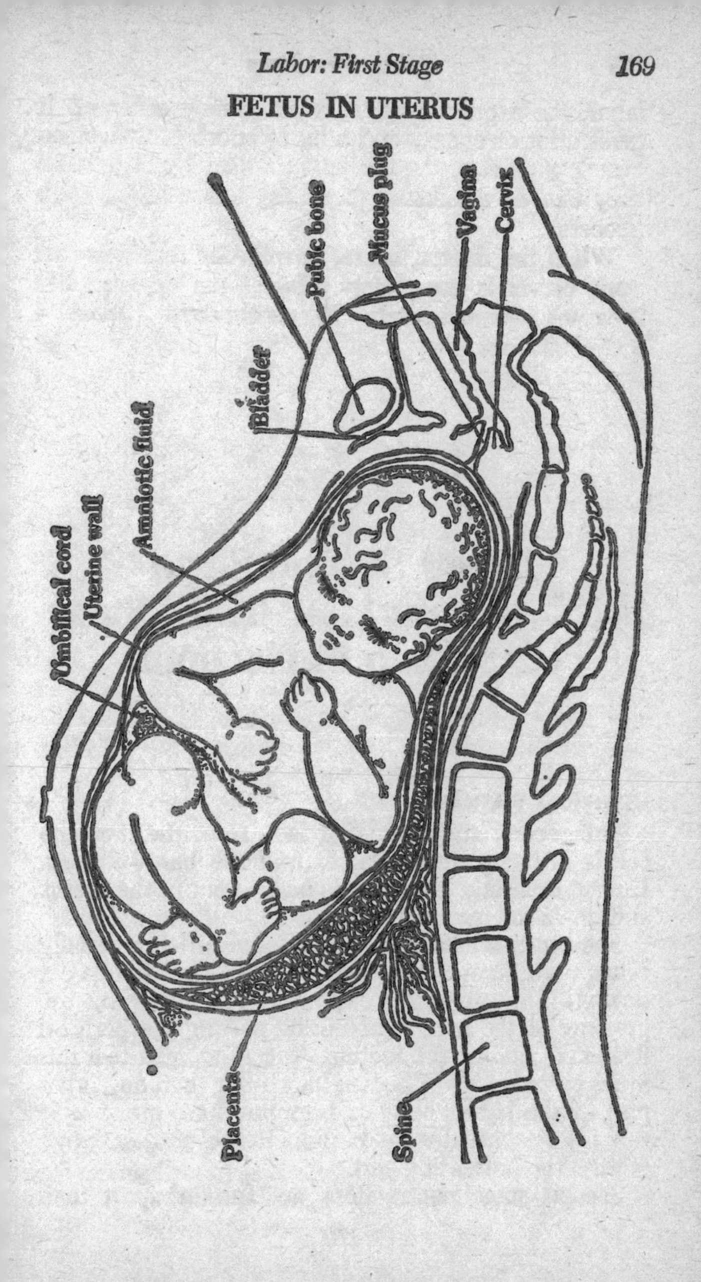

Labor: Second Stage [Birth of Baby] and Third Stage [Expulsion of Placenta]

STAGE 2 LABOR

The second stage of labor lasts from the time the cervix is completely dilated until the baby is born. During this stage the baby is pushed out of the uterus and down the birth canal.

The contractions during this stage of labor usually bring with them a tremendous urge to push (or bear down). This urge is instinctive; it's caused by the pressure of the baby's presenting part on the perineal floor and against the rectum. Not all women feel this urge, but most do. The head is harder than any other part of the baby's body and applies more pressure so the urge is usually more pronounced if the baby's head is the presenting part.

Second stage contractions are further apart than

those of transition. They are usually 4 or 5 minutes apart, but they can be as little as 2 minutes or as much as 8 minutes apart. The contractions are usually between 60 and 90 seconds long. The expulsive stage typically lasts between 1 and 3 hours for first-time mothers, and between 30 minutes and 1 hour for multiparas. In some cases it takes only one contraction to push the baby out.

It is very important that you don't accept the presence of the urge to push as a positive indication that your cervix is completely dilated. Sometimes the urge to bear down comes prematurely and to push along with it is dangerous. Premature pushing can cause the cervix to swell or you can end up with painful lacerations. As soon as you feel the urge to bear down, let your coach and nurse know what you are feeling. The doctor, nurse or midwife will examine you and tell you whether it is okay to push. If the cervix is not yet fully dilated, you will have to use panting or blowing techniques taught in childbirth education classes to avoid pushing along with your body. The coach is vitally important at this stage of labor, and s/he shouldn't be far away if you are anywhere near transition and full dilatation.

When you are given the go-ahead to push, much of the discomfort you may have been feeling will probably disappear. Most women feel greatly relieved when the expulsion stage starts. The transition symptoms disappear and a woman often feels she has regained some control over the situation. The pushing is very active and very strenuous. It can be a great relief after trying to be completely passive during the first stage of labor. Pushing usually doesn't hurt if the baby is in a good position.

In most births, the head is the presenting part and it enters the pelvic basin turned to one side. From that position it rotates to either a face up or a face down position. Most rotate to a face-down position so that when the baby emerges, s/he is looking at the floor. This face-down position puts the baby's soft facial structure next to the mother's sacrum during labor.

This is the normal position, and usually the least painful and the shortest kind of delivery.

On the other hand, if the head rotates to a face-up position so that when the baby emerges s/he is looking up at the ceiling, the hard bones in the back of the baby's head press against the mother's sacrum during labor. This pressure can produce severe backache throughout first and second stage labor. This position can make the whole process, including the delivery, longer. Posterior positions (face up) and back pain in labor are discussed more thoroughly in the chapter on special labors. Many women find that the back pain and pressure lessen as the baby progresses down the birth canal.

As second stage begins, some women become very concerned about just how the baby manages to come out of such a seemingly small opening. A couple of things make the somewhat unbelievable seem more realistic. The vagina is composed of folds of skin which fan out to allow the baby to pass through. Even the mother's pelvic bone structure is altered slightly at the coccyx and the area of the pubic symphysis; the hormone relaxin produces a natural softening which causes some mobility of the bone structure.

This stage is nice because the mother tends to be quite sociable and happy between contractions if the baby is not in a pain-producing position.

Exactly when, in terms of labor progress, that the mother is moved to the delivery room differs from hospital to hospital, but usually first-time mothers do some pushing in the labor room before they are transferred. Some doctors prefer to move even first-time mothers to the delivery room as soon as the cervix is completely dilated, but this is not too common. Multiparas are moved to the delivery room as soon as the cervix is completely dilated, or sometimes even when the cervix is at 7-8 centimeters. The speed of labor as a whole and the speed of any past labors are considered when the physician or midwife decides just when to transfer the individual mother.

A good rule of thumb is that first-time mothers are

moved to the delivery room when a patch of the baby's head the size of a 50-cent piece shows during a contraction, and multiparas are moved to the delivery room when dilatation is complete.

After you are told that you can push, it usually takes several contractions before you are doing really effective pushing. It is important that you practice the pushing techniques taught in your childbirth education class; this "pretend" pushing will make your pushing during labor just that much more effective. The more effective the pushing, the shorter your second stage will be.

A wide variety of positions can be utilized for pushing in the labor room. A kneeling position, a squatting position, a side-lying position, a back-lying position or a down-on-all-fours position can be used effectively. It's a good idea to practice pushing in all of these positions before labor starts because you won't know until you are in labor which position you find the most comfortable and effective for pushing. If you're familiar with all of the positions, you will have all of them available when you need them.

The general pushing techniques remain the same no matter which position is used. Two or three deep breaths are taken, then the breath is held and the expanded lungs push down on the diaphragm. The pressure of the diaphragm pushing on the fundus of the uterus helps to move the baby down the birth canal. It is important for the coach to be thoroughly acquainted with the pushing techniques because the breathing and the pushing efforts can be difficult to coordinate without instructions to follow. By the time the mother reaches the second stage of labor, she has been concentrating for a long period of time on relaxation and various breathing techniques; suddenly she is asked to perform completely differently. Not only that, she is asked to perform this different task just as she comes out of the confusion and intense work of transition. Simple, explicit instructions can be a big help to her as she adjusts to the change and becomes effective at pushing.

If you choose a back-lying position, it is possible to adjust most labor room beds so that the head of the bed is at a 35° to 50° angle to the rest of the bed. If this source of back support is not available, it is possible to use several pillows to produce much the same effect.

Sometimes it is easier to miss the beginning of a second stage contraction than it is to miss the beginning of a first stage contraction. In order to catch the contraction at its very beginning, it is a good idea to keep your fingertips on on your uterus; as the contraction begins, the uterus becomes harder and seems to lift up.

It's a common misconception that the same muscles are used to push out a baby as to push out a bowel movement. The two kinds of pushing are not the same. Pushing for a bowel movement originates much lower in the body than does pushing for a baby. Pushing for the bowel movement involves muscles in the buttocks; pushing for a baby involves use of the lungs and diaphragm. When the lungs are expanded, they push down on the diaphragm which pushes down on the fundus of the uterus. The fundus of the uterus exerts pressure on the fetus and it is pushed down into the birth canal and out the vaginal opening. So if a relatively uninformed nurse comes in and tells you to push just like you're having a bowel movement, ignore her. If, on the other hand, a supportive nurse offers a suggestion for pushing that indicates she understands the difference between the two kinds of pushing, try taking her advice. If you feel more effective doing it the way you were, you can always revert to your own technique.

The pushing urge is often accompanied by a feeling of pressure in the vagina and rectum. This pressure is caused by the baby's presenting part moving down the birth canal.

In order to make pushing really effective, the pelvic floor and the area around the anus should be relaxed. It is easy to tense the anus as a precaution against letting any fecal material slip out. Remember that the enema that you probably had when you arrived in the labor room cleaned out your lower bowel tract, so there's nothing to push out anyway. Relax everything and exert as much force with your diaphragm as you can.

If you're pushing in the labor room, the nurse may allow the coach to come around to the foot of the bed to see the tiny view of the baby that shows during each contraction as you push. After each contraction, the baby recedes a little; it is important not to relax too quickly at the end of the contractions. The baby will tend to retain more of its forward progress if the mother relaxes slowly and gently. It is easier for each coach to visualize the process if s/he is able to see the presenting part appear and disappear as contractions come and go. Often the mother prefers that the coach lift her up during the contractions to get her in a better position for pushing; if the coach doesn't fully understand the mechanism of expulsion s/he may lower the mother too rapidly after each contraction and progress can be slowed.

If you are in a birthing room, you will labor and deliver in the same room as long as there is no problem or suspected problem. If you are using traditional facilities, you will be moved to the delivery room shortly before the birth of the baby.

When it is determined that you are ready to be taken to the delivery room, things really start happening. You will be wheeled to the delivery room on either your labor room bed or a guerney (a table with wheels). When you arrive in the delivery room, don't let its appearance intimidate you. It is a sterile, functional room with lots of stainless steel and strange-looking instruments. Everything in the room is geared to caring for you and your baby in the safest manner possible. If you wear glasses and have taken them off in the labor room, don't forget to take them to the delivery room with you so you can see what is happening.

You will be either asked to crawl onto the delivery

table by yourself, or you will be lifted onto the delivery table if you need help. The transfer can be quite awkward. You will probably be quite tired from the efforts of labor, and the baby will be far down between your legs by this time. The delivery table itself adds to the awkwardness because it is quite narrow. The move is much easier for you if it is undertaken between contractions instead of during a contraction. Sometimes the hospital personnel seem to forget things like that in their hurry to get you properly situated for delivery. If you are being asked to move, or if someone is moving you from bed to delivery table, during a contraction don't feel shy about pointing out that you still need to concentrate during contractions, and that you are unable to cooperate fully at that time. This switch to the delivery table can cause you to temporarily "forget" your pushing routine, and it may take several contractions before you are doing effective pushing again.

The coach must gown while you are being transferred from labor to delivery if s/he hasn't done so earlier. This absence of the coach can make the transfer and the regaining of control more difficult. It is a good idea if the coach puts on the sterile clothing early in your labor; this avoids the last-minute rush and allows the coach to be with you during the transfer. If the coach does gown early, s/he will not be able to leave the labor/delivery area unless s/he dons a new set of sterile gowns before entering the delivery room.

How you will be positioned on the delivery table depends upon what position you and your doctor or midwife have chosen for delivery. The most common position in American hospitals is the lithotomy position. If you do not discuss delivery position with your doctor or midwife ahead of time, it is safe to assume that you will deliver your baby in the lithotomy position. Even though there are a number of very different delivery positions used in many cultures, few physicians in America offer their patients a choice. In addition to the lithotomy position, positions that are commonly used include dorsal, side-lying, semi-sitting, squatting, and hands and knees.

Lithotomy Position

The lithotomy position is the one most often seen in movies about childbirth. The mother lies flat on her back and her legs are held up and wide apart by stirrups. It is basically the same position as that used in the doctor's office for pelvic examinations. The two positions do differ somewhat though, because the stirrups on the delivery table include trough-shaped leg rests, or slings, so the legs are supported from the knee to the foot. After the mother's legs are positioned in the leg supports, the delivery table is "broken"; this consists of the section just at the bottom edge of the mother's buttocks being pushed down and back under the main section of the delivery table.

The main advantage of the lithotomy position and the broken delivery table is the convenience that's afforded the physician.[1] S/he has direct and immediate access to the perineal area. The lithotomy position came into almost universal use in America when general anesthesia was widely used in childbirth. Obviously a completely anesthetized woman is unable to position herself in any manner whatsoever, so it had to be done for her. In addition, she couldn't push her baby out in her drugged state, so the physician had to pull the infant out. For these purposes the lithotomy position worked very well.

However, the position itself is not physiologically sound for childbirth and it lessens the mother's ability to push effectively.[2] The position is certainly of use in an abnormal birth, or during a medicated birth in which the mother has no control over the movement of her legs. But in a normal birth where the mother is unmedicated, or minimally-medicated, the lithotomy position is unnecessary and perhaps counterproductive. The force of gravity doesn't help the birth process when the mother is in this position, blood circulation and blood pressure are altered because she's flat on her back, and the contractions are less intense.[3]

Be aware that all American doctors were trained to deliver their patients in the lithotomy position. Some are willing to try something different; many are not. Often a midwife will allow her patients more freedom in the choice of delivery position than will a physician.

Dorsal Position

In the dorsal position the mother lies flat on her back, bends her knees and places the soles of her feet flat on the bottom section of the delivery table. The delivery table is not broken in a dorsal delivery. The dorsal and the lithotomy position share many of the same drawbacks, including interference with the mother's blood circulation and alteration of her blood pressure, reducing the strength of the contractions and hindering the mother's ability to push most effectively.[4] However, the contraction intensity and the pushing ability are not altered as much in the dorsal position as in the lithotomy position.

The dorsal position is much more comfortable than the lithotomy for most women, and it allows the woman more freedom. The feet are not spread so far apart in the dorsal position, and tension on the pelvic floor is less in the dorsal position. Increased tension on the pelvic floor, such as that produced in the lithotomy position, increases the need for episiotomy because the perineal muscles are not allowed to stretch in the natural manner.[5]

When giving birth on a broken delivery table, many women have the subconscious fear that the baby will fall on the floor because there's nothing between the vaginal opening and the floor except the birth attendant's hands. Many women are concerned that the attendant's attention could be diverted at the moment of expulsion, and the baby not caught. In the dorsal position, with the unbroken table, the baby would just slide out onto the table if the birth attendant were not there.

The legs can easily and quickly be inserted into the stirrups after the birth so that the physician or midwife can inspect the cervix, vagina and perineum and make any necessary repairs.

Side-Lying (Left Lateral) Position

In this position, the woman lies on her left side; again, the delivery table is not broken. Either the mother, her coach or a nurse holds up the mother's right leg during the pushing contractions. Or, if desired, the right leg can be laid in the stirrup normally used for the left leg. Many women have found this method of leg support to be more comfortable and less tiring than supporting the leg physically during each contraction.

The left lateral position does not reduce the strength of the contractions, nor does it reduce the mother's pushing effectiveness. Some claim that fewer perineal lacerations occur when the left lateral position is used.[6] Many women find this to be the most comfortable position during first stage labor and prefer to retain the position during second stage.

Some women who have delivered in this position complain that it is difficult to watch the birth in the overhead mirror because the upper (right) leg is in the way. If this is a problem for you, experiment a little with exact positioning and you can probably solve the problem without too much difficulty.

Semi-Sitting

In this position, the mother's upper torso is propped up at about a 45° to 50° angle, her knees are flexed, and her feet are flat on the delivery table. In some hospitals the delivery table will adjust to the angle, and in others it is necessary to use pillows to achieve the semi-sitting position. The table is not actually broken, but some delivery tables are designed so that the bottom section will drop down several inches and secure in that position without pushing back under the main section. This allows the physician or midwife good access to the vaginal opening, and leaves the protection of the table under the baby.

This position is physiologically very good for birth. The strength and effectiveness of the contractions is not lessened, the perineal skin is not stretched unduly by the position itself (as in the lithotomy position), and the force of gravity aids the descent and expulsion of the baby. The mother can be inspected and repaired in this position, or her legs can be raised into the stirrups after the birth.

Squatting

This is the most commonly used position in many areas of the world. The force of gravity is used to its best advantage, the contractions are not interfered with in any way, nor is the mother's blood pressure and blood circulation altered. However, in the cultures where this position is most frequently used, birth is considered much less pathologic, the mother often delivers her own baby, and sterile conditions are not observed. It is very difficult for the birth attendant to manage the birth if the mother is in the squatting position, and very few doctors will even consider this position. The semi-sitting position is usually considered a good alternative to the squatting position because it combines the advantages of both.

Hands and Knees

The main advantage of this position is that it gets the baby off of the mother's spine. In cases where the baby is pressing very hard on the sacrum and tailbone of the mother, such as in a posterior presentation, the only way to relieve the pressure and discomfort is to get the baby off and away from the spine. This position is hard for the birth attendant to manage and for the mother to comfortably maintain when she is on the narrow delivery table, and it is almost never used in American hospitals.

DELIVERY POSITIONS

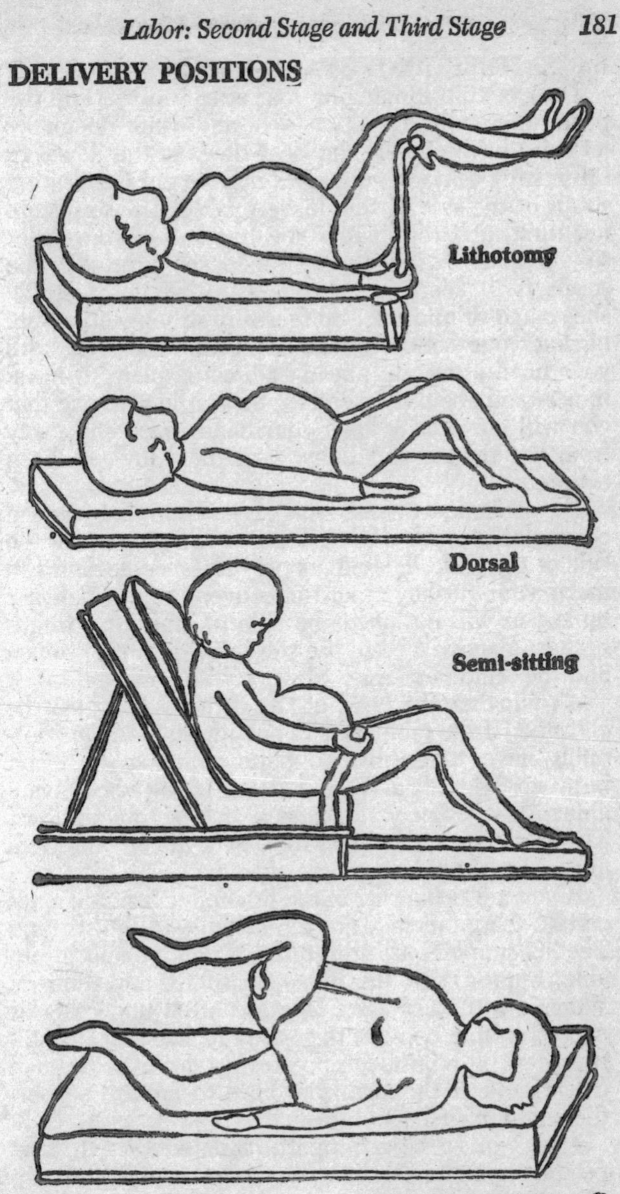

BACK TO SECOND STAGE LABOR

The exact positioning of your arms and legs will depend upon what position you and your doctor or midwife have chosen ahead of time. In the dorsal or lithotomy positions, your arms may be put into leather straps at the side of the delivery table. The straps are not tight, and they allow you freedom of movement so you do not feel really restrained; the purpose of the straps is to keep your hands away from the sterile sheets and draping. If you feel very strongly about not having your hands restrained at all, discuss it with your birth attendant ahead of time. Explain that you understand about the need for the sterile field and that you will voluntarily keep your hands back and away from the drapes and baby until the baby has been checked.

If your hands are restrained, be certain that you can comfortably reach the handbars or stirrup posts at the side of the table. These bars provide leverage, and can make your pushing more effective. On the delivery table you will no longer be able to grab your thighs because they will be in the sterile field. Many women find the handbars easier to work with, anyway.

Ask whether the head of the delivery table can be elevated. If the table itself is not adjustable, some hospitals have removable supports available to insert between the table and the pad. If nothing else is available, ask whether you can have two or three pillows. The elevation of the upper torso gets you off your back and makes the pushing more effective.

If you are delivering in the lithotomy position, make certain that your legs are comfortable in the stirrups. The leg supports are adjustable; if you are uncomfortable, request that the nurse do something about it. Women with very long legs are often unnecessarily uncomfortable because they don't realize that the stirrups can be adjusted. The stirrups seem to be most comfortable if the legs from knee to hip are perpendicular to the delivery table.

After you've been properly situated for whatever position you've chosen, your perineum will be swabbed with an antiseptic solution. This can be a very minor discomfort in that it seems very cold, even though it is usually room temperature. Then you are draped around the perineal area with sterile sheets and towels. Bear in mind that it is important that you don't touch the sterile field that has been created because you will contaminate it and the whole antiseptic process will have to be done over again.

It's usually about this time when the coach has rejoined you. Everyone in the delivery room, except the mother, wears a surgical mask. This includes the coach so don't be surprised when the one really familiar face doesn't even look familiar any more!

Several minutes after you've been positioned, draped and swabbed, you should be back in control and pushing with maximum effectiveness. Pushing and expulsion are much more effective when the pelvic floor is relaxed. If the perineum is tense and acting to hold the baby back, it is naturally going to be more difficult to expel the infant.

Most hospitals require that the coach remain at the head of the delivery table, but some birth attendants allow the coach to come around to the bottom of the table and view the birth from the doctor's eye view. Hospitals want the coach to stay at the head of the table because everyone in the delivery room has a job to do. It is important for every member of the team to know what every other member is doing and where each member is. It can unnecessarily complicate matters if a coach is wandering around looking here and there. The concern that the coach will touch sterile equipment is also considered. In any case, the coach can watch the birth in the mirror that is attached to the ceiling. It's easier for the coach to remember to keep up the coaching if s/he is right next to the mother's head. It is easy to get so involved in the birth that the coach can forget just why s/he is there and unintentionally leave the mother to fend for herself. Many hospitals provide a stool for the coach to sit on.

The mirror should be adjusted so that the mother can see the birth. The mother's position is rather stationary, whereas the coach can move around a little, so the mirror should be positioned for the mother's convenience. Don't hestitate to tell the delivery room staff if it is tipped at an inappropriate angle. Even if you aren't sure that you want to watch the actual birth, take a peek. Then you can decide whether you want to watch the rest or not; but if you don't look at all, you may be sorry later. This is the only time that this baby will ever be born.

If your doctor or midwife has not yet arrived, the nurses may get you all set up on the delivery table and ask you to pant or otherwise refrain from pushing along with the contractions. Controlling the urge to push at this late stage is very difficult, and strong coaching is extremely helpful. Even with the best coaching, it is doubtful that you will last more than 5 or 10 minutes; if the doctor or midwife hasn't arrived by then, chances are the nurse will deliver the baby. Today's nurses are fully qualified to deliver a baby unless there is some major complication. **The old practice of the nurses forcibly holding a woman's legs together to delay the birth was extremely harmful and could lead to brain damage in the infant. If anyone tries to do this to you, don't let him get away with it.**

During the last few minutes, the doctor or midwife will probably tell you how hard to push and when to stop pushing. When the baby's presenting part reaches the perineum, it is important to ease the baby out instead of pushing it out with full force. If the infant comes out slowly and in a controlled manner, it is easier on the mother, the baby and the birth attendant. The chance of maternal laceration is reduced in a controlled birth.

The baby's presenting part is crowning when it bulges the perineum and does not recede from sight between pushing contractions. As the baby crowns, the birth attendant may perform an episiotomy. This is a surgical incision of the skin and tissue of the perineum done to enlarge the vaginal outlet. This eases the baby's passage and lessens the chance of vaginal and perineal tears. The straight surgical incision heals better than does a jagged tear if it occurs. As with many routine obstetric practices in modern hospitals, there are arguments for and against routine episiotomies. It's not a clear-cut matter.

Proponents of routine episiotomies claim that the surgical incision is controlled; the direction of a tear, if it occurs, is not. The straight incision, as well as being controlled, is easier to repair.

The enlarging of the vaginal outlet shortens the second stage of labor because the infant does not have to fight so much resistance while opening the perineum. Saving the baby this amount of work can be important if the child is premature, especially small, or in some sort of fetal distress.[7] However, it has not been proven that a shortened second stage benefits the baby if s/he is term and has shown no sign of fetal distress.[8]

Some claim that the incidence of unwanted pelvic floor relaxation in later life is reduced if the woman had episiotomies when she had her children. This has certainly not been proven, and facts seem to point to some genetic factor as being the cause for pelvic relaxation.[9] In fact the Kegel muscle (the muscle structure of the pelvic floor) cannot be properly reconstructed if it is cut improperly.[10]

Another argument is that the reconstruction of the vaginal opening can restore the original tightness to the vagina, thereby assuring continued sexual response and enjoyment for both the woman and her partner. There is no evidence that this is the case, and a properly exercised Kegel muscle probably does as much to assure vaginal tone as an episiotomy does.[11] In addition, an episiotomy can actually harm the sexual relationship because the stitched area is often very tender and can make resumption of sexual relations difficult if the woman is afraid of discomfort from penetration.

Episiotomy is certainly a useful and necessary procedure when it is medically indicated. In cases where tearing is inevitable, it can prevent dangerous lacerations and needless suffering. Episiotomies are commonly needed when the baby is especially large, or is in an unusual position for delivery. However, it has not been established that routine episiotomy on every woman in childbirth is the best course. Unnecessary episiotomy and the resultant stitches for the repair cause unnecessary pain and discomfort during the postpartum period.

If you would prefer that your doctor or midwife judge the necessity for an episiotomy on the situation at hand rather than on the theory that everyone needs an episiotomy, be sure to discuss the matter with your birth attendant well in advance of labor. There is just not enough time in the delivery room to debate the relative merits of the incision. Remember that it is not a good idea to decide ahead of time that you will not have an episiotomy, no matter what. That approach is being unfair to both your baby and yourself. All throughout a prepared labor and delivery, you are asking your medical care-takers to be flexible and consider you as an individual. You are asking them to base their decisions on the situation as it pertains to you personally, rather than treat you as a routine, assembly line baby-producer. If you would rather not have an episiotomy, discuss it ahead of time with your doctor or midwife; if the attendant understands your need for individuality and is supportive, then don't fight it if s/he tells you at the time of delivery that the episiotomy is necessary. Ask why, but accept it in good spirit.

Physicians frequently administer an injection of novocaine or a similar drug before the episiotomy is performed. This practice is entirely unnecessary because of the natural anesthetic action of the baby's presenting part pressing against the perineum. If the episiotomy is given at the proper time (during a pushing effort), the mother cannot feel it. If the novocaine is not given before the episiotomy is performed, it will be given after the baby is born. After the birth the natural anesthetic action is no longer present, and the repair work would be very painful with no drug relief. If you wish to have the episiotomy given without the use of a drug before the baby is born, let the birth attendant know ahead of time.

As the baby's presenting part is born, you will feel a release of tension. With the next few contractions, the rest of the body will be born. If the head is the presenting part, the delivery is more straightforward and quick than if the breech is the presenting part.

It's not uncommon at all for a baby to cry before it is competely born. This happens more frequently with unmedicated babies (babies whose mothers have received no medications or drugs during labor and delivery) than with medicated babies.

The coach should be sure to look at the delivery room clock and note the exact time of birth. The delivery room personnel often round it off to the nearest five minutes because no one thought to look at the clock at the exact moment the baby was born.

After the birth, both you and the coach (particularly if the coach is the father) can have a lot of different emotions. You can feel exultant, humble, relieved, tired, sweaty, talkative, excited, depressed, hungry, thirsty, and countless other ways. The point is that there is no "right" way to feel or act. Let out whatever emotions you have at the time. No matter how you feel, it is probable that you will be fascinated by the appearance and the sound of the brand new creature you have produced.

Some birth attendants will place the baby on the mother's abdomen immediately after birth; it's nice to be able to touch and experience the baby as soon as s/he's born. The closeness of the newborn can help the uterus to contract and make the third stage of labor shorter. After the umbilical cord is cut, the nurses will take the baby and check its APGAR score and clean it up. If you want the baby on your abdomen immediately after birth, talk to the doctor or midwife about it ahead of time. Some medical people refuse to handle the birth in this manner. Of course, even if the birth attendant had agreed to such a plan before the birth, the stipulation will always be made that the mother's abdomen will have to wait until later if the baby shows any sign of respiratory distress, or any other problem. Only a baby who looks healthy, acts healthy and is breathing well would be placed on the mother's stomach.

Ask about the health and appearance of the baby. If you are afraid something is wrong, voice your fears. Chances are good that your concern is unfounded, but it is ridiculous to lie there and stew about it when you have professionals available to answer your questions. Do read the chapter on The Newborn and be prepared for the strange appearance and funny color of most new babies. Be sure to ask about the baby's APGAR score. S/he will be rated at 1 minute and at 5 minutes. If you don't know what the delivery people are doing with the baby, ask.

Remember that the baby may seem very bloody to you. If you've had an episiotomy, most of the blood will have come from passing directly over the open incision.

Hospitals vary in their precise identification procedures, but those listed below are fairly common. As soon as the baby is born, both you and the baby will receive matching bands that include the mother's surname, the baby's sex, the time of birth and possibly the name of the mother's doctor or midwife. Your band will go around your wrist and the baby's will be fastened to his/her arm or ankle. In many hospitals, it is a standard procedure that whenever the baby is brought to the mother, the two bands are compared to make sure that the right mother is getting the right baby. Other methods, such as recording the baby's footprints and the mother's thumb print are often used in addition to the banding.

The umbilical cord is usually not cut until it quits pulsating. This practice is thought to provide the infant with some extra placental blood. The cord is clamped in two places and cut between the clamps.

The delivery room nurses are responsible for several aspects of immediate care for the newborn. The first order of business is to make sure the baby is breathing properly. If the infant does not start breathing immediately, the nurse will probably suction the mucus from the baby's mouth with either a bulb syringe or a small catheter. In some cases the baby may require more drastic methods of resuscitation such as an electric infant resuscitator. If the delivery personnel are using equipment on your baby, ask what they are doing, but don't be impatient if they can't answer right away; they will explain everything you want to know as soon as the baby is breathing adequately on its own. Even if the baby is breathing fine on its own, the nurses may do some suctioning.

It is a statutory requirement in all states that an antibacterial agent be placed in the baby's eyes as a protection against infection from venereal disease. Penicillin and silver nitrate are the most common substances used.

Many doctors prescribe an injection of a water-soluble form of Vitamin K_1 for the infant to guard against neonatal hemorrhage.

STAGE 3 LABOR

While all of these things are going on, your uterus is probably still contracting. It must still expel the placenta. These contractions are usually not nearly so strong as your earlier contractions; they are much milder because of the drastic decrease in the size and amount of contents of the uterus. When the birth attendant tells you to, give a little push and the placenta will plop out. When the placenta is delivered, the third and final stage of labor is completed. The third stage of labor can take from a few minutes to an hour or so. The placenta should separate from the uterine wall spontaneously; it's dangerous to pull it out.

After the placenta is born, ask to see it if you are interested. Most doctors and midwives are happy to show it to their patients. At the end of the third stage of labor the birth attendant will examine both the uterus and the placenta to see whether any part of the placenta has been left behind. If anything remains in the uterus, it can cause dangerous hemorrhage later, so scrupulous examination is essential.

IMMEDIATE POSTPARTUM

The uterus normally tightens into hard ball and closes the raw area where the placenta was attached. When this action is effective, as it usually is, it stops the bleeding from the placental site. Many physicians give an injection of an oxytocic substance to stimulate the uterus to contract after the birth. If you are planning to nurse your baby, be certain that you are not given an injection to dry up your milk supply. The oxytocic substance will not affect your milk supply. Ask what any injection is for.

After the immediate care of the baby is completed, it may be possible for you to nurse the infant on the delivery table. This is a controversial matter and many hospitals and physicians simply do not allow it, but many do, too. The infant's sucking on the breast can be extremely beneficial; it stimulates the uterus to contract because it causes the body to release an oxytocic hormone. The early sucking also helps stimulate milk production.

Opponents of delivery table nursing claim that the baby has too much mucus and is unable to nurse properly (and that if the baby refuses the breast the mother's feelings will be hurt), that the nursery staff must complete a "test feeding" with glucose water first in order to make sure that the baby is hooked up properly from top to bottom, that the mother is in no condition to hold her own baby immediately after delivery, and that the baby is not kept warm enough if s/he's not in the hospital's baby warmer.

In truth, some babies want to nurse minutes after birth and some do not. Most prepared mothers are more than ready and able to hold their babies immediately after delivery, and the baby is kept warm enough if s/he's wrapped tightly and held close. This early contact may affect early infant-parent bonding in a very positive way. If the mother is allowed to nurse on the delivery table, the coach is able to get much more involved directly with the infant than if the infant remains in the corner of the room in the warmer.

If you wish to have the opportunity to nurse your

baby on the delivery table, you will have to discuss it ahead of time with your doctor or midwife. Sometimes if the hospital does not routinely allow it, the physician can stretch the rules and let you anyway. Having written orders from the pediatrician can help your cause.

In some delivery rooms, the coach (if it's the father) is allowed to hold the baby. Often the father can hold the baby if he requests to do so, but if he doesn't mention it, neither do the nurses. Sometimes all the excitement of birth is a bit overwhelming, and it may be later before the new father realizes that he's the only one who didn't get to hold the infant. So, if the father would like to hold him/her in the delivery room, be sure to ask.

It's common for the mother to shake, sometimes quite violently, after the birth. This is a perfectly natural phenomenon; it's caused by the adrenalin in her system, the sudden change in her circulation patterns (due to the detachment of the placenta), the tremendous adjustments her body is making, and the great amount of energy she's expended in such a short period of time.

The baby is usually weighed in the delivery room, but sometimes this is done in the nursery. Some hospitals measure the baby in the delivery room, and some wait until the baby is in the nursery being cleaned up.

From here on out procedures differ greatly from hospital to hospital. Be certain that you know in advance just what to expect so you won't be disappointed. Some hospitals allow the mother, the coach and the baby to be alone for a while after the birth. This is a good time just to be alone and be amazed at what has happened. It's a nice, quiet way to begin parenthood together. It's nice if the three of you can be completely alone; the nurse is only as far away as the call button if there is a problem.

In some hospitals the mother, the baby and the coach can all go to the maternity recovery room where the mother and the baby will be watched very closely by the recovery room personnel. This, of course, is not quite so private, but is still a time for you to be together as a family.

Sometimes the mother, the baby and the coach can go directly to the mother's room and visit together. This allows for some privacy, unless the room is semi-private or a ward; in that case, the curtains can be drawn to offer a little more privacy.

In most hospitals, however, the mother has no choice but to spend the first hour or so in the maternity recovery room under the watchful eyes of the nurses. Sometimes the coach (father) can stay for a while and visit, but that is usually up to the individual nurse in charge. If you want the father to stay, explain to the nurse that you have just shared the labor and the birth and that you'd like to be together a little while longer.

In situations where the baby cannot stay with the mother during the recovery period, the infant goes to the central nursery where it is cleaned up, weighed and measured (if that hasn't been done previously) and maybe given a test feeding of glucose water. If there is reason to suspect a blood incompatibility in the baby, blood will be drawn from the baby soon after birth.

The father may be able to follow the baby to the nursery to help with the weighing and measuring (or just to watch). This, too, is more or less up to the individual staff involved in most hospitals, so if he would like to do this it is best to ask very nicely.

Some fathers first see what's happening in the nursery, and then join the mother in the recovery room or in her room.

In some hospitals the mother or the father is allowed to carry the baby from the delivery room either to the nursery or the recovery area (maternity recovery room or the mother's room). If your particular hospital offers all of the above options (and many don't), remember that what actually happens in your individual case will depend upon the baby's condition, your condition, how much medication you have had, what medications you have had, and probably the time of day or night. As with every other aspect of the birth, try not to be too disappointed if things don't go exactly as you had planned. Keep in mind that the most important thing to come out of the total experience is having a healthy baby to take home with you.

During the immediate recovery period (usually 1-3 hours) the nurses will take your pulse and blood pressure frequently. They will also knead your uterus in order to make sure it is remaining hard. Your sanitary napkin will be checked to see that you are not passing large clots and to see that you're not hemorrhaging.

Chances are good that you will be very hungry following delivery, particularly if you were unmedicated or minimally medicated. Let someone know how hungry you are, and keep complaining if no one brings you anything to eat. After the tremendous amount of work you have done, you deserve something to eat, even if it is 2 a.m. If all else fails, rummage around in your goody bag and see whether you can find any of the snack items you brought for the coach or any of the lollipops you brought for you.

If you want to, and if your physical condition is good enough, try to spend as much of the immediate postpartum period with the baby as you can. Research indicates that early maternal-child separation can affect later maternal behavior.[12] Maternal-child separation during the 24 hours postpartum tends to interfere with normal maternal responses to the infant. This early period can be crucial to establishing a bond; it's even been suggested that there may be a biochemical mechanism involved during this period that produces an increased sensitivity toward the newborn.[13]

If you plan to have rooming-in, it's a good idea to start the plan as soon as you feel like it. The earlier you begin to establish your relationship with your baby, the sooner you will be able to tune into the baby's life rhythms. The earlier the nursing process is begun, the easier it will be to establish the supply and demand arrangement that governs your milk production.

Whatever your feelings are during the immediate postpartum period, accept them. Examine them and understand them for what they are. Love simply does not just "happen." It grows and develops. If you are having thoughts or feelings that you don't understand, by all means discuss them with someone. Several good candidates for appropriate listeners include the father, your childbirth instructor, other mothers in your childbirth class and friends. Women who have recently given birth or women who deal with the birth experience frequently (such as childbirth education instructors) are usually the most helpful while you are attempting to sort out your feelings. Women who have never given birth are probably among the least helpful. Some women can discuss their postpartum feelings effectively with their mothers, some can't. If the person you talk to is judgmental, the whole purpose is defeated.

Discussion with the appropriate people is a good way to help you realize that what you are thinking and feeling is not uncommon, nor strange. Unfortunately, most physicians do not have the time nor the inclination (nor sometimes even the understanding) to discuss these sorts of problems. Of course, there are a special few who are excellent for this purpose, and if you have one of these, you are very fortunate. Midwives are normally much better sources of moral support and understanding than are physicians.

SOME ADDITIONAL NOTES ON DELIVERY

Fundal Pressure

In some cases, the mother's pushing efforts are not adequate to expel the baby. This may be due to medication the mother has received or to an especially large baby or a particularly small pelvis. It is the practice in some hospitals to apply fundal pressure to aid the pushing efforts of the mother. The nurse will push down on the fundus of the uterus at the same time the mother is pushing in order to make the contraction more effective. This is a poor practice for several reasons; it is possible to cause uterine damage or rupture of the uterus if the pressure is severe,[14] and the fundal pressure can cause a depressed oxygen saturation in the newborn.[15]

Forceps

If the mother's pushing is not adequate to expel the baby, or if the baby must be removed quickly because of signs of fetal distress, the birth attendant may use an instrument called forceps to pull the baby out. Forceps must be used routinely in medicated births where the anesthesia has made the mother's pushing impossible or ineffective. The forceps are large curved pieces of metal that are slipped into the vagina around the baby's head, and then locked together at the intersection of the two pieces. When they are fastened together, the two blades form an instrument that resembles a large set of salad spoons. A forceps delivery can be either a low forceps delivery, a midforceps delivery or a high forceps delivery. Some sort of medication to relax the birth canal is given if the mother has not already received a regional anesthetic.

In the low forceps delivery the baby's head is down very far in the birth canal and is either visible or almost visible on the perineum. Midforceps delivery indicates that the head of the fetus is into the birth canal, but not far down past the cervix. A high forceps delivery is one in which the baby's presenting part has not yet cleared the ischial spines. A high forceps delivery is extremely dangerous to both the mother and baby and is rarely attempted.

The lithotomy position is always used for a forceps delivery. A forceps delivery is never attempted until the cervix is completely dilated.

Some doctors do forceps deliveries routinely, especially on all primiparas. Although it rarely happens, the pressure applied by the forceps can cause intracranial hemorrhage and damage to the facial nerve of the infant.[16] It's not uncommon for a baby delivered with the use of forceps to have bruises on the head. There's no scientific evidence which indicates the routine use of forceps during birth should be adopted.[17] Certainly forceps have their place in obstetrics, but not routinely for every primipara. **Ask ahead of time how your doctor feels about the routine use of forceps. If s/he feels very strongly that forceps should be used on all first-time mothers, consider the implications of that viewpoint as it relates to all aspects of your birth experience.**

Vacuum Extractor

Another way to get the baby out is use of a vacuum extractor. In this process a metal cup is affixed to the fetal head by use of vacuum. The metal cup has a chain attached to it, and the physician can pull the baby out. Vacuum extractors are used much more rarely than are foreps.

Birth Without Violence

A fairly recent development in delivery room techniques is the idea of birth without violence. The technique, or series of practices, is really an attitude and atmosphere created in the delivery room.

A French obstetrician, Dr. Frederick Leboyer, has examined birth from the baby's point of view. He points out the tremendous adjustments the infant must make during the first minutes of life and recommends minimizing those changes that are not absolutely essential. For instance, Dr. Leboyer is in favor of lowering the noise level and the light level of the traditional delivery room. He, of course, does not suggest turning off the lights, he just would like the infant to be able to enter a dimly-lit room rather than one with intensely bright lights. The baby has been in darkness for all of its intra-uterine life. Full lighting for emergency situations is as close as the panel of light switches.

A hushed atmosphere in the delivery room, according to Dr. Leboyer, can also make the infant's entrance into the world more peaceful.

Dr. Leboyer also recommends that the baby not be held upside down, because of the trauma to the spinal cord as the infant is abruptly forced to come out of the fetal position. He suggests that the baby be put on the mother's abdomen and massaged for the first minutes. He also requests that the baby's body be submerged in a basin of lukewarm water; this is to make the transition from the wet intra-uterine life to the dry outside life easier on the infant.

If you are interested in having a "Leboyer birth" the best thing to do is to talk it over with your birth attendant much in advance of your due date. It is a new procedure, and even though it is more of an attitude change than an actual change in delivery technique, members of the medical profession are slow to change. In a Leboyer birth the basic procedures and techniques normally used in deliveries are used; the biggest differences occur in the handling of the infant during the first few minutes of life.

The safety and health of the infant and mother must always be considered, and if the mother or the baby is in trouble, of course the Leboyer techniques would be abandoned in favor of emergency techniques designed to bring the situation under control as quickly and as efficiently as possible.

THE PROCESS OF BIRTH

Those who understand the process of labor and birth cannot help but be awed by it. It is truly a miracle that we can reach out and touch.

> My pushing urge came at about 7 centimeters. It just shocked me! I couldn't believe how my entire body took over control to push.

> They kept saying not to push. I wanted to push so bad that I would grab Mike and almost cry. It was the hardest thing I've ever had to do and as hard as I tried not to, I snuck a push or two in there, I just couldn't help it.

The doctor said, "You can push with the next contraction." I told them when it was starting and Randy and the nurses held my shoulders up while I gripped the handles on the table. Everyone said, "Push, push, push" and I felt like a member of a team.

The pushing was not uncomfortable; it was hard work, but gave the feeling of doing something very active.

What a wonderful feeling to push the baby out.

I tried several ways of pushing; using the bed rails, the method taught in class, and pushing from my side. I spent three hours doing this. It was the most work I have ever done in my life.

I anxiously awaited the next contraction. It felt so good to push.

After a night without sleep, being very drowsy and nervous, I was surprised at the way entering the delivery room seemed to refresh me. All of a sudden I was wide awake and alert, everything happened so fast!

Once we left the labor room everything moved so fast, but I'll never forget when the doctor said, "It's a boy!" and we heard his first cry. There were three nurses as well as the doctor and Tim, and I felt as though they were all working as hard as I was and cheering me on.

Looking back on the labor and delivery, I feel that only toward the end of labor did I really have uniform contractions. I had expected very defined and regularly-spaced contractions with beginnings, endings, and peaks; this just wasn't the case.

After about four pushes, at 9:22 p.m., we saw and heard a wiggling pinky-purple baby come into our world. They placed her in a warming bassinette right next to the delivery table where we could see her really well. It was so incredible. She was sucking her thumb and looking all around at us. Then they wrapped her in a warming blanket and handed her to Rich. It was explained that this is a symbolic gesture, the father gives the baby to the mother. After I got to hold her, the three of us returned to the same labor room to have some time together. This was also when I was able to nurse her for the first time.

How wonderful to have been an active member in the birth of my baby.

We chatted with the doctor while he stitched the episiotomy and we both felt relief and pride in having successfully completed a wonderful cooperative physical experience. Knud was such a help to me. I feel so grateful to him for making this birth a happy memory.

I felt great, like I could jump off the delivery table and run to my room.

Special Labors and Births

Each labor and delivery is unique; no two are identical. Because of the differences, words such as "usually," "frequently," "often," "most," and "probably" are essential in describing what happens during a "typical" labor and delivery. When a labor, or some part of a labor, does not conform to what "usually" happens, it is no longer a typical labor; it is a special labor. Prepared childbirth techniques are especially helpful in these special labor situations because the special circumstances sometimes bring with them special problems and discomforts.

PRESENTATIONS

The presentation of the fetus indicates which part of the fetal body will enter the birth canal first. The presenting part is the part which lies over the cervix during labor. The three basic presentations are cephalic presentation, breech presentation and transverse presentation.

Cephalic Presentations

In a cephalic presentation, the fetal head leads the way down the birth canal. Cephalic presentations account for about 96.3 per cent of all births.[1] The fetus normally assumes this head-down position because of the size and shape of the uterus; there is more room for the breech of the fetus in the upper portion of the uterus. The three cephalic presentations are:

1. **Vertex:** The top of the head is the most common presentation of all and 96 per cent of all births are vertex.[2] Normally the baby is facing the mother's back, so in a dorsal, lithotomy or semi-sitting delivery the baby is looking at the floor as it is born. This is an anterior vertex presentation, and is usually the easiest presentation barring factors such as an extremely large baby or an extremely small pelvis in the mother.
   A variation of the vertex presentation is the posterior vertex presentation. Again, the top of the head is the first thing born, but instead of facing the mother's back, the baby faces her abdomen. This places the hard, bony part of the baby's head against the mother's sacrum. This can produce severe back pain. A posterior labor is usually longer than an anterior vertex presentation.
2. **Face:** In this presentation the face, instead of the top of the head, leads the way down the vagina. This is a rare presentation and only about .2 per cent of all babies come out this way.[3] Forceps are often required to deliver a face presentation. The baby's face is often quite swollen and discolored for the first few days of life, but this is only temporary.
3. **Brow:** When the forehead comes first, it is termed a brow presentation. This, too, is quite rare; approximately .1 per cent of all infants present in this way.[4] If the presentation is persistent, and will not spontaneously convert to a face or vertex presentation as the fetus moves down the birth canal, a Cesarean delivery may be necessary. In

a brow presentation the difficulty is caused because the largest diameter of the head is presenting.

Breech Presentations

In breech presentations, the fetus has settled into the pelvic basin bottom-first. Breech births account for just about 3.3 per cent of all term births.[5] The breech labor may be longer than a vertex labor because the baby's buttocks do not provide as efficient a dilating wedge as does the top of the head. In a vertex presentation the largest part of the baby's body leads the way through the cervix and down the birth canal; in a breech presentation the three major parts (head, shoulders and buttocks) come through in the reverse order so a breech birth is sort of three births in one. First the buttocks pass into the birth canal, then the cervix must open wider to allow the shoulders to pass through, and then it must open wider to allow passage of the head. The most common breech variations are:

1. Complete breech: In this presentation, the fetus is sitting cross-legged in the bottom of the uterus.
2. Frank breech: In a frank breech position, the legs are straightened and the feet are up near the face of the fetus.
3. Footling breech: This position is similar to the complete breech position, but instead of having crossed legs, one or both feet present. It looks as if the baby is trying to jump out. This is a very rare presentation.
4. Knee breech: In this presentation a knee, instead of a foot (or feet), is at the os. This is an even rarer presentation.

Transverse (or Shoulder) Presentation

About .4 per cent of all term births are shoulder presentations.[6] If the fetus persists with the head to one side of the cervix and the breech to the other side with the shoulder over the cervix, the only way to get the baby out is by Cesarean delivery.

CEPHALIC PRESENTATIONS

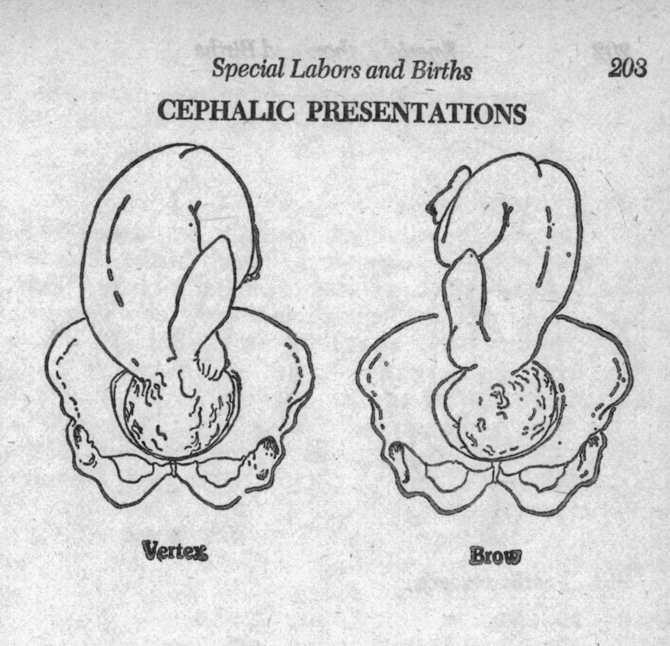

Vertex

Brow

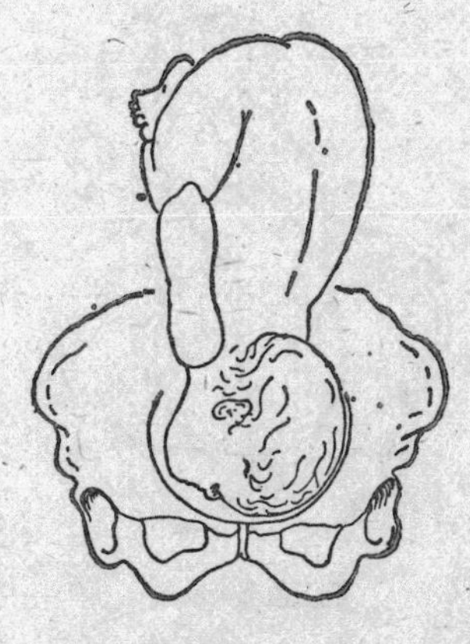

Face

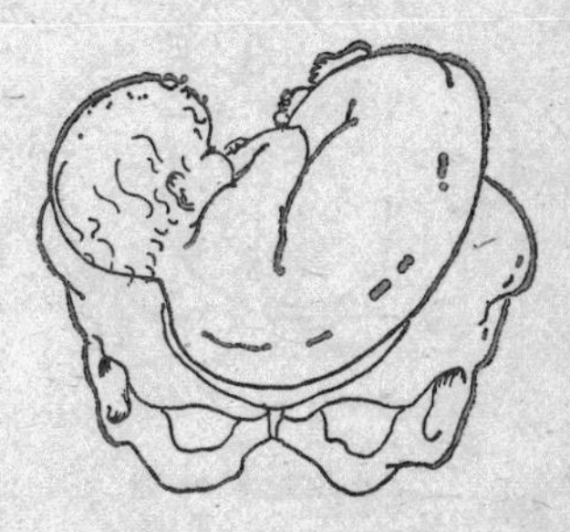

Transverse (Shoulder)

BREECH PRESENTATIONS

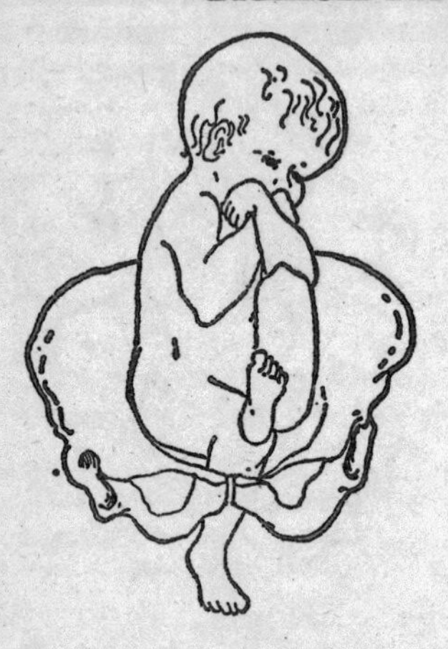

Footling breech

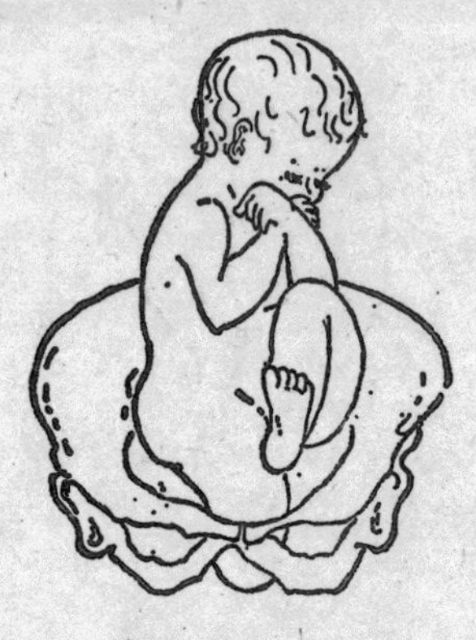

Knee breech

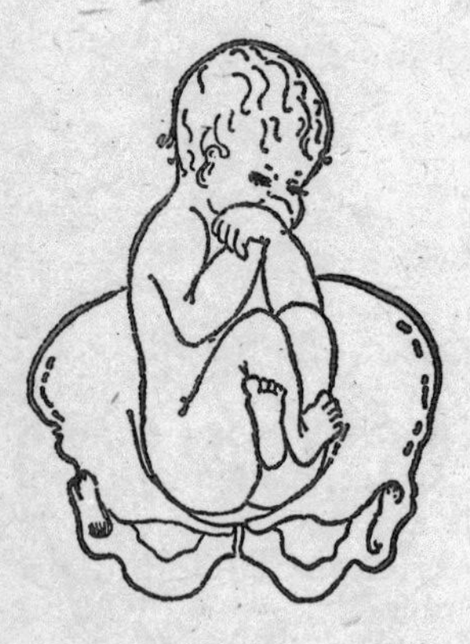

Complete breech

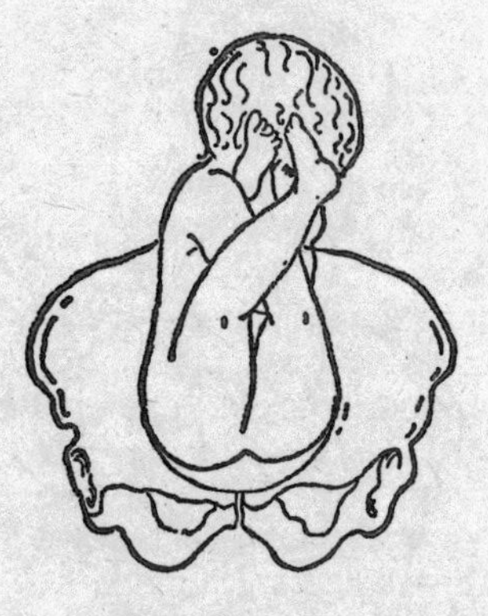

Frank breech

BREECH DELIVERIES

A breech presentation may or may not be known before labor begins. It is sometimes difficult to determine if the fetal lump felt at the top of the uterus is a head or breech. If a breech is diagnosed late in pregnancy, some doctors feel the best course is to try to turn the fetus into a cephalic presentation by external manipulation of the abdominal and uterine walls. This maneuver is called external version.

This procedure is usually most successful if it is attempted about a month before the due date. Sometimes the fetus refuses to turn at all, and sometimes it returns to the breech position within a few hours of the version. In some cases it is a success. However, some doctors frown upon use of the procedure at all and question whether the version was a success, or whether the fetus would have turned on its own before labor.

Some doctors do an x-ray pelvimetry on each first-time mother who is carrying a baby in a breech presentation. The x-ray is done to determine the exact measurements of the pelvis. A problem with breech births is that sometimes a cephalo-pelvic disproportion (when the baby's head is too large to pass through the mother's pelvis) is not discovered until the body of the baby has been born.

A breech labor is frequently felt chiefly in the back, above the waistline, instead of in the low back and low abdomen as is the typical cephalic labor. It is not uncommon for meconium (the dark, tarry substance found in the large intestine of the fetus) to be expelled from the mother's vagina after her membranes rupture. This is because the rectum of the fetus is directly over the cervix. The presence of meconium during the first stage of labor is a sign of possible fetal distress and should be reported to the doctor at once. Presence of meconium is particularly alarming in a cephalic presentation.

Some mothers don't realize that the meconium is coming from the baby, and are embarrassed. If this happens while you are still at home, wear a sanitary napkin or clean cloth next to the vaginal opening on the way to the hospital because more meconium is likely to be expelled with each contraction.

Your doctor will probably want you to be at the hospital a little sooner if you have a diagnosed breech presentation and s/he will give you appropriate instructions regarding when to call and when to go to the hospital.

Unless other complications exist, such as cephalopelvic disproportion, it is frequently possible to give birth vaginally to a baby in a breech presentation. Effective pushing by you can be most helpful in a breech birth, and many doctors prefer that mothers be unmedicated, or minimally medicated so that they can push more efficiently. Sometimes the doctor will have to carry out an obstetrical maneuver to get the baby down the birth canal; s/he may use forceps, for example. In this case the doctor would probably prefer that the birth canal be completely relaxed, so s/he may wish to use an anesthetic during late second stage labor. If you have decided positively ahead of time that you don't wish to have an anesthetic, try not to be too disappointed if the doctor decides to use one. Keep an open mind. Remember that the safety and health of the baby are of utmost priority. If that is the only way the baby will come out, take advantage of the procedure and the anesthetic.

Breech babies sometimes have rather odd-looking legs for the first few days. In a frank breech presentation, the baby's legs have been held in a relatively straightened position in the uterus. Thus the baby's legs do not curl into the familiar fetal position as most newborns do. Don't worry about it, because it is not a permanent situation.

BACK PAIN IN LABOR

Back pain to one degree or another is quite common in labor. However, some women experience fairly severe, fairly extensive pain. The pain can come with the contractions or it can be constant during all of labor or during all of a particular phase of labor. Back pain frequently shows up during transition even if it has not been experienced earlier in the labor.

All of the causes of back pain in labor are certainly not understood, but a commonly-accepted cause is a posterior vertex presentation or a breech presentation. If the hard back of the baby's head presses against the nerves surrounding the mother's spinal column at one time or another during labor, as it is likely to do in these presentations, back pain is often the result.

In most cases it is helpful to assume a position that gets the baby off the mother's spine and lessens the pressure on the sacrum. Semi-reclining positions, standing positions and forward-leaning positions are all helpful. Some women find it most comfortable to lie on the side toward which the baby is rotating (usually the left side). Try tailor sitting. Some women find a knee-to-chest position brings relief.

Pelvic-rocking in the hands and knees position, or while leaning against the wall often brings some relief. It is helpful to change position frequently because if the muscles become tense and stiff from remaining in one position for long periods of time, it can intensify the pain. Walking keeps the circulation patterns functioning as well as helps to exercise muscles. If you walk, remember to rest frequently, too.

Back massages or firm counter-pressure applied at the point of pain is often helpful. The coach can apply the pressure, or you can lie on your own fists or on small hard objects such as tennis balls. If the nursing staff doesn't object, try applying a hot water bottle, a heating pad or an ice pack to the lower back region.

Try very hard to stay alert; concentrate on anything other than your back. If you feel like talking, let your coach know. Your coach is there to offer you the emotional support that you need, and to do whatever will make you the most comfortable.

If you have back pain in labor, it is particularly important that the coach have something to eat while you are at the hospital in the labor room. It takes a lot of energy to apply the firm counter-pressure that you will probably demand almost constantly.

The following signs are often present in a posterior labor. Having one or all of them is not, of course, positive proof that the baby is in the posterior position. Likewise, it is possible to have a fetus in the posterior presentation without experiencing these signs.

1. Low backache during, and possibly even between, contractions
2. Slow progress, especially during early labor
3. Contractions that are irregular in character, strength and length
4. Contractions that do not settle down into a pattern
5. Restlessness and inability to relax

Ask your birth attendant ahead of time what his/her approach is to posterior presentations. If s/he recommends trying to rotate the posterior baby into an anterior presentation by use of maternal positioning, try the following positioning instructions. This routine has been found to be very helpful in encouraging a posterior fetus to rotate.

1. Use positions that get the baby off the mother's spine and encourage it to rotate. Hands and knees positions and forward-leaning positions are particularly helpful. Sitting on the edge of the bed and leaning onto a chair is good. Standing and leaning over a table is another possibility. The worst possible position is flat on your back.
2. Change positions at least once every 30 minutes. Do pelvic rocking during the contractions. Keep this up as long as you can, even after the contractions get quite strong.

Back pain in labor is something that generally can't be predicted, and is hard to train for. The most important thing you can do is be aware of the possibility and know what comfort measures to try if you have back pain. If one labor involves back pain, it does not necessarily mean that your next labor will. If a posterior presentation was the cause, it does not mean that all of your children will present that way.

INDUCTION OF LABOR

An induced labor is one which is started artificially by either chemical or physical stimulation. Induction is indicated in cases where continuing the pregnancy would adversely affect either the mother or the fetus. Mothers with toxemia or diabetes are likely candidates for induction. If the mother's due date has come and gone, and the placenta is aging (and thus not nourishing the fetus as it should be) an induction will probably be done. If the baby is very near term and the doctor fears cephalo-pelvic disproportion if the fetus gets larger, the doctor often induces in order to reduce the chances of a Cesarean delivery. Another common reason for induction is labor not starting spontaneously within 24 hours after the membranes rupture. Sometimes induction is done merely for the convenience of the doctor and/or mother.

Induction is a valid and useful medical tool when it is done for a medical reason; when it is done merely for convenience it becomes an unnecessary risk to both the mother and the fetus.

Castor oil is one of the oldest, and least successful, approaches to induction. It was used in the belief that the peristatic waves produced by the castor oil would somehow spread to the uterus and induce contractions to start. This is a highly unsuccessful method of induction and the woman who tries it can be fairly uncomfortable for several days.

One sort of pre-induction method that the doctor may use is called stripping the membranes. This consists of the physician running a finger around the inside of the partially dilated cervix between the cervix and the amniotic sac. This loosens the amniotic sac from the uterine wall and irritates the amnion.

A physical method of inducing labor is artificially rupturing the membranes. In this procedure the physician introduces a long hook-like instrument into the partially dilated cervix and tears the amniotic sac. This is completely painless. The procedure is officially called amniotomy. Because of the risk of infection to the fetus after the membranes are ruptured, if this method does not bring about the start of contractions within 24 hours, some chemical means of induction will have to be employed.

Another way to induce labor is to administer an oxytocic drug. The most common way of introducing the oxytocic drug into the body is through the use of an intravenous drip. The drug (often pitocin) is added to an IV bottle of glucose water and administered through plastic tubing into the patient's vein. A needle is inserted into a vein in the patient's forearm or the back of the patient's hand and taped in place; plastic tubing is then connected to the needle. The other end of the plastic tubing is attached to the IV bottle which contains the pitocin diluted with sugar water. The solution drips into the patient's hand and taped in place; plastic tubing is then connected to the needle. The solution drips into the mother's system at a carefully controlled rate. The amount can be easily adjusted by the medical personnel. If the contractions are not coming often enough, or are not strong enough, the number of drips per minute can be increased; if the contractions are too strong and too close together, the number of drips per minute can be decreased. Once the IV needle is inserted, the whole IV mechanism is painless; even insertion is either painless or only a minor discomfort. If a woman has an IV "pit drip" she is kept under constant supervision by either a doctor or a nurse.

Another use of the IV pit drip is augmentation of labor. If a woman's labor has reached a plateau, or has stopped altogether, the doctor may use an IV pit drip to start the contractions again or to speed them up and make them stronger.

A second way to chemically induce labor is by the use of tablets in the mouth. The tablets are put in the patient's mouth either under the tongue or between the gums and the cheeks. The tablets dissolve slowly. This is called a buccal pit induction. The strength and frequency of the contractions can be controlled by the number of tablets in the mouth. Tablets can be added or removed to adjust the contractions to whatever intensity and frequency the doctor deems appropriate. It can be very difficult to do the various breathing techniques with several of these little pills dissolving in the mouth.

The third way to induce labor chemically is by use of an injection. In this case the oxytocic drug is injected intramuscularly in small doses. It is difficult to predict exactly how a patient will react to even small amounts of the oxytocic drugs, so this method is less controllable than the other two chemical means.

Induction, particularly by one of the chemically-produced methods, has some drawbacks. These drawbacks must be judged against the possible benefits of induction in order to determine whether induction is the best course to follow. It is clear that in the case of medically-indicated inductions there are benefits, and an induction should be done; it is equally clear that inductions for mere convenience do not have enough benefits to outweigh the risks. If your doctor suggests an induction, be certain that you find out why s/he is suggesting the procedure. Ask about the possible risks, and ask about which method s/he intends to us. If it is an induction simply so you'll deliver before the doctor goes on vacation, and there is no medical reason for the induction, consider refusing it. We simply do not know exactly what causes labor to start; why take any unnecessary chances?

Induced contractions tend to start out much stronger than normal contractions. Quite often the induced contractions will peak at the very beginning of the contractions instead of near the middle of the contraction as a regular contraction usually does. This makes the labor very difficult for a couple to handle. If you are being monitored electronically, you will be able to tell when a contraction is just about to start so you can be ready for it. If there is no fetal heart monitor, the coach will have to watch the time very closely and let you know just before another contraction is due.

The supply of oxygen to the fetus is decreased during a contraction. It has been suggested that perhaps the fetus builds up some sort of tolerance to the contractions if they are allowed to begin spontaneously and gradually increase in strength as with a normal labor.

If the mother receives an overdosage of an oxytocic substance, it is possible that the placenta can separate from the uterine wall before the baby is born. This disrupts the baby's oxygen supply, and is a grave complication and necessitates a Cesarean delivery unless a vaginal delivery can be effected almost immediately.

Another problem with induction is that it is not always possible to determine the exact gestational age of the fetus. Unless the date of conception is positively known, or x-ray or ultrasound studies have been done, it is possible to induce a premature fetus.

Because of the sudden and strong way the contractions start in an induced labor, the induced labor is often quite short. An induced labor of two or three hours is not uncommon. Woman pay for this shortness by having to handle intense contractions that may come very close together right from the very beginning. Some women have described the induced labor as being much like one long transition. A shortened labor has not been shown to be of benefit to the fetus unless there is some sign of fetal distress.[7]

The use of Pitocin (or other oxytocic substance) for either inducing or augmenting labor has been associated with neonatal respiration problems and an increased incidence of newborn jaundice.

PRECIPITOUS LABOR

A precipitous labor is a spontaneous labor which progresses particularly rapidly. A labor of this sort usually starts out almost immediately with very strong, very frequent contractions and can last anywhere from a few contractions to a couple of hours. As with a chemically-induced labor, things are happening so fast that it is often very difficult to handle the contractions during a precipitous labor.

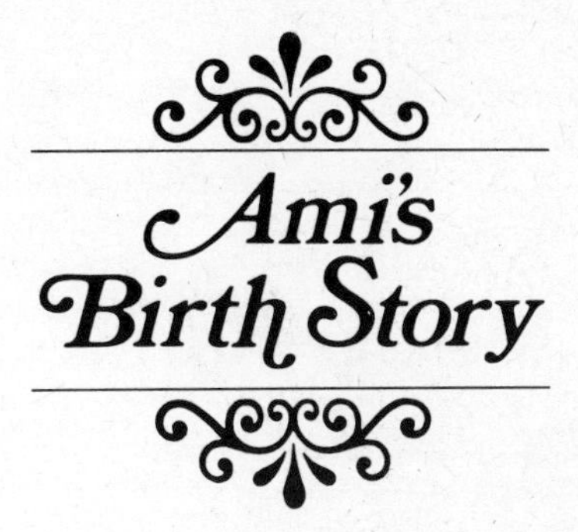

Ami's Birth Story

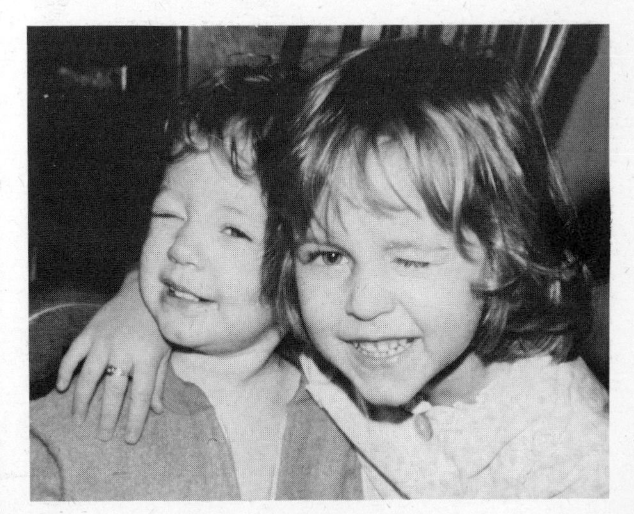

Ami (1½) and Alisa (3½).

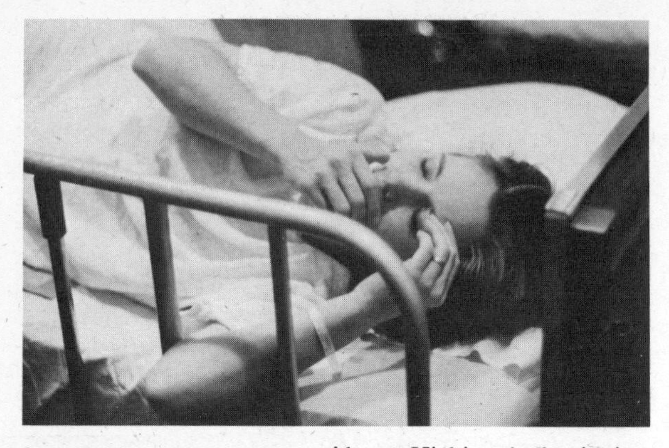

Above: Vicki at the beginning of the second stage of labor; sucking on a wet washcloth between contractions.

Opposite, top: Ami's head crowning. Vicki is in the dorsal position, undraped. The delivery table is not "broken." Only the hair around the vaginal opening has been shaved—a "mini" prep.

Middle: Vicki panting to avoid pushing. The nurse's direction to stop pushing was so Ami would ease out.

Bottom: Ami's shoulders being born. The umbilical cord is over Ami's shoulder, in the nurse's left hand. Ami was 21 inches long and weighed 7 pounds 10 ounces at birth.

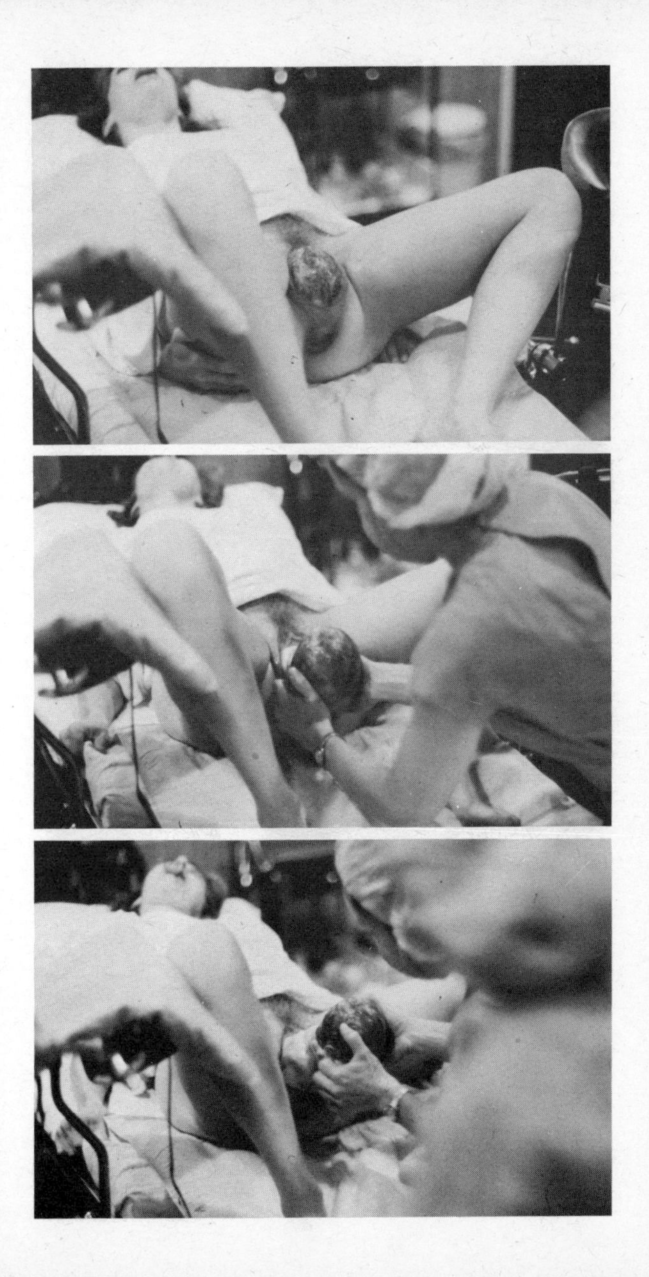

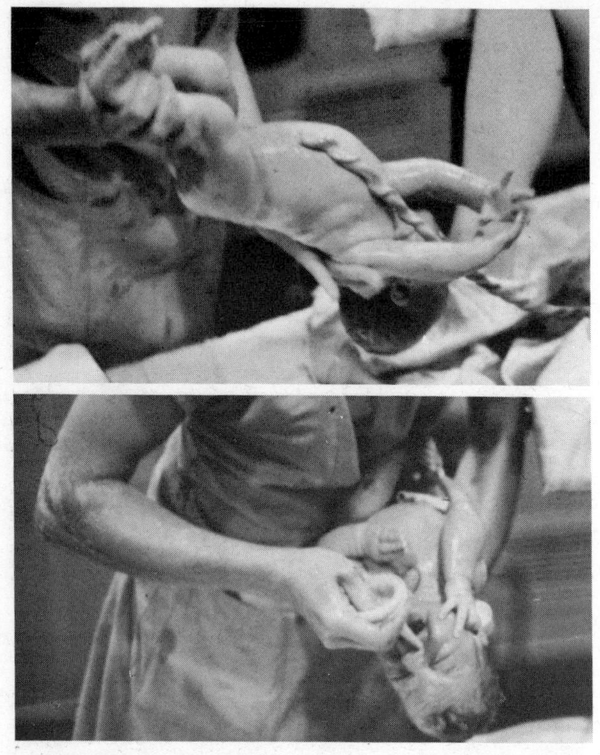

Top: Ami immediately after birth. Placenta has not yet been expelled.

Bottom: Nurse suctioning Ami's nose with a bulb syringe. The blood on Ami's leg is from the umbilical cord.

Opposite, top: Ami 5 minutes after birth. her nose is a little off-center because of her position in utero. It straightened completely by the time she was 2 weeks old.

Middle: Doctor doing repair work —one stitch was necessary.

Bottom: The placenta.

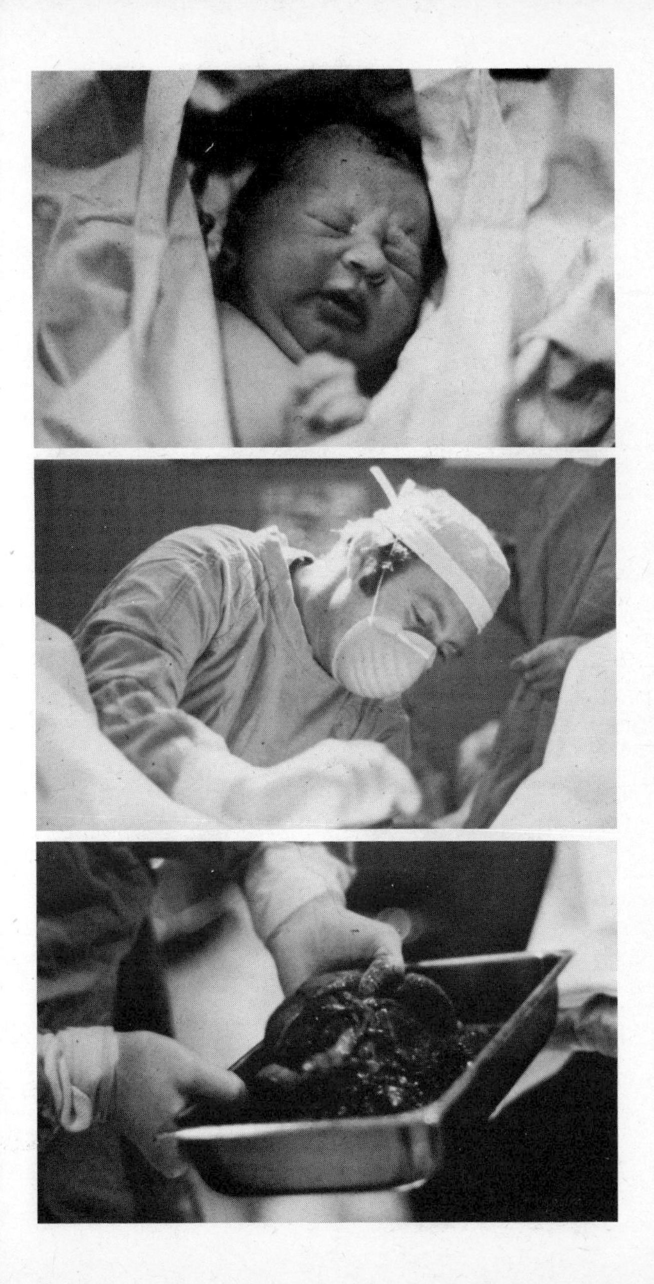

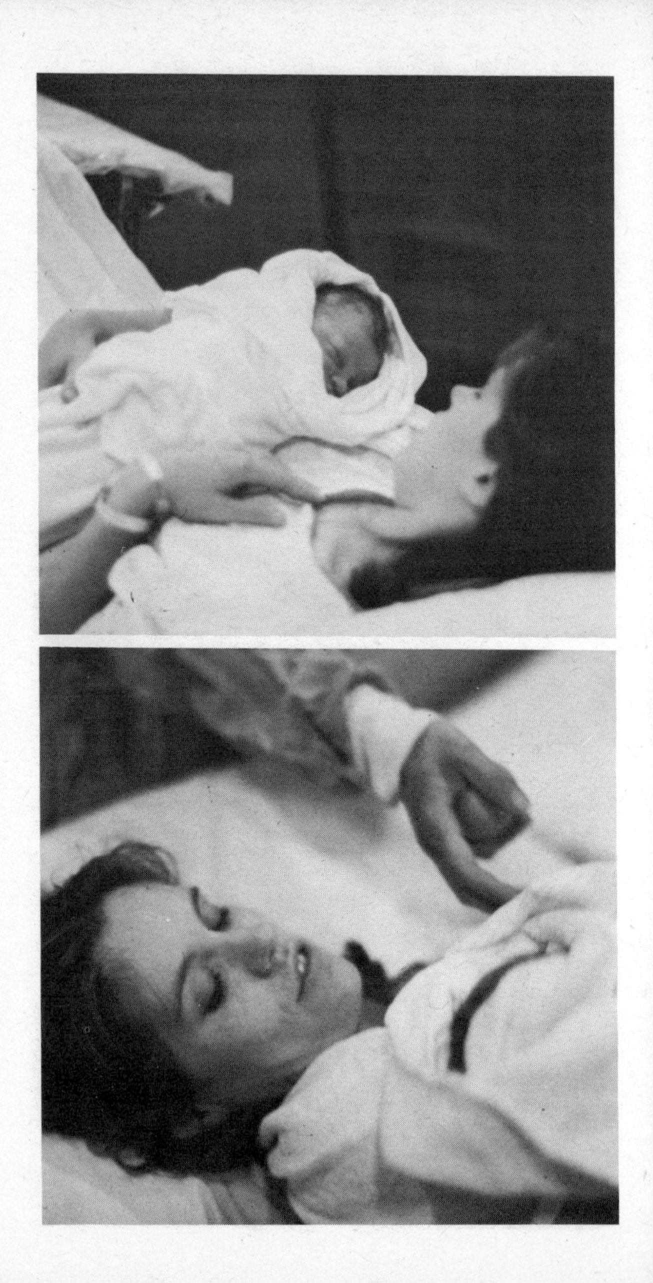

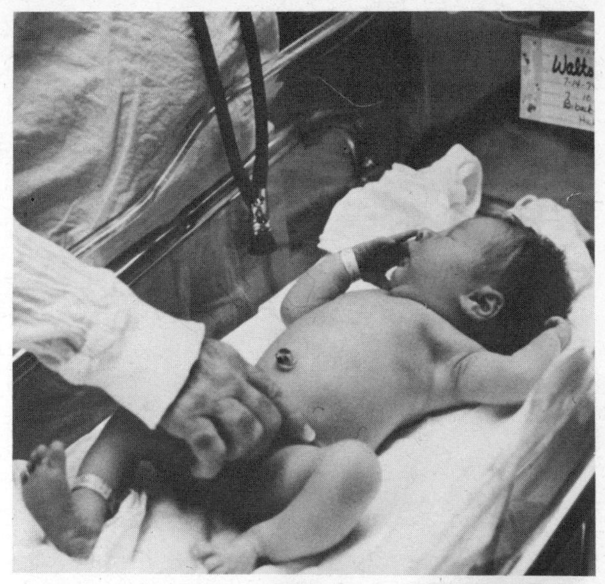

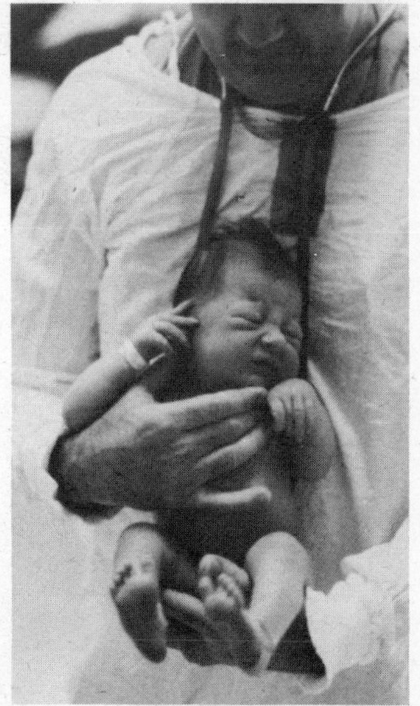

Opposite, top: Ami and Vicki 10 minutes after Ami's birth. Doctor has finished the repair work.

Opposite, bottom: Ami and Vicki on the way to the recovery room about 10 minutes after the birth.

Above and right: Pediatrician examining Ami the next morning. Ami is 15 hours old.

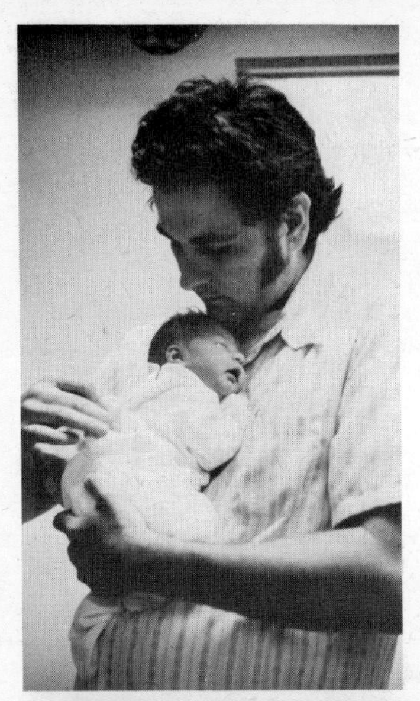

Left: Philip dressing Ami for the trip home. Ami was sleeping in her own cradle by the time she was 16 hours old.

Below: Ami two weeks after her birth.

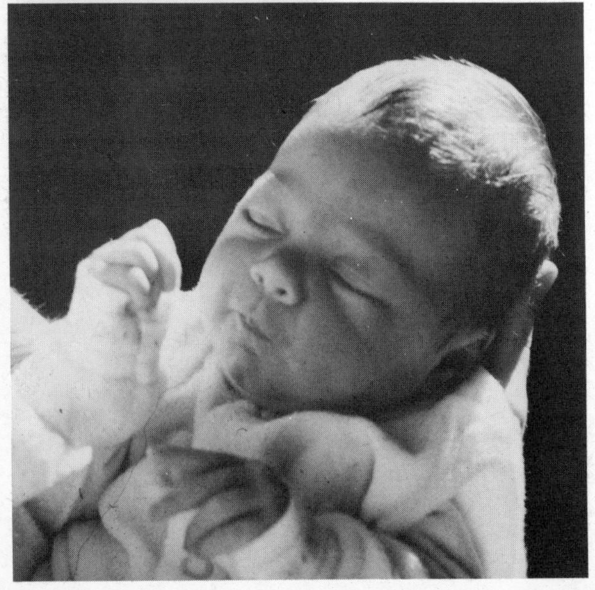

Any delivery should be gentle and controlled. This is a little harder to effect in the case of a precipitous labor and delivery. Controlled delivery lessens the chance of cerebral trauma in the infant and vaginal lacerations in the mother. For this reason, doctors sometimes attempt to slow the progress of labor through use of medication, but this is done less with prepared mothers than with Ostriches who do not know how to control the pushing contractions.

If you are in the hospital, and suddenly feel that the birth is imminent, have your coach contact the nurse immediately. The nurse is qualified to deliver the baby in the labor room bed if there's no time to get you to the delivery room and if there is no doctor near. If it is so sudden that the nurse can't get there in time, let the baby be born. Do not hold your legs together, and do not push with the contractions. The baby will ease out into the world by itself because of the tremendous force that the uterus is exerting. It's best if the head is born between contractions in a precipitate delivery.

If you are still at home, or in the car, do not panic. Just let the infant be born as naturally as possible, and call for medical aid as soon as you can. Instructions for handling an emergency birth can be found on pages 108 and 109. The most important thing to do is to to remain calm and handle the baby very gently. If it is not breathing, stimulate it gently; do not spank it. Call the police, the fire department or emergency aid units if you need help in resuscitating the baby.

The reasons for a precipitous labor and birth are not entirely understood; but the pelvic size and structure may have something to do with the chances for having such a labor. If a woman has had one precipitous labor, her chances for another are very good. So she can be ready for the second one!

MULTIPLE BIRTHS

When there is more than one fetus in the uterus, the pregnancy is termed a multiple pregnancy. Most pregnancies are diagnosed ahead of labor, but not all of them. Sometimes a woman goes into the delivery room expecting one baby and comes out with two; and sometimes a woman goes into the delivery room expecting two babies and comes out with three.

Of course, the most common type of multiple birth is twins. Twins can be either identical or fraternal. Identical twins develop from one ovum that was fertilized by one sperm. Early in the development, the ovum divides into two identical parts and each part develops as an individual fetus. Identical twins carry all of the same genes, so are always of the same sex.

Fraternal twins develop from two eggs fertilized by two separate sperm. Since these twins do not develop from one egg, each fetus has its own individual genes. The two babies may or may not be of the same sex. They will look no more alike than siblings usually do.

The normal discomforts of pregnancy are usually increased with a multiple pregnancy due to the tremendous size of the mother's abdomen. Rest is so hard to get during the latter stages of pregnancy, but so important.

Some doctors send all of their patients with multiple pregnancies to childbirth education classes as a routine matter. This is because a spontaneous delivery, either unmedicated or minimally medicated, is safer because of decreased blood loss and because the babies are more likely to be healthy and undamaged. Multiple babies are usually smaller than single babies, even at term, and twins commonly weigh about a pound less than an average single baby. It is also common for multiple babies to be somewhat immature at birth. Great amounts of labor and delivery medications could prove deleterious to the infants, especially to their initial respiratory efforts.

After the first baby is born, the birth attendant usually has to rupture the membranes surrounding the second baby. If the second baby is in a transverse presentation, the birth attendant will probably try external version combined with vaginal manipulation to turn the baby into a breech or cephalic presentation. The second twin is usually slightly smaller than the first twin born. The second twin is usually born within a few minutes of the first.

If you are diagnosed as having a multiple pregnancy, be especially sure that you know how to push effectively. The uterine walls are stretched so thin that contractions may not be as effective as they should be; your knowing how to push properly could make the birth easier on both you and your babies.

CESAREAN BIRTH

A Cesarean delivery (or C-section) is the method of birth employed when a vaginal birth is impossible or highly dangerous to either the mother or to the fetus. When a Cesarean delivery is performed, an incision is made in the abdominal wall and the uterus. The baby is removed through these incisions.

A Cesarean delivery is major surgery and is only performed if it is necessary. Sometimes the need for a Cesarean can be ascertained prior to the start of labor, and sometimes it is an emergency operation. Cesareans are done in cases where the baby simply can't be born vaginally. Some examples of this situation are cephalo-pelvic disproportion, transverse presentation and placenta previa. In a cephalo-pelvic disproportion the fetal head is too large to pass through the bony structure of the mother's pelvis and there's no way to get it out vaginally. If the fetus is in a transverse presentation, and refuses to turn, the baby can't get out of the uterus unless a Cesarean is performed. In a placenta previa the placenta has implanted low in the uterus and either partially or wholly covers the opening to the cervix. Again, the baby cannot enter the birth canal. Placenta previas happen in only about .5 per cent of all pregnancies; the placenta normally implants in the upper portion of the uterus.

Some Cesareans are performed when fetal distress is detected by monitoring the fetal heart tones. If the fetus is in trouble, it must be removed from the uterus as soon as possible or its life may be in great danger. For instance, if the placenta separates from the uterine wall before the baby is born (abruptio placentae), the baby's source of oxygen is impaired and the fetus may try to breathe in utero. Another situation which may necessitate a Cesarean is the prolapsed cord. A prolapsed cord is when the umbilical cord slips down in front of the baby's presenting part and becomes compressed, thereby cutting off the baby's blood and oxygen supply.

In cases of prolonged labor where the uterus is functioning ineffectively or the cervix is not dilating properly, the doctor may perform a Cesarean for the safety of the fetus. Or if a fetus is well past term, and the placenta shows signs of aging, a Cesarean may be done, especially if induction does not start contractions. If the mother has diabetes or severe toxemia, a Cesarean may be performed.

These are some of the more common reasons for birth by Cesarean, but there are others. If the doctor feels a Cesarean is the safest way for your baby to be born, accept that the surgery must be performed to save either your life or your baby's life.

The abdominal incision can be either vertical or horizontal. The vertical incision is located in a line between the navel and the pubic hair. The horizontal incision (the "bikini" incision) is located parallel to the pubic hair line and low on the abdomen.

The kind of incision on the abdomen is not necessarily the same as the kind of incision on the uterus. The uterine incision may be either vertical (classical incision) or horizontal (lower uterine or lower cervical incision). The lower uterine type of incision is used more frequently than the classical incision. In cases of emergency Cesarean, the vertical cut on both the abdomen and the uterus may be used because it is faster.

When it is determined that a Cesarean is necessary, the mother's body is shaved from just below the nipple line to mid-thigh. The abdominal area is swabbed with an antiseptic solution. A urinary catheter is inserted into the urethra to insure that the bladder remains empty throughout the operation. The catheter may be left in place for 24 to 48 hours following surgery.

An IV of glucose water will be inserted in the patient's forearm or the back of her hand. This, too, is often continued for 24 to 48 hours after surgery. Diet is normally limited to liquids at first, because the intestines do not function properly after abdominal surgery. The mother's diet is increased when either bowel sounds are heard, or intestinal gas is passed.

An injection of atropine may be given to dry up respiratory secretions. A cardiac monitor may be attached.

The anesthesia employed is chosen by the anesthesiologist, but the choice may be made in consultation with the mother. The spinal is the most commonly used anesthetic for Cesareans, but epidurals are also used. In some cases, a general anesthetic is required. Sometimes other anesthesia is used, depending upon the preference of the anesthesiologist. The Cesarean mother who is given a spinal or an epidural is able to remain awake and see her baby as soon as s/he is born. After the baby is born, some doctors administer a general anesthesia for the repair work; others continue only with the spinal or epidural. If you have strong feelings about remaining awake for the repair procedure as well as for the birth, talk to your physician.

Remember that a Cesarean is major surgery and maintenance of a sterile field is of utmost importance. A screen is often placed in front of the patient's face; some physicians feel that the screen is essential in maintaining the sterile field. However, the screen may be there in part to "protect" the patient from the sight of the operation, because other doctors do not see the necessity for the screen in the preservation of the sterile field. This, too, is something you can discuss with your doctor. If you wish to see the operation (which is the actual birth of the baby), ask whether the screen can be skipped.

Sometimes when a Cesarean is being performed, a

silence is maintained that's punctuated only by necessary requests. Other times the medical people tend to discuss rather trivial things in an apparently offhand manner. In the former case, the patient can feel that the situation is very grave, and in the latter case can feel that her surgery is really of little importance to the people performing the operation. If you should find yourself in either situation, and you are not happy with the verbal atmosphere, tell them how you feel. It is your body that they are operating on.

From the time the patient enters the operating room until the time she leaves is about an hour. The first 5 or 10 minutes is spent in administering anesthetic, making the incisions and delivering the baby. The rest of the time is spent in suturing the incisions. Clamps or stitches may be used to close the abdominal incision. Some doctors use the stitches that dissolve and do not require removal. It's a good idea to ask your doctor to check to see whether you are allergic to any of the various materials used for the suturing; an allergy of this sort can make the recovery period much more uncomfortable than it need be.

Because Cesarean babies are more likely to have respiratory problems than vaginally born babies, the Cesarean baby is often rushed away from the operating room to the Special Care Nursery where s/he is closely observed. The normal process of labor helps to prepare the baby to breathe by the coming and going of pressure produced by the contractions; the Cesarean baby has often not had such an advantage, and is thrust into the world and asked to breathe without this preparation. Many Cesarean babies go to the Special Care Nursery unnecessarily just because that is the hospital's procedure. If the baby is not in respiratory distress, ask whether you can hold it for a minute before s/he's taken to the nursery. If you feel like it, some doctors will allow you to nurse the brand new baby on the operating table or in the recovery room a few minutes later.

In some hospitals the baby is required to stay in the SCN a minimum number of days or hours no matter what its condition. If your baby is healthy, yet still in the SCN, make every effort to have it released either to the central nursery or to you so you can start rooming-in. If that attempt doesn't work, try to make arrangements to visit the baby (including touching as well as looking) in the SCN until the staff will release him/her.

Some doctors will allow the parents to be together during the Cesarean. This is something that can mean much to parents, particularly prepared parents. Prepared parents have usually looked forward so much to sharing the birth experience that it can be crushing if the doctor or hospital won't allow the father into the operating room. If the doctor's choice is not wholly governed by hospital rules, do stress your preparation and your deep desire to share the experience, even if a Cesarean must be performed.

After the operation the mother will go to a recovery room to be observed carefully for the next few hours. Some hospitals will allow the father into the recovery room. If he isn't allowed into the operating room, at least maybe the father can join the mother in the recovery area to celebrate the birth of the baby.

If you and your doctor know ahead of time that you will need a Cesarean to deliver the baby, talk to the doctor about making the birth as family-centered as possible. If s/he does not see the necessity of father participation, and says s/he will forbid his presence in the operating room, seriously consider changing doctors. Find someone who will allow the father to be present. If you do change doctors, be certain that you write a letter to the first doctor detailing why you felt compelled to go elsewhere for medical service.

The Cesarean mother can certainly go ahead with rooming-in plans; in fact it's an especially good idea because of the extended hospital stay for a Cesarean. Lifting the baby and caring for it will certainly be more work for the Cesarean mother than it is for the other mothers, but the nursing staff will be happy to help you until you can handle the baby by yourself. Sometimes special visiting hours can be arranged for you so you can have a friend or relative (ideally the father) stay with you and help you with the little one. This arrangement helps a lot of people: you, the baby and the nursing staff.

The Cesarean mother can also nurse successfully. Because her mobility is somewhat hampered at first, the early days may not go quite so smoothly as she might like, but with some effort a good nursing relationship can be established. Cesarean mothers may find that placing a pillow over the abdomen and placing the baby on that during the nursing may lessen pain from the incision. Having the baby in the SCN at first may make nursing more difficult, but perhaps the staff will let you nurse the baby in the SCN. Or maybe you can hand-express your milk and the SCN staff will feed it to the baby for you.

Pain and itching around the abdominal incision are common for several months following the operation. In most cases, the scar fades during the few months following delivery. If the mother has another Cesarean later, the same scar is normally used.

The Cesarean mother has the vaginal flow, lochia, following delivery just as does the woman who delivered vaginally. The Cesarean mother's flow may be lighter, however, because the physician cleans out the uterus manually at the time of the Cesarean.

Many women have a fever after surgery, but it is possible that the mother and baby do not have to be separated because of it.

In order to promote faster recovery and avoid decrease of muscle tone, Cesarean mothers often are required to walk the day after surgery. After the first walk, the mother is encouraged to go on short walks frequently. Bladder and intestinal function are both helped if the mother walks. Coughing and deep breathing are encouraged to lessen the chances of lung congestion. Some of these activities can be quite painful, and pain relief medications are available. Take advantage of them. If you are nursing, be sure your doctor knows that you are. Some medications are safe to take when you are nursing; others are not.

Most Cesarean mothers remain in the hospital for about a week after surgery. This can obviously be a problem if the mother has other children at home. Special arrangements might be possible for you to see your other children while you are still in the hospital. A week or so is a long time, especially for the little ones.

If beds are available, many hospitals make an effort to keep Cesarean mothers together. Women who were unmedicated, or minimally medicated, for their vaginal deliveries are often quite active immediately after the birth. This can seem very unfair to the Cesarean mother who has had major surgery as well as a birth.

Once the Cesarean mother goes home, the people around her should remember that her body is recovering from surgery as well as making the normal postpartum adjustments. That in itself can take a great deal of energy, without even considering taking care of a new baby. If it fits anywhere in the family budget, it would be a good idea to hire help with the cooking and housework. Don't get help with the baby unless you absolutely need it. It's better to have the other people, grandmothers included, doing the housework. Lifting should definitely be avoided for several weeks. Some mothers feel healthy and rested again within a week or so; others don't feel really good for several months. The amount of help at home, general health before the operation, personal attitude, the baby's disposition, and a multitude of other things enter into determining the length of the recovery period.

Some doctors will let Cesarean mothers attempt to deliver vaginally in a subsequent pregnancy. This is a medical question that depends upon many factors. Discuss it with your doctor.

Unfortunately, some mothers feel as though they've somehow failed if they need a Cesarean delivery. This attitude is particularly prevalent among prepared mothers. Prepared mothers have spent a great deal of time and effort preparing for the birth of the baby. The mother and father look forward with great excitement to sharing the experience of birth. Of necessity, childbirth education classes must focus on the normal birth process; this is what most parents anticipate, and what most parents experience. This bias helps produce some rather mixed emotions if a Cesarean becomes necessary.

Some Cesarean couples seem to feel that if the mother had just been able to relax more efficiently, or breathe more rapidly, a Cesarean would not have been necessary. Some coaches feel responsible; if the coach had only coached more effectively, or if s/he hadn't left the mother to eat that sandwich, things would have turned out differently. Cesareans are not performed because the mother is not breathing fast enough, or because the coach got hungry and had to eat a sandwich. They are performed to save the life of the mother and/or baby. Self-recrimination is damaging and pointless. The need for a Cesarean is beyond the control of both the mother and father. A Cesarean birth should not be viewed as a failure.

A Cesarean is, about all, the birth of a baby. Coping with the disappointment of not being able to breathe and push your way through childbirth can be a lot easier if you remember that. With appropriate planning, a cooperative doctor and a good attitude on your part, the Cesarean, too, can be a family-centered experience that celebrates the birth of your child.

If you feel that you do not know enough about the Cesarean after you complete your childbirth education classes, discuss it with your instructor. If she doesn't have more information for you, she will be able to direct you to appropriate sources. The incidence of Cesareans is on the rise in America; more babies are being saved and more women are being spared the possibility of a really difficult vaginal birth. A Cesarean birth, just like a vaginal birth, is easier to handle and cope with is the couple is educated ahead of time. In some areas of the country, it is possible for couples to take classes designed especially for couples who know ahead of time that a Cesarean will be necessary.

Cesarean support groups have come into being with

the goal of making Cesarean birth as pleasant and meaningful as possible for each couple. The groups offer support, encouragement and information to couples that are prepared for the possibility of a Cesarean. Another very useful and valid function of the groups is providing support and concern to couples who have experienced a Cesarean and feel frustrated and cheated by the experience.

Local groups that offer this special support to Cesarean couples are forming all over the country. Some of these groups are listed in Appendix C. Check with your local childbirth education groups to see what is available in your area.

Especially for the Labor Coach

In most cases the labor coach is also the father of the baby, so this chapter is directed toward the labor coach in general and the father in particular. Most of the information applies to anyone who is a labor coach, but some of it applies only to the father.

It is difficult to explain how important a labor coach is to prepared childbirth techniques and a positive birth experience. It's possible that only a woman who has been through a prepared birth can fully understand the impact that you, the coach, can have during labor and delivery.

Labor coaching elevates you into a position of importance not possible in a traditional birth. Your most important function during labor is no longer getting her to the hospital in time. It's your job to provide the mother with constant support and affection throughout the childbirth experience as well as perform specific tasks designed to make labor more comfortable and efficient.

One of the most valuable aspects of your labor coaching is your presence. You are the one person in the world that she most depends upon; she needs your understanding and support in all areas of life, but most particularly in areas relating directly to the baby. Helping her to give birth to the child that you both created can add a great deal of meaning to both her life and your life. Being together during the labor and birth is a good way to start your life as a family. Meeting the baby in the delivery room is an incredible experience; much more personal than meeting the little one through the glass of the nursery room windows.

It's natural for a father to be a bit hesitant about accompanying his lady into labor, and especially into the delivery room. Years and years of exposure to the traditional view of childbirth has probably created some rather mixed feelings about childbirth in your mind. It may seem like a waste of time to attend childbirth education classes. A couple of classic comments from fathers are "Why should I learn anything about childbirth—it's not going to happen to me" and "What is there to learn anyway—the doctor will be there and handle everything." The value of childbirth education can only be understood through participation. Since there is no way the mother can avoid going through childbirth, most fathers are willing to do what they can to make her experience as positive as possible.

Even if you are absolutely against attending classes, it's good to consider going to the first one or two classes just to see what it is you are so against. **Childbirth is a great adventure; if you can, experience it with your lady.**

The total childbirth experience demands your support and encouragement to make it truly positive. Labor coaching is just the natural extension of this caring attitude. For example, during the latter part of pregnancy, she'll appreciate help with the household chores much more than you realize. Even something so simple as carrying a laundry basket full of clean clothes can be very difficult when her center of gravity has changed and she is contending with a distended uterus. One area that demands special consideration is sex. Due to her expanding abdomen, it if often hard to find a position for lovemaking that is comfortable for her. Try to be understanding and realize that it is not you she may be rejecting; it is the awkward positions.

Sometime during the pregnancy the two of you should tour the hospitals that you are considering for the birth. If for some reason you don't have a choice of hospitals, make certain that you still take the time to go on an orientation tour of her hospital. It is very helpful to know in advance where the appropriate entrances are for daytime and nighttime admissions. It's also good if you are somewhat familiar with the labor and delivery facilities; it will help both of you to feel more at home when she arrives in labor.

Meeting her doctor or midwife ahead of time is another thing that makes the birth, and the time spent in the hospital in labor, more familiar. All you need do is accompany her to one of her prenatal appointments; the doctor or midwife will be happy to speak with both of you. If she visits several doctors or midwives early in the pregnancy in order to choose the one she likes best, it is a good idea if you can arrange to go with her. It's always helpful to have two of you asking questions and expressing concerns; what one of you forgets to ask, the other one may remember. In any case, it is easier for you, the mother and the birth attendant if you have talked with the birth attendant ahead of time. If a medical emergency arises during the labor and delivery, it is easier for you to have confidence in someone you have met before.

STAGE 1 LABOR—PRE-LABOR PHASE

When it becomes apparent that labor may have started, encourage the mother to rest. If it is a normal sleeping period for her, try to convince her to sleep as long as she can. If it is not a time when she usually sleeps, encourage her to limit her activity and to ignore all of the things that she still has to do "before the baby comes." Remind her that this is the only time that she will ever have the baby and that she owes it to herself, the baby and you to do whatever will produce the best birth experience possible. If the dishes in the sink, or the one last load of dirty laundry is really upsetting her, it might be a good idea to go ahead and do whatever it is that's bothering her. Not only will it make her quit worrying about the task, it will mean a lot to her that you were considerate enough to do the task so that she could rest. Psychologically it is a very good way to start labor.

If it looks as though she still has a fair amount of time before the birth, have her take a shower or a warm bath to help her relax. She should not take a bath if her membranes have ruptured or if her doctor has advised against tub baths. It's good if you can help her into and out of the tub or shower area in order to minimize the chances of her falling.

If she has the doctor's permission, she may want to give herself an enema at home. This will help her avoid having one later in labor when she arrives at the hospital. The later in labor the enema is given, the more uncomfortable it may be.

Throughout labor, offer moral support and physical assistance in every way you can think of. If she doesn't like something that you are doing, she'll tell you. If she does like what you are doing, she probably won't tell you at the time, but she will after labor is all over. It's good to practice the breathing techniques some during these early contractions, but don't use them seriously until she feels that she needs them. The longer she can last without going on to each level of breathing, the better off she will be in late labor.

You should record the interval between contractions and the length of each contraction so that you can report accurately to the doctor or midwife. It's also good to note when in the contraction the peak comes. Both by communicating with her and by observing her, evaluate the strength of the contractions and make a note of when they seem to be getting more intense.

During this early phase of labor is a good time to

tell her how much you love her and how excited you are about the baby. Going into labor is exciting for both of you because suddenly the whole thing gains an aura of reality. However, the next hours are hard work so it's good to get the giggles and the "this is really it!" feelings out now so you can both concentrate later on the work at hand.

Unless she is feeling nauseous, she should eat something light during the pre-labor phase. Remind her to stick to high carbohydrate, high protein foods such as gelatin or toast and honey and to avoid dairy products. The dairy products digest too slowly to be eaten during labor. Encourage her to drink fluids: fruit juices are particularly good because of the natural sugar content.

You should get something to eat, too. Labor coaching is strenuous work, and there's no way for you to know how long the labor will be. Pack something to take with you to eat at the hospital. Be certain that it is something with a very non-offensive odor. The sense of smell is heightened during labor, and something with a strong smell, such as salami or tuna fish, could be unpleasant for her to deal with.

Sometime during all of this it is easy for you, too, to realize that this is really it. You are about to become a father. When these thoughts hit you, if they do, remain calm. Above all, retain confidence in yourself as a labor coach. The most important thing to her is that you are sharing the experience with her from beginning to end. You're not expected to be an expert labor coach.

The doctor or midwife will have given the mother instructions about when to call. It is nice if you can do the actual calling, but she should be close at hand; sometimes the birth attendant will prefer to talk directly to the laboring woman. If the instructions say to call when the contractions are 5 minutes apart, and the contractions start out every 3 minutes, do not wait until they are 5 minutes apart, because it just isn't going to happen. That may sound silly, but some couples have actually waited for the contractions to space out.

When the doctor says to go to the hospital, it is up to you to get your other children to the pre-arranged sitter or to get the sitter to your home. Don't make the mother worry about these details. Another thing that you should do is check the list taped to the outside of the suitcase and the goody bag to see what last-minute items you must collect from around the house. After everything is in, put the bags in the car and come back into the house to get the mother. That way you can pay full attention to her on the walk to the car. Let her lean on you if she has a contraction on the way to the car. If you are planning to take pictures, be sure to grab the loaded camera and extra film. You should have an adequate supply of film ready to go at least a month before the due date.

Know several routes to the hospital and choose the one that is most appropriate for the time of day or night. Try to take roads that have a minimum of bumps, lumps and stoplights. Drive safely. Obey all traffic laws. If you feel there is not time to get to the hospital without speeding, call an ambulance.

STAGE 1 LABOR—ESTABLISHED LABOR PHASE

Once you arrive at the hospital, the admitting procedure should be relatively simple if you have preregistered. Most hospitals encourage pre-registration, and filling out one of the forms ahead of time allows you and the mother to avoid a lot of unnecessary hassle when she is entering the hospital in labor. After she's signed a paper or two, she will be taken to the labor/delivery area and you'll be left to complete any remaining paperwork. Someone will probably meet the mother at the admitting desk and escort her; in some hospitals she will be allowed to walk if she wishes, and in others she will have to ride in a wheelchair or on a stretcher.

While she's being examined, prepped and given an enema, you will most likely be asked to wait in the

Fathers' Waiting Room. The procedures shouldn't take any longer than 20 to 30 minutes, and if your wait there becomes what you consider excessive, find a nurse, identify yourself and ask when you can join the mother. It is possible that the mother could be all set up in the labor room and just waiting for you to come in. Sometimes the nurses forget to come and get the coach. This isn't too common, but it has been known to happen, especially if the staff has several women laboring at the same time.

If she is having difficulty handling the contractions when you arrive at the hospital, sign your name on one or two dotted lines and go immediately to the labor area. It is not legally necessary that you complete the admission paperwork before the baby is born. If she is having a hard time with the contractions, she obviously needs your presence more than the admitting clerks do. Don't be obnoxious with the nursing staff, but do make it very clear that the mother has prepared herself for the labor experience and that it is much easier for her to handle the contractions when you are with her. You will very likely still have to stay outside of the room while she is being initially examined and prepped, but you'll probably be able to join her sooner than if you were waiting in the Fathers' Waiting Room.

Because you are in a hospital, and hospitals try to maintain cleanliness as much as possible, it's a good idea if you wash your hands when you enter the labor room. If you leave the labor room, be sure to wash your hands before re-entering the room.

The mother may have some difficulty in maintaining her breathing and relaxation techniques during the hassles of being admitted. Unless she is extremely far along in labor, she will probably get back on the track within a few minutes after you have rejoined her. You would not believe the difference that just your presence can make. After you have helped her regain control, if, indeed, she lost any, you should take stock of the labor room. Peek outside the room and locate it in relationship to the other rooms in the immediate vicinity. Find out where the bathroom that you will use is. You probably won't be allowed to use the one in the labor room. Look in the drawers and closets in the labor room so you can find out what supplies are immediately available to you. If you can't find any extra pillows or blankets, ask for some. Don't be shy about asking for things and using things; you are paying for the use of the facilities. Ask the nurse to bring some ice chips, a pitcher of water, a glass, a straw and a couple of washcloths. Depending upon how far along the mother is in labor and upon the hospital's policies, you may not get everything that you ask for, but it doesn't hurt to ask.

Ask the nurse where the nearest phone is. Find out where the cafeteria is and where the Fathers' Waiting Room is (if you haven't been there already) in case you aren't allowed to eat your lunch in the labor room. Find out where the call button for the nurse is. Be sure to tell the mother where it is.

Find out how the labor room bed operates. Most hospital beds can be adjusted so that the head of the bed is at an angle to the rest of the bed; and the total bed can be raised and lowered in relationship to the floor. If the bed is raised some, it may be easier for the coach to give back rubs. Adjust the bed to a good angle for the mother, and arrange pillows and blankets around her so that she is as comfortable as possible.

Another job that is yours throughout labor is running interference for her. If there is a hassle with the staff, it should be you who does the hassling. If the nurses keep asking questions right in the middle of contractions, for instance, explain to them that the breathing and relaxation techniques that the mother is using require a great deal of concentration and that it is impossible to maintain that concentration and answer questions at the same time. Ask them to please wait until between contractions to speak to your lady. Let every new staff person that you see know that you are trained parents.

Offer the mother ice chips, sips of water, back rubs,

back pressure, anything that you can think of to make her more comfortable. Ask whether the room is the right temperature, offer to open or close the windows. Offer to get another blanket, or to rearrange those that she has.

Both of you should relax between contractions, but remember that it is easier for you to relax than it is for her to relax. Watch her very carefully for signs of creeping tension. It often shows up first in the forehead, the neck, the shoulders or the feet. Stress use of relaxation techniques that you've learned. Have her use relaxation both during and between contractions.

Encourage her to maintain each breathing level as long as she can. Each successive technique is more tiring, and demands more of her. Each is more effective distraction. When one technique is no longer effective, move on to the next. If she's using a more advanced level of breathing than you think she should be (and you are afraid that she might "run out" of new techniques before the first stage of labor is over), have her drop back to the previous level for a few contractions. Then when she again advances to the same level, it is possible that it could have regained effectiveness. It is certainly worth a try.

Some women find it very helpful if the coach calls off the time at 10- or 15-second intervals throughout the contractions. Or you can say "the contraction is ¼ over, ½ over, etc." Some women find this extremely annoying. Try it and find out whether she likes it or dislikes it.

If you become hungry, eat your lunch in the labor room if you can. If the nurse makes you leave, hurry down to the Fathers' Waiting Room and eat as fast as you can without getting indigestion. Try not to leave if it looks as if the mother is anywhere near transition. She will need you very much when that phase of labor comes.

Remind her to empty her bladder once an hour. If her membranes haven't ruptured, she'll probably be allowed to walk to the bathroom. Help her get there if she needs help. There are bars on the wall next to the toilet, so she should be able to manage getting up and down by herself. Quite often the activity of getting up and walking will bring on more intense contractions, so do stay by the door and coach her, even though there is a closed door between you. Once her membranes have ruptured, she will probably have to use a bedpan. It's an awkward maneuver for her and is bound to make the contractions temporarily more intense. If either the nurse or the mother asks you to leave, offer lots of encouragement before you leave, and let her know that you will be just outside the door. Emptying the bladder is very important because a full bladder can interfere with the expulsion of the baby and the progress of labor. If she has a full bladder, it is possible that she will have to be catheterized to remove the urine. Remember that she may not recognize the need to urinate, so you will have to remind her. Start her toward the bathroom or onto the bedpan just at the end of a contraction so she'll have the maximum amount of time before the next contraction.

Without sacrificing your other coaching duties, try to keep as complete a record of the frequency, duration and intensity of the contractions as you can. Each time she is checked for dilatation by the nurse, doctor or midwife, ask what it is-in centimeters, and record the time and dilatation. So much happens in such a short period of time that details will be hard to remember later. The record you keep of labor will help you both to go back over the labor in years to come; it's a good addition to the baby book. If the examining person does not automatically tell you both what the dilatation is after each exam, be sure to ask. It is possible that the mother is depending on you to get that information.

Ask her whether she wants some lip balm or some of the hospital's glycerine lemon swabs. She might prefer to suck on a wet washcloth instead. If it doesn't annoy her, or detract from her concentration, it is possible to put a damp washcloth on her face so that part of it falls over her lips; this will help keep her mouth and lips moist. Offer her lollipops and remove the candy from her mouth as each contraction starts.

Praise and a positive attitude on your part are extremely helpful to the mother. Even if she is normally rather independent, your praise and constant encouragement are important during labor.

As she tires, and as the contractions become more intense, it is sometimes hard for the mother to anticipate accurately the beginning of each contraction. Even though contractions often do take on a pattern, they very seldom space themselves out at exact 3-minute or 4-minute intervals. You can help her anticipate each contraction by placing your hand on her abdomen. When you feel the uterus start to harden and begin to rise up, have her take a deep breath and start her breathing. That way she will be ready when the peak comes. If she is attached to some kind of fetal heart monitor, you will be able to tell when a contraction is coming by looking at the read-out or print-out. Be careful that you do not become so involved with watching the machine that you don't pay attention to the mother. If the machine is between the two of you, move the machine, the bed or you so that you can get beside her.

Throughout labor, follow her lead regarding activity between contractions. If she wants to talk, talk to her; if she wants to play cards, play cards; if she wants to lie quietly, then let her lie quietly.

Watch her closely, especially as labor progresses. Look for changes in her attitude, the frequency of contractions, for apparent discomfort and the like. If she begins to exhibit any of the signs of transition, let the nurse know immediately.

If the bed rails must be kept up, adjust your positioning so that they don't interfere with your coaching any more than they have to.

If she shows signs of hyperventilating, (dizziness, tingling of the nose or limbs, numbness, restlesness), have her breathe into a paper bag or her own cupped hands so she will re-breathe her carbon-dioxide. If she has trouble holding the bag, or holding her hands in front of her mouth during contractions, cup your hands over her nose and mouth for her.

If she is offered a medication, or if she requests one, be sure to discuss it with her. This is especially important if she has indicated a desire to remain unmedicated throughout the childbirth experience. If the doctor is recommending a particular medication, find out exactly what it is for, how long it will take to become effective, and how it may alter the mother's behavior. If she indicates that she would like to accept the medication, be certain that she knows the answers to the questions listed above. Ask the nurse to check her for dilatation. If she has progressed a great deal since the last examination, perhaps she will want to change her mind about the medication. If she can, have her wait another 15 minutes or ½ hour and be checked again. Sometimes just this length of time can produce a great amount of dilatation. The attempt here is not to avoid medication completely, it is to avoid unnecessary medication. If the mother truly wants medication, then she should have it, by all means. An unfortunate byproduct of childbirth training is that sometimes women set unrealistic sights before labor and decide that they want no medication whatsoever, under any circumstances. If medication becomes necessary, or if they just decide they'd like something during the stress of labor, these same women may be bitterly disappointed in themselves later. If the mother has a little time to think about her decision to accept the medication before she actually accepts it, she is usually happier than if she accepts it as the result of a sudden decision.

In some cases medication is definitely indicated. For instance, if contractions continue but dilatation, effacement and descent of the baby do not, the doctor may prescribe something to help. Another example of medically-indicated medication is when the doctor has to perform a delivery maneuver with forceps and wants the tissues of the vagina completely relaxed.

There is absolutely no reason to refuse medically-indicated medication. But, again, do find out what it is and discuss it with the mother before it is administered.

STAGE 1 LABOR—TRANSITION PHASE

As the mother enters transition, she will probably become decidedly more uncomfortable. This is when she most needs strong coaching and simple directions. Breathe along with her if that approach makes it easier for her to keep her breathing rhythms on course.

Try very hard to get her to relax. Have her change position if she seems terribly uncomfortable. See whether the room temperature is comfortable for her. If she seems warm, wipe her face with a cool, damp washcloth. Do not ask questions that require verbal answers; don't force her to talk. Now, more than any other time during labor, express your affection, praise and encouragement both verbally and non-verbally. Use words and actions that mean something to just the two of you. If she doesn't want you to talk at all, don't. Have a system of coaching worked out ahead of time that involves no touching, and no speaking. If your speaking does not irritate her a great deal, continue with simple, firm commands. She may seem very confused at this time, and it may be hard for her to understand anything but the most simple directions.

As transition progresses, she may act ungrateful and quite crabby. It is transition, not you, that she is mad at. Don't be hurt; just stay with her, coach for all you are worth and realize how much she needs you. If she doesn't want to be touched, and tells you to go away, she only means for you to not touch her; stay very near the bed.

Even if she hasn't had any back pain before this, she may have some now. Offer to apply counter-pressure to her lower back. Offer to massage her back.

Don't carry on any unnecessary conversations. If someone in the hall outside of the door is being particularly noisy or bothersome, politely tell them that your lady is in transition and is having a hard time concentrating.

If she gets cold, bring her blankets and don't be surprised if she is too hot by the time you get there with the blankets. The changes going on inside her body at this time are absolutely incredible.

Try to keep her alert with cool cloths on her face or an ice pack on her back. If she persists in falling asleep between contractions, keep your hand on her abdomen and let her know when a contraction is beginning. Remember that the rest period between transition contractions is shorter and that each contraction may have two or three peaks. It is essential that she is ready for each contraction.

Coach her to take one contraction at a time. If she thinks about the possibility of coping with an infinite number of transition contractions, she will become overwhelmed. Remind her that transition is the shortest phase of labor and that each contraction may be the last one in first stage labor. Remind her that it won't be long until the baby is born. Show her pictures of the dilatation chart and help her visualize her progress.

If she complains that her feet are cold, help her put on the warm socks from the goody bag. If her legs begin to tremble, cover them with blankets, hold them firmly and stroke them. Remind her constantly of the progress she is making.

Not too many women actually become sick; however if she experiences nausea or vomiting, get an emesis basin from the nurse to catch the vomit.

If she grunts, or starts to make pushing movements in the middle of a contraction, call a nurse immediately. Coach her to use whatever "don't push" techniques you've learned. She will need extremely strong coaching here if she is experiencing an intense urge to push. Tell her that it won't be long before she can begin to push the baby out.

STAGE 2 LABOR—EXPULSION

She will probably welcome the contractions of second stage labor after those of transition. These contractions are farther apart and bring with them a strong urge to push rather than the discomfort of the first stage contractions. When she starts pushing, the mother is being asked to do something completely different from what she was doing during first stage labor. It is up to you to help her remember the pushing techniques you learned in class. It will probably be a few contractions before she is doing really effective pushing; the clearer and more precise your instructions, the sooner she will become comfortable with the pushing techniques. Talk her through each contraction. Help her get into a comfortable pushing position; if you have practiced several at home before labor, it should be fairly easy for her to find an effective position. Remind her to relax her pelvic floor. Have her take two or three deep breaths as the contraction begins, then as it reaches its peak, have her hold a breath and push. The pushing will be more effective and less tiring if she exerts her greatest effort with the peak of the contraction. The pushes should be long, strong and steady.

If she has no urge to push, but has been told to push by the staff, she will need more coaching. Talk and encourage her through each contraction. After a few contractions she should be able to pick up the rhythm pretty much for herself, but if she doesn't feel the urge to bear down it is more difficult for her to make the adjustment from first stage labor to second stage labor contractions.

Reassure her that the sensations of pressure and stretching that she feels during the second stage are normal. Some women interpret these as pain sensations, but most women find the pushing to be an extremely satisfying experience.

Second stage usually brings about a change of attitude and she may be very talkative between contractions. Again, follow her lead. Transition is over and she will probably want you to touch her again. The confusion of transition will also be gone.

Don't be at all upset if her face turns red and she seems to be grunting during the pushing contractions. If she looks, and sounds, like a weightlifter who is trying to press 300 pounds, that's fine. She is exerting a tremendous amount of energy. She is probably not feeling pain; if she is, she will let you know. Don't be embarrassed for her. Just be lavish and frequent with praise for the good job she is doing.

While she is being transferred to the delivery room, you will be shown where you can change into the sterile clothes necessary for delivery room participation. To avoid this last-minute rush, it's better if you can change earlier in the labor; when you first arrive is a good time, but some hospitals won't allow that. If you must change now, do hurry. In some hospitals you will just be given a gown to slip on over your street clothes. In other hospitals, you will have to remove your outer garments and put on hospital pants and a top. If you aren't sure what size will fit you, ask the nurse to help you guess. That way you will avoid having to get dressed twice in case the first one is much to big or much too small. Of course, none of the outfits will fit right, but some will be closer to right than others. In addition to the pants and top or gown, you will be given a hat, a mask and paper shoes to put on over your shoes.

If you are not going into the delivery room, you will be asked to wait in the Fathers' Waiting Room. It may be an hour and a half before you are contacted, because it can take that long for the birth and the episiotomy repair. In many hospitals you can decide to go into the delivery room up until the last minute, even if you have said ahead of time that you do not wish to accompany her to delivery.

When you join her in the delivery room, you may be surprised to find that she is not pushing as effectively as she was in the labor room. She may seem to have lost some control. Remember that while you were getting dressed, she was being moved from room to room, and onto the delivery table. It's very hard for her to keep all of her attention on the contractions when so much else is being demanded of her. And remember that she was handling those contractions alone; you weren't there. Do the same thing that you did at the beginning of second stage; talk her through each contraction. Within a few contractions, she should be back in control and pushing as effectively as possible.

If she is delivering in the lithotomy position, her legs will be in the stirrups. Be sure to ask her whether they are comfortable. If they are not, ask the nurses to adjust them. If she is planning to deliver in a side-lying position, either help her hold her right leg up during the contractions or help her put it into the left stirrup.

If she is in the lithotomy position, or the dorsal position, ask the nurses whether the bed can be cranked up or tipped at an angle. If not, ask whether they have a removable support that you can slip behind her back. Ask whether you can put several pillows behind her to prop her up. If you can't do any of these things, lift her up with each contraction in order to make the pushing more comfortable and more effective. Lifting her up also improves her blood circulation. Get her as close to the semi-sitting position as you can. If her legs are up in the stirrups, follow her guide as to how far to lift her up. At the end of the contractions, put her down gently.

In all the bustle of delivery room activity, your voice is the most important thing she hears. It is you that she will be listening to. It is up to you to be sure that she is following the doctor's instructions. The doctor may use different terms than you've practiced with. You translate the instructions into terms she is familiar with. If the doctor wants her to push differently, or do anything else differently, than you've practiced, help her make the adjustment.

It's good to touch her shoulder, or stroke her hair, but remember to stay at the head of the delivery table unless the birth attendant invites you to come to the other end. If you do leave the mother's head, don't forget to coach her from wherever you are standing. Keep your hands off the sterile sheets and drapes at all times. Do not wander around the delivery room touching things.

Be sure to remember to watch the birth in the mirror provided for the purpose. Remind the mother to look, too. She may be so involved in pushing the baby out that she forgets to look.

If you are asked to leave the delivery room at any time, do so without question. In the case of a medical emergency, the medical team must be allowed to perform at peak efficiency without having to worry about you and your reactions to what may be happening. If you are sent out of the room, however, stay very near. It's a possibility that the situation may be cleared up very quickly and the staff shouldn't have to hunt all over for you to tell you that you can come back in.

THE BIRTH AND AFTER

Don't be embarrassed to share whatever feelings you have when the baby is born. Ask about the baby's appearance and health. Congratulate your lady and tell her what a good job she did. Remember that all newborns are funny-looking little creatures that are a very strange color.

If there is a problem with the baby, for example s/he doesn't breathe immediately, let the staff proceed with necessary emergency measures without interference from you. And if a problem does exist, what better place for you than with the mother? It would be a lot easier for her to handle the uncertainty with you right there.

When the nurses hand the baby to the mother, ask whether you can hold it, too. But in the excitement of the baby's arrival, don't forget to continue your coaching. The placenta still has to be expelled, and there is probably repair work to be done. The best thing you can do is keep the mother occupied while the birth attendant is examining the cervix, vagina and perineum for lacerations. Remind her to relax the pelvic floor. She may not hear the doctor if s/he tells her to push the placenta out, so you should be listening for instructions to relay to the mother. If she feels any discomfort, have her do one of the early breathing techniques.

New parents, particularly those who shared the birth experience through classes and participation, have a tendency to look upon the birth of their baby as the first really meaningful birth in the history of the world. And that's certainly not an unreasonable viewpoint. Participating fathers have a pride in the birth that goes far beyond the macho attitude of the Ostrich father. It's suddenly more important to tell other expectant fathers about this "new" way of having a baby than it is to pass out cigars with pink or blue labels on them.

Of course, immediately after the birth, the first impulse is to go directly to the nearest telephone and call all of the numbers on the list in your pocket. That's a good idea, but don't just abandon the mother at this point. When she is moved to the recovery area, whether it is her room or a maternity recovery room, stay with her as long as you can. If she's all alone, or with a couple of Ostriches who are moaning and groaning about how awful labor was, she can be very lonely during this period of time. Many hospitals won't let her have the baby for the first couple of hours at least, so she is just in a sort of limbo. She's all hyped up with no one to share her excitement with. It's easier if she is in her room with a phone, but there's no phone in the recovery room for her to use. If she must remain in the central recovery room for a period of time after the birth, and you cannot stay with her, provide her with some reading material to occupy her in case she doesn't feel like sleeping.

If she is able to go to her room, the two of you can make the announcement phone calls together; that's more fun, and it lets her be a part of it. It also surprises Ostriches that she sounds so cheerful and bright such a short time after the birth.

Sharing the birth can be a tremendously exciting and powerful experience. If other people don't understand what you did to help during the birth, hand them this chapter or spend some time telling them. Many fathers who were not prepared for the birth of their first child take classes or read a lot before the second child is born because they wanted to help the mother through labor the first time, but they didn't know what to do. There are so many things that a labor coach can do to make labor easier and more comfortable that it boggles the mind; however, the most important thing s/he can do is be there with love and understanding of what is happening, and what she's feeling.

If you enjoy sharing the experience when your baby is born, let people know. Let other expectant parents, particularly fathers, know. If the hospital staff was particularly helpful and supportive, write a letter to the hospital administrator praising the staff. Mention individual personnel by name if you can. The spread of family-centered maternity care owes its momentum to satisfied and excited parents. Hospitals will be likely to institute more and more family-centered practices if consumers make their needs and desires known. A heartfelt thank you makes it just that much nicer for the next prepared couple. Hospital administrators are particularly impressed when they hear from fathers.

First, and most important, I can't imagine going through this experience without John being there to help me and give me the constant encouragement that he did. One of the nurses said afterwards that he had restored her faith in men, and did I know how lucky I was to have him? I DO!!

Curt coached me very well. I don't think I could have done it without him. When I started to get excited and breathe too hard, he was afraid I would hyperventilate. He did the breathing with me and it helped me keep a steady breathing pattern. He

reminded me to relax and stayed very calm and worked right with me.

I could never have made it without Dwight. He gave me great moral support.

Jenny's birth was really the most exciting moment of our lives and an experience we'll always remember and cherish. The coach plays such an important role and is such a big help. It's wonderful to be able to share something as miraculous as childbirth.

The total experience was satisfying, especially because of the "sharing" aspect with Josh. His being there filled a real need for me. He was at no time ever upset or worried, or a hindrance to anyone; just a help to me.

I've never seen Dave so beaming with pride before; we were both so very happy with our experience together in having our little girl. It was a wonderful experience.

Being one of the first to see him and the first to hold him (even before Shirley) really makes me feel more a part of the creation of my son. I feel as though I really helped him into the world.

I felt very happy and fulfilled and very much in love. When our son cried, I felt closer to John than at any time. I am looking forward to my next prepared birth.

My feelings about the birth of Craig are nothing but positive. I felt in excellent spirits immediately afterwards and am exceedingly pleased that I did not need medication. However, I must confess to having doubts before labor began that I would be able to tolerate the birth without it. John was my great source of strength and without him I could not have succeeded.

The contraction monitor proved to be helpful here because John could see how the strength of contractions was differing and could suggest different breathing accordingly.

I would have been lost without David. He was out of the labor room for two very short periods of time. At those times I felt very alone and a little panicked. It was easier, and I was calmer when he was there.

David's voice kept me from losing more than one contraction. I was so tired and hazy that it would have been easy to just give it all up.

My mother drove us to the hospital which we hadn't planned on, but I was glad she did. I wanted Larry by me and helping me the whole time.

Labor without Michael would have been impossible. His verbal and physical support was a definite necessity. The thought of his leaving my side at any time sent me into a panic.

Boy, was I glad to see him after two hours of going it alone. Physically I had control, but psychologically I was a little discouraged. Now everything was fine and with focal point established we proceeded to tackle each contraction by itself.

Part of our silent communication was that I would place my arms at my sides, palms up with fingers open, to show him that I was relaxing. If I started to reach for the bed rails, John would gently replace my arms at my sides.

At this point everything started to move very fast. The caudal was not taking effect and the contractions were getting harder to stay on top of, especially without Don in the room. I really depended on him to help me stay calm.

Dennis's constant presence and reassurance was all that kept me in control. I did lose several contractions, but was able to regain control as long as I knew Dennis was there to help me.

I think the greatest thing about our prepared childbirth classes was that John was able to be with me as a constant encouragement throughout my entire labor and delivery.

One thing that really helped in the delivery room was Bill's encouragement. His excitement really showed in his urging me to push. It seemed to give me an added strength.

I picked mother and son up at the hospital 48 hours after delivery. In the bed next to Sandi, there was an 18-year-old girl who suffered the side-effects of a saddle block. She had gotten out of bed the day after delivery and, being dizzy, she fell and hit her head on a metal rail. She had been bedridden for 7 days! No childbirth training, of course.

My doctor gives his patients a copy of their prenatal records to carry to the hospital. When she arrives, the staff will know precisely what she wants and doesn't want. My doctor also had his patients make a little "contract" as to the patient's wishes. My list included no anesthetics that would affect me after delivery or that would affect my baby, only a mini-prep, suppository instead of enema, and Rich in delivery if he chose to be there.

Medications Used in Childbirth

Medication is definitely the most misunderstood aspect of childbirth education. Some members of the medical profession, as well as a large segment of the population as a whole, equate childbirth education simply with unmedicated birth. As previously stated, this erroneous notion has probably stopped countless women from taking advantage of the prenatal education available to them.

The childbirth education movement is not against the use of medication. Childbirth educators support the use of necessary medications in proper dosages. There is a great deal of difference between being totally against the use of all medication in childbirth and urging judicious use of medications. The misunderstanding is partially based in, and perpetuated by, the fact that it is not uncommon for a prepared woman to require less medication during childbirth than an Ostrich does. Some prepared women simply feel less need for medication because of reduced fear, and the effectiveness of breathing and relaxation techniques; some prepared couples attempt to remain unmedicated or minimally-medicated because they are concerned about the risks that medications may subject the fetus and newborn to; and some prepared couples are self-motivated for personal reasons to take as little medication as possible.

Couples are taught during the classes that drugs and anesthesia sometimes play a vital role in a positive birth experience. They are also taught that the decision to accept any particular medication should be made jointly by the physician and the couple. It is the doctor's responsibility to recommend medications that s/he deems appropriate and to tell the couple why those medications are recommended; within reason, it is the couple's responsibility to accept or reject those medications. Despite this consumerist attitude, couples are encouraged to accept medication if the doctor recommends it for a specific medical reason. Determination of the true need for medication requires medical knowledge and judgment. If medication is recommended for a purely medical reason, she should accept it for her safety and the safety of her baby.

During childbirth education classes, expectant parents are told about the various medications that are commonly used in childbirth. As consumers, the couples are entitled to an explanation of all aspects of medical care related to childbirth; this includes information regarding medications. Many physicians do not have the time, nor the inclination, to explain the risks and benefits of each medication in detail to their patients. And many patients, unfortunately, do not care to know about the medications, particularly about the risks related to each drug and anesthetic.

This consumerist attitude on the part of expectant parents, partially instilled by childbirth education classes, spreads to other aspects of the childbirth experience. Birth attendants frequently find more resistance to routine procedures from prepared couples than from Ostriches. Prepared parents know more about the entire childbirth process and are more likely to complain about, or reject completely, procedures that are performed merely for the convenience of the medical attendants. Induction of labor, forceps delivery and routine medication all fall under this heading unless these procedures are medically-indicated. Some medical people find this particular patient perspective difficult to deal with.

The medical personnel that support childbirth preparation and are truly patient-oriented offer medication to prepared women in a way that offers the mother a choice. These supportive doctors and nurses make an effort to let mothers know that pharmaceutical aid is available, but do not make the decision for her, nor express disappointment and disapproval when medication is refused. The prepared woman has responsibility for her own decisions; she also has the responsibility to accept medications if they become necessary for the well-being of either herself or her baby. For instance, a great deal of tension on the mother's part can actually slow labor and produce undue hardships on the baby; appropriate medications can reduce the tension. It is extremely important for the parents, as well as the birth attendant, to enter the childbirth experience with a flexible attitude.

An inflexible attitude on the part of the parents can ruin their perception of the birth experience. Unfortunately, some couples enter labor with the attitude that it is a contest with an unmedicated birth as the ultimate goal. Couples with this outlook tend to lose the ability to accept the fact that medical intervention is sometimes necessary for the safety and health of the mother and/or baby. If medication becomes necessary for some reason, these couples are likely to consider themselves failures. This inflexibility can be dangerous and unhealthy. Just as prepared parents are asking the medical community to offer alternatives, the medical community has the right to expect a responsible attitude on the part of prepared couples.

There are some things that parents have a responsibility to know about medications in childbirth. Medications do, indeed, affect the fetus and the newborn child; the degree to which the baby is affected depends upon the kind and amount of medication administered.

T. Berry Brazelton, M.D., an eminent pediatrician, has expressed his views on the excessive use of childbirth medication in the following way, "I am frankly pro-baby. And I do not like what drugs administered to a woman in labor do to her baby."[1]

Dr. Brazelton outlines his views regarding the effects of excessive doses of childbirth medication in an article which appeared in the February, 1971, issue of *Redbook Magazine*. He is concerned about the effects of heavy medication on both the infant and on the early mother-infant interactions. According to Dr. Brazelton, "After a normal, nonmedicated delivery infants are alternately sleepy and overexcited, disorganized and difficult to reach for 24 to 48 hours . . . When the mother has been medicated, there is a lengthening of the baby's depressed period; it can continue for a week after delivery, rather than for two days."[2]

He explains why the medications affect the baby for such a long period of time by pointing out that the baby is at a comparative disadvantage. The medications administered to the mother just before delivery promptly cross the placenta and enter the baby's system. If the mother has drugs in her system at birth, so has the baby. The mother can rid herself of the medications within several hours because her kidneys and liver function efficiently. The kidneys and liver of a newborn, even a healthy term baby, are immature. This immaturity means that it takes longer for the baby to break down the depressant drugs. If large doses of the drugs have been used, the drug substances may be stored in the baby's body for several days after birth. These stored drugs are concentrated in the midbrain, the section of the brain that governs much of the newborn's behavior.

Because s/he's in this drugged state, the baby of a woman who was heavily medicated during labor, is likely to be very sleepy and unresponsive for the first week or so. Dr. Brazelton is very concerned about how this can affect the parent-infant relationships. It can confuse and hurt new parents when the baby does not respond as they think s/he "should." Certainly newborn babies cannot walk, nor talk, nor read; no one expects them to do that. But they are capable of responding positively to cuddling and attention if they are not under the effects of heavy medication.

Throughout the article, Dr. Brazelton shows that he understands the need for medication in some cases; however, his contention is that medicated mothers should be the exception rather than the rule.

Aside from being told what effects the medications could have on her baby, the mother is entitled to information regarding how the medications affect her own labor and ability to cope with it. All of the medications may alter the mother's ability to work alertly with each contraction. If she is not fully in control of her body and brain, it lessens her capacity for concentration. In many cases, obstetrical help such as forceps is required to deliver the baby because the medicated mother is less able to push her baby out on her own than is the unmedicated mother. Some of the major anesthetics eliminate the bearing down reflex, so the mother doesn't know when she is having a pushing contraction; this makes it very difficult for her to work with the contractions. The baby must rotate on the pelvic floor; this is most easily accomplished on a somewhat firm base. When the pelvic floor is relaxed to the degree that it is when it is completely anesthetized, it is hard for the fetus to rotate properly. The mother should also be told of any possible postpartum effects, such as headache.

Many doctors leave fairly standard orders with the labor room staff to give a particular medication when his/her patients are at a given number of centimeters of dilatation. This is grossly unfair and does not take into account the individuality of each patient. It considers neither the physical nor mental differences that affect different patients' labors. John J. Bonica, M.D., author of **Obstetric Analgesia and Anesthesia**, has said that "the type of analgesia and anesthesia must be tailored to the needs of the individual patient."[3] This certainly seems like a much more valid approach than administering a particular drug in a particular dose just because a woman's cervix is dilated to a particular number of centimeters. Some nurses can pressure a woman into taking a medication that she really doesn't need, nor want, simply by insisting that "the doctor ordered it." The doctor did order it, of course, but not necessarily for that particular patient; rather for all of his/her patients.

It is possible for doctors to leave orders at the hospital for nurses to make certain medications available upon the patient's request. All the nurse need do is let the patient know that the medication has been ordered by the doctor and that when (and if) the patient feels a need for it, the nurse will give it to the patient. This method of offering medication leaves the decision up to the parents. This arrangement, of course, demands communication between the doctor and the patient prior to labor.

In order for the mother, doctor and coach to be fully satisfied regarding the use of medications, it is necessary for a good deal of honest communication to take place. The mother must express her expectations and concerns to her doctor, and she must be willing to accept the doctor's judgment regarding medication. If she has chosen a supportive doctor who is willing to determine her need for medication on a truly individual basis, she does not have to worry that she will receive unnecessary medication.

The doctor's views on routine medications for all patients are extremely important to consider when choosing health care. Some doctors routinely give a particular anesthetic at delivery and pull the baby out with forceps. A doctor who is supportive of childbirth preparation will not hold such an inflexible attitude. It is important that the doctor is fully aware of the mother's wishes regarding medication and that such information in written on her chart. If it is on her chart, it is there for the hospital staff to see, and it is there in case an alternate doctor attends the birth.

Communication between the mother and the coach is also necessary. Advance communication can help the coach determine whether the mother's request for medication during labor is a real need for medication or a passing desire. Sometimes a few encouraging words from the coach can get the mother past a really rough time, and she will not need medication. If the mother really does want, or need, the medication, she certainly should have it. However, many mothers have taken medication on the spur of the moment and regretted it later. The coach can be very helpful here. If there are any particular medications that you wish to avoid completely, such as scopolamine, it is good to let the coach know about it ahead of time. Then the coach can make certain that you aren't given those particular medications.

Tell each new nurse and staff person you come in contact with that you are a prepared couple. It will help the staff give you care more suited to your individual needs. If a certain nurse is especially insistent that you take medication that you do not want, remember that you have the legal right to refuse any medications. Tell the nurse that you must discuss it with your doctor before you will take it. Try to stay relaxed.

If medication becomes necessary, a smaller dose may do the job if you are totally relaxed. The more tense a patient is, the more medication is necessary for the same effect. If you decide that you want some medication, ask for the smallest suitable dose.

If you begin to feel a need for medication, it is particularly important to stay informed about your labor progress in terms of effacement and dilatation. If you are progressing quite rapidly, that knowledge can be as much of a boost as can an injection of a drug.

Some women have found the following guidelines to be helpful in deciding whether or not to request medication. These guidelines are not, of course, appropriate in every case; they are especially not appropriate if the medication is medically necessary. When you feel a need for medication, have your dilatation checked. If you are dilated less than 6 centimeters, wait 30 minutes and be checked again. If there's been no progress, or if you still want medication, try to wait another 30 minutes and be checked again. Then decide whether or not to take the medication.

If, when you feel the need for medication, you are dilated more than 6 centimeters, wait 15 minutes and be checked again. If there's been no progress, or if you still want medication, try to wait another 15 minutes and be checked again. Then decide whether or not to take the medication.

In other words, if you are dilated to less than 6 centimeters, you wait one hour after you first feel as though you might like to have medication until you request the medication. If you are dilated to more than 6 centimeters, you wait one-half hour from the time you first feel as though you might like to have medication until you request it. Remember that this is only a guideline; it may or may not work in your case. If you reach a plateau, and show no progress over a long period of time, medication may be advisable to relax you. Tension could be causing the lack of progress. In any case, don't ever make the decision to accept medication during a contraction.

Do not accept any medication without asking what it is, how soon it should take effect, what it will do for you, and how long its effects will last. You are legally entitled to such information. Different drugs in different doses have different effects.

Remember that the transition phase of first stage labor will be the roughest to handle. During all of labor, but particularly during transition, it is essential that you deal with each contraction as it happens. Take one contraction at a time. Remember that transition is the shortest phase of labor and that when transition is over, the second stage of labor begins.

Accept the fact that there is no "failure" in childbirth. Realize that you have not failed if you accept medication. Make your decision deliberately, and with thought. It can be difficult to remain cool-headed in labor, but the coach is there to help. Do not suffer needlessly just to prove something. Once you've made your decision, be happy with it. If the doctor tells you that medication is truly necessary, accept it. Above all, don't regret whatever decision you have made. It is impossible to go back in time and do it over again. There is no failure in childbirth.

ANALGESIA AND ANESTHESIA

The difference between analgesia and anesthesia is quite simple. Analgesia is what is used during labor to relieve pain. Anesthesia is what is used during late first stage labor and during expulsion to block sensation either in a particular area of the body or to block consciousness totally, causing complete unconsciousness.

Anesthesia, because it blocks sensation entirely, is very effective in providing pain relief. Conduction anesthetics are anesthetics which are injected into the body in a particular location of the body to block nerve impulses to the brain from that portion of the body. Because anesthesia blocks sensations entirely, the mother does not feel the urge to push the baby out. This often necessitates the use of forceps during delivery. A trained mother can often help to push the baby out if she is told when to push; an untrained mother usually finds it very difficult to even help.

ANALGESIA

Tranquilizers, barbiturates and amnesics are really sedatives instead of analgesia medications, but they are commonly used in labor, so they are usually grouped under the analgesia heading.

Tranquilizers (for example Miltown, Vistaril, Phenergan, Largon, Sparine) are often used to relieve anxiety. Tranquilizers may have little effect on the fetus, and it is a good idea to try a tranquilizer alone at first. The drug can help to relieve tension without confusing the brain. Tranquilizers are good for long labors if tension is building. A drawback of tranquilizers is that too much of the drug can hamper the mother's alertness and, therefore, her efforts to deal with the contractions. This reduced control, and difficulty in maintaining breathing rhythms, can make it difficult for the mother to work with the contractions, and strong coaching is helpful.

Barbiturates (for example Seconal and Nembutal) are given to sedate the mother and produce sleep. Barbiturates do not relieve pain. If it is suspected that the mother is in false labor, she may be given a barbiturate so she can go to sleep. Barbiturates cross the placenta within 1 minute if administered intravenously and within 5 minutes if administered intramuscularly.[4] Barbiturates are not handled well by the newborn, and are stored in the midbrain of the infant. Barbiturates are not used near the time of delivery.

Scopolamine is an amnesic. In the past, it was used quite commonly for women during labor, but today it is seldom seen. Scopolamine itself does not stop the pain sensations, but it is normally used in combination with some drug that does relieve pain. Scopolamine actually alters thought processes; results are very unpredictable. A woman who has been "scoped" must be watched constantly because she may become physically violent. It can produce the nightmarish sleep known as Twilight Sleep. It is possible that a woman's request for pain relief may go unheeded because she can't be considered responsible for her actions when she is under the influence of scopolamine. Women who have been scoped feel all of the pain sensations of labor (unless another drug is administered to relieve pain), they just aren't supposed to be able to remember the pain later. Unfortunately, it is possible that something may cause the woman to remember her labor, and her behavior, later. That situation can produce a great deal of embarrassment. Scopolamine is a drug to avoid.

Narcotics (Demerol, Nisentil, Dolophine) act to relieve pain to some degree, produce sedation and decrease anxiety. Narcotics have a depressant effect on neonatal respiration. Newborn depression is most severe if the infant is born between one and four hours of administration of the narcotic.[5] Some women have found that Nisentil helps them relax, but allows them to stay in control of the contractions. Most women find that Demerol, especially in high doses, makes it very difficult to stay with the contractions. It can cause dizziness, sleepiness, difficulty in concentrating; it can easily sabotage efforts at control. When Demerol has been administered, women frequently fall asleep between contractions and wake up just in time for the peak of the contraction; then it is too late to catch up with the breathing techniques. It's possible that Nisentil will produce the same effects, but the effects may be somewhat less. Narcotics, too, reach the fetus within 1 minute if administered intravenously and within approximately 5 minutes if administered intramuscularly.[6]

Inhalation Analgesia

Inhalation agents can be used during the first stage of labor to produce an analgesic effect. These agents, when used for labor analgesia, are in a much lower concentration than those used for general anesthesia. The gas (for example, nitrous oxide, Penthrane, Trilene) is inhaled during the contractions; the gas can be self-administered because a protective device is built in—when the patient begins to feel light-headed, the inhalation mask will fall away because her arm will no longer be able to hold it. Within a few seconds she will again be fully conscious.

The inhalation analgesia has advantages over the other analgesics because it does not cause any "clinically significant respiratory depression or other side effects on the mother, fetus and newborn," nor does it interfere with the uterine contractions or labor progress.[7]

The patient and the inhalation apparatus must be watched closely so the concentration of gas can be adjusted as her needs change during labor. Inhalation analgesia is sometimes used through delivery.

GENERAL ANESTHESIA

These anesthetics are inhaled by the mother, and produce unconsciousness. The only real advantage of general anesthesia is that it is fast-acting, and if the birth attendant needs an anesthetic which takes effect immediately, a general inhalation anesthesia will probably be used. A general anesthetic is only administered very close to delivery.

Deep general anesthesia interferes with the contractions and slows labor. The anesthesia crosses the placenta within a very short time and causes neonatal depression which can be eliminated by giving the newborn oxygen. Chances of postpartum hemorrhage are greater if the mother has had a general anesthetic. Of course, the mother's capability for pushing is completely gone, so the baby must be removed by the use of forceps. The mother is not aware of the birth.

It is essential that the mother's stomach is empty when a general anesthetic is administered. If there is any food in the mother's stomach, it is possible that she will vomit, and then aspirate the vomitus into her lungs. This is extremely dangerous.

General anesthesia is seldom used in a normal birth situation; the regional anesthetics are safer for the mother and the fetus, and they allow the mother to be conscious at the time of the birth.

REGIONAL ANESTHESIA

Caudal

The caudal is administered in the lower back at the tail of the spine in the caudal space. The caudal anesthetic does not mix with the spinal fluid. The mother is normally turned on her side while a small catheter is inserted and taped into place. The anesthetic solution is then injected into the catheter as needed. The process of inserting the catheter and administering the proper dosage takes about 10 to 20 minutes. The caudal can be given after about 6 centimeters of dilatation if the contractions are strong, long enough, and the baby is well down into the pelvis.

The caudal blocks sensation, but does not have much effect on motor nerves, so a woman can normally move after a caudal is given. If too much anesthetic is administered, the uterine contractions can slow and become weaker; however, in proper doses, the caudal has very little effect on the length and strength of the contractions. Women who have been given caudals do not get "spinal headaches" because the spinal dura is not punctured.

The caudal can produce a drop in maternal blood pressure, and the mother will be monitored closely. The mother's lowered blood pressure can affect the amount of oxygen that the fetus receives.

If the caudal is given too early, or in strengths too great, it can cause labor to be prolonged because of the effect on uterine contractions. The mother who has a caudal does not experience the urge to bear down, and she must be told when to push. Trained women can sometimes help push the baby out, but untrained women often cannot help, even though the motor nerves are not affected too much. The unprepared mother does not know how to push, and she hasn't got the urge to push to help her figure it out. Forceps are often required. The anesthetic used in the caudal transfers to the fetus rapidly.[8]

Epidural

An epidural is quite similar to a caudal. This method of anesthesia, like the caudal, does not mix with the spinal fluid. A catheter is placed in the mother's back a little higher than the caudal catheter is; again, the anesthetic solution is injected through the catheter as needed. The anesthetic is injected into the tissue that surrounds the spinal fluid. An epidural may be given when the cervix is dilated somewhere between 6 and 8 centimeters; contractions must be strong, and the fetal head must be down a good distance into the pelvis before it is given.

The mother may continue to feel pressure after the epidural is administered, but she does not feel pain.

However, an epidural often does not stop the intense back pain that some women feel during labor.

According to John J. Bonica, M.D., in **Obstetric Analgesia and Anesthesia**, the advantages of an epidural over a caudal are: less drug is required for the epidural, the epidural takes effect more rapidly than the caudal does, there's less risk of infection because it is easier to keep the skin clean in the region that the epidural is given than in the area where the caudal is given, and there's no risk of puncturing the rectum or the head of the fetus when administering the epidural.[9] Perineal relaxation is less likely to result from the epidural than from the caudal; perineal relaxation can produce difficulty in rotation of the fetus.

Dr. Bonica also points out the disadvantages of the epidural as compared to the caudal. Administration of the epidural requires greater skill, and risk of puncturing the dura (membrane surrounding the spinal cord) is greater with the epidural than with the caudal; this puncture would produce total spinal anesthesia and possibly cause postpartum headache.[10]

Advantages of the epidural over spinal anesthesia, according to Dr. Bonica, consists of the greater control of the duration and intensity of the anesthetic action in the epidural, less chance of maternal blood pressure being lowered, and that when the epidural is properly administered, there is no chance of a postpartum headache as there is with the spinal.[11]

The mother's blood pressure can be lowered with the epidural, as with the caudal. The lowered blood pressure can affect the amount of oxygen that the fetus receives.

The epidural is not always available because of the skill necessary for proper administration and because the mother must be closely observed after the epidural is given. The epidural produces a loss of the pushing reflex, and the mother must be told when to push. Forceps are frequently required for delivery of the baby. The anesthetic used in the epidural crosses the placenta rapidly to the fetus.[12]

Spinal

The spinal is injected into the spinal fluid. For administration the mother may be asked to lie on her side with her knees pulled up; this position allows maximum space between the vertebrae for injection of the anesthetic solution. In some cases the anesthesiologist may have the mother in a sitting position instead. The spinal may be given after the mother's cervix is dilated to about 8 centimeters, but is often not given until the mother's cervix is fully dilated. In this case, no relief of first stage labor discomfort is offered by the spinal. Sometimes the anesthetic is administered when a patch of the baby's head about the size of a 50 cent piece shows during the pushing contractions; sometimes it is administered just before the last contractions, when the head is crowning, to afford complete perineal relaxation.

A spinal is simple to give and takes effect rapidly. The spinal is sometimes used for a mother who is extremely tired and can push no longer; it allows the doctor to use forceps to deliver the baby. The spinal can relax a tense perineal floor. It can also serve to delay the birth if the doctor deems it advisable. The mother loses the urge to push, but she can still push, with somewhat reduced efficiency, if she has practiced ahead of time and knows how to control her diaphragm and surrounding muscles for appropriate pushing. However, forceps are usually used for delivery.

The mother's blood pressure may be lowered after the spinal is administered.

To guard against possible headache, the mother will be required to remain flat on her back for a period of time after the anesthetic is given. This can range from 4 to 8 hours in most cases. The so-called spinal headache is caused because of leakage of spinal fluid through the puncture in the dura; this hazard has been lessened with the use of finer gauge needles in administration. The leakage of fluid causes pressure changes within the spinal cord.

There is no placental transfer of the anesthetic when a spinal is given.[13]

True Saddle Block

Spinals are often called saddle blocks, but a true saddle block is injected into the spinal fluid lower than a spinal is. The woman is in a sitting position for the administration of the saddle block. This anesthetic gives perineal analgesia and relaxes the muscles. It also anesthetizes the legs to some extent. Its name was derived because it deadens the approximate area of the body that would come in contact with a saddle if the woman were riding a horse. Less drug is required for the saddle block than for the spinal.

The true saddle block, like the spinal, can lower the mother's blood pressure. It also requires that the mother remain flat on her back following the administration of the anesthetic in order to guard against postpartum headache.

When a saddle block is given, the anesthetic used does not cross the placenta.[14]

Saddle blocks, like spinals, are given quite close to delivery. Both spinals and saddle blocks are being used less and less frequently as the use of caudals and epidurals becomes more widespread.

Paracervical Block

A paracervical block is an anesthetic administered on the side of the cervix. A long needle is inserted through the vagina and one of the "caine" drugs (i.e. Xylocaine, etc.) is injected on the side of the cervix at approximately 3 o'clock and 9 o'clock on the cervical rim. The needle is guided through the vagina by the use of a long hollow tube called an Iowa trumpet; the needle barely penetrates the cervical rim. Because the cervix is a landmark for the paracervical block, it must be administered while there is still enough of the cervix left to find. However, the paracervical block, as with other methods of anesthesia used in labor, cannot be administered before active labor is well under way.

A paracervical block interrupts pain in the pelvis

from uterus and cervix, and is good for a cervix that is not dilating well. The paracervical block does not affect the perineal area, so if perineal anesthesia is desired, an additional anesthesia is necessary. Paracervical blocks are easy to give and may be administered by the doctor rather than by an anesthesiologist.

The effects of a paracervical block last about an hour, and wear off rapidly. The coach should watch the time very carefully, because it is easy for the mother to become overwhelmed when sensation is returned to the area of the cervix. The paracervical may be given repeatedly. The anesthetic crosses the placenta rapidly and can affect the fetus within 2 to 4 minutes of administration. The fetal heart rate sometimes slows quite obviously after the paracervical block is administered.

Paracervical blocks can cause a temporary decrease in the intensity or frequency of uterine contractions, but rarely slow labor. Five or ten per cent of patients are not helped when a paracervical block is administered.

Pudendal Block

In giving a pudendal block, the doctor injects a caine drug into the pudendal nerve in the vagina. The pudendal block numbs the vagina and perineum, so it is good for a forceps delivery which requires complete relaxation of the vaginal tissues. The pudendal block, like the paracervical block, is easy to administer and can be given by the doctor rather than by an anesthesiologist.

When she has a pudendal block, the mother usually does not feel the desire to push,[15] and she may have to be told when to do so. She may feel the baby move down the birth canal because of the pressure exerted by the fetus. The anesthetic used in the pudendal transfers to the fetus rapidly through the placenta.[16]

Local infiltration for the episiotomy

Just before the baby is born, the birth attendant may inject a substance such as Xylocaine or procaine into the perineum to deaden it in preparation for the episiotomy. The injection will affect the baby to a slight degree because the baby's head is very vascular and is very near to the point of penetration. In any case, this injection is really unnecessary if the episiotomy is given during a pushing contraction because there is a natural anesthetic action produced by the pressure of the baby's presenting part against the perineum. If this injection is not given prior to the birth, it will be given after the baby is born, so the repair of the episiotomy will not hurt. After the baby is born, the natural anesthetic action is no longer in effect.

POSTSCRIPTS ON MEDICATION

If you have questions about analgesia and anesthesia used in childbirth, ask your doctor. S/he should be willing to tell you which medications s/he prefers and why. Be sure s/he points out the risks as well as the benefits associated with each medication. Much is still not known about exactly how the fetus and/or newborn is affected by each substance, but the knowledge we do have can help doctors and parents to make the best decisions possible.

Unnecessary medication subjects the baby to unnecessary risks. Necessary medication contributes to the safety and well-being of both the mother and the baby. Parents have the responsibility to provide the baby with the best possible start in life; a flexible, informed attitude toward medication can help them make appropriate decisions regarding medication.

The choice to accept or reject medication is important; it should not be made lightly. Knowledge of the alternatives available will enable you to make an intelligent decision for whatever situation you find yourself in. In any case, effective use of breathing and relaxation techniques will make smaller doses of medication more effective than if you were as tense as the typical unprepared woman.

The Newborn

Newborn babies are sort of odd-looking little creatures. That's not to say ugly, or unappealing, just odd-looking. The babies whose pictures we see on television and in Grandma's wallet are usually 4 or 5 months old; they've had time to get it all together and present a cute little dimpled smiling face to the world. A newborn hasn't had all that time, and s/he has just finished the long and difficult trip from the uterus to the outside world. As a result s/he may look much different from what the parents expect. Many new parents have never seen a newborn until they have one of their own. Few people, except medical personnel and brand-new parents, spend much time with brand-new babies.

The enormous amounts of both physical and mental energy the mother has expended during labor and delivery are obvious. People around her can see it in both her words and her actions. The hardships of the baby's journey are sometimes overlooked, because his/

her journey is invisible to the spectators. The uterine contractions during labor exert approximately 50 pounds of pressure on the baby, and the pushing during the expulsive phase exerts nearly 100 pounds of pressure.[1] **The baby's head must even reshape itself to fit the mother's pelvic measurements during the trip down the birth canal.** Another thing to remember when you first see the infant is the tremendous adjustments s/he must make during the first minutes of life.

Amazing and awesome things happen as the baby's body starts functioning as an entity separate from the mother's. **The baby must start breathing for the first time.** This is a very big step, and requires a great deal of effort on the part of the baby. The first breaths must expand the tiny uninflated sacs of the lungs (called the alveoli); it has been estimated that the first time the baby breathes in, the effort required is five times that of the effort required for an ordinary breath.[2] In utero the fetus receives oxygen from the blood circulating through the umbilical cord and placenta. As the baby emerges, s/he receives the last oxygen from the placenta. When the umbilical cord is born, the exposure to the air causes the jelly-like substance which surrounds the vessels in the cord to expand. This expansion compresses the vessels, cutting off circulation. The baby's air passages are filled with fluid before delivery, and, in addition to expanding the alveoli, the first breaths must clear mucus from the respiratory tract. The mucus is a reminder that the baby has spent the last few months in a liquid environment. It is two or three days, possibly more, before the baby's breathing is regular because of the mucus which is accumulated in the air passages. Early breathing is typically shallow, uneven and irregular. As the baby adapts to life outside the uterus, its respiration usually ranges from 35 to 50 breaths per minute.[3] Given the facts, it is understandable that the medical personnel and parents alike are relieved when the baby starts breathing on its own.

As soon a blood circulation is cut off by the Wharton's jelly in the umbilical cord, the baby's entire circulatory system changes drastically. As the baby starts breathing, its heart must start pumping blood to the lungs to pick up oxygen for circulation throughout the body. And a major opening in the heart, the foramen ovale, must close to complete the proper separation and circulation of the blood. The newborn's pulse rate is normally between 120 and 150 beats per minute when the baby is in a moderate state of activity. The rate can drop to as low as 70-90 beats when the infant is sleeping and can go to 180 or more beats per minute when the baby cries for prolonged periods of time.[4]

Aside from these major internal adjustments, the infant must contend with its radically changed physical environment. The baby has been completely surrounded by liquid during its entire intra-uterine life. Suddenly, instead of the floating, gentle support of the amniotic fluid, the baby can feel the full effects of gravity. The baby's movements are no longer the slow graceful gestures s/he is used to; they are jerky and unpredictable. The amniotic sac and fluid have been protecting the baby from direct contact with outside stimuli for a long time. Now the protection is gone. When the pregnant woman bumped her tummy, all the fetus felt was a gentle rocking motion. Now the baby feels poking, prodding hands and rubber syringes removing mucus.

The uterine environment is warm. At birth the baby is thrust from the 98° uterus into a delivery room that is probably 25° cooler. That is a startling difference in temperature to the baby, particularly because s/he is wet. It can be compared to stepping out of a hot shower into a cold bathroom at 6 a.m. This initial change in temperature may serve to help the baby start breathing, but it is important to warm the baby immediately after birth in order to raise the temperature to normal body temperature. The baby's temperature, taken rectally, is approximately 96° at birth. It takes a while for the baby to develop temperature control, but when this control is established, the normal reading is approximately 99.6° rectally.

The inside of the uterus is a comforting darkness. Most delivery rooms are incredibly bright, and the baby's eyes are immediately assaulted by brilliant lights. This must be similar to having someone awaken you by suddenly turning on the bedroom light. The new babies can distinguish light and patterns.

The sounds heard in the womb are nothing like the sounds of the delivery room. During the pregnancy, the sounds the fetus heard had been diffused through the amniotic fluid and are "heard" as felt vibrations. Delivery rooms contain only essential equipment, have no carpeting and are quite empty. In such a "hollow" environment, sounds are magnified, not diffused. Stainless steel instruments and stainless steel surfaces combine to produce a clatter. The baby's hearing mechanisms are mature at birth and, after its first cry, the infant can hear. Hearing appears to become acute within a few days as the eustachian tubes and the middle ears become cleared of mucus.

Conversely, a sound the infant has lived with all during its life in utero, the mother's heartbeat, is gone. Experiments have indicated that newborns find the "sounds" of the mother's body to be soothing. Recordings of the sounds seem to comfort the infants. Suddenly these soothing, rhythmic sounds are replaced by sharp, loud, harsh, metallic noises.

Something else the newborn must learn to cope with is hunger. The fetus in utero is constantly nourished by the placenta through the umbilical cord. Even though the newborn doesn't need food for approximately the first 48 hours after birth, s/he may start feeling an unfamiliar gnawing in the tummy.

The infant's physical condition is evaluated by using a scale developed by Dr. Virginia Apgar. **The APGAR rating is done one minute after birth and again at five minutes after birth.** The scale is a gross evaluation of the baby's physical condition, and does not take into account physical abnormalities such as club foot or cleft palate. Five criteria of the infant's condition are rated 0, 1 or 2 points each for a total of 10 points possible. An APGAR score of 7 to 10 points indicates that the infant is in good condition; a score of 4 to 6 points signifies that the baby is in fair condition; and a score of 0 to 3 points means the baby is in extremely poor condition and that emergency measures must be taken immediately.

APGAR SCORING CHART

SIGN	0	1 point	2 points
Heart Rate	Absent	Slow (less than 100)	Over 100
Respiratory Effort	Absent	Slow, irregular	Good, crying
Muscle Tone	Limp	Some flexion of extremities	Active motion
Reflex Irritability	No response	Cry	Vigorous cry
Color	Blue, pale	Body pink, Extremities blue	Completely pink

One of the first things to strike the new parents is the small size of the newborn. Before the baby is born, the newborn-sized clothes look so tiny that it is hard to imagine that the baby could possibly be that small. Fathers-to-be, especially, are usually fascinated with the tiny clothes and frequently end up pretending the T-shirts are hand puppets. When the parents dress the baby for the first time, they realize that the same T-shirt is actually too big for the infant. It's a sobering realization. The average newborn is between 18 and 21 inches long and weighs between 7 and 8 pounds. It is not uncommon for a baby to lose up to about 10% of its weight during the first few days after birth. This weight is usually regained within the first two weeks, although it can take up to a month for a baby to gain back up to its birth weight. A baby that weighs less than 5 pounds 8 ounces at birth is classified as premature, regardless of fetal age.

Most babies do gain weight at similar rates, but remember that each baby is a unique individual. It is not important that your baby gains as much per week as your neighbor's baby does. If your baby has frequent wet diapers and a generally bright-eyed, healthy look, and is gaining weight steadily, the chances are good that s/he is getting enough to eat. The charts of weight gain and development in books and doctors' offices are abstracts of data received on children who were studied. The really useful charts give the ranges and extremes of normal, as well as the "average." It is not important that your child is right on the average. What is important is that your child is healthy. Adults come in different sizes; so do children. If you are worried about your baby's size, weight gain and health, talk to your pediatrician.

Newborns aren't the color most people think they should be, and unless parents are prepared for it, the color of the baby at birth can be frightening. The baby may be a grayish-blue or a mottled red. The skin will become pinker as the baby breathes. This change in color starts with the head and trunk, and moves to the fingers and toes last. In some cases the hands and the feet remain bluish for a longer period of time, maybe even for several days after birth. The race of the child does not affect its color at birth; all come in the same nondescript color. Some start to develop their own racial color immediately, but most will remain a very light color for at least several hours after birth.

The baby's skin may have a marbled look to it, as if s/he were cold. The skin may seem very transparent, and blood vessels can often be seen just under the surface of the skin. The skin is usually wet, and can be streaked with blood. However, large amounts of blood, especially on the baby's head (or presenting part) are usually from passing directly over the mother's episiotomy. The baby may be covered with a cheesy substance, vernix caseosa, that protected the baby's skin from the liquid environment in utero. If the baby hadn't had the protection of the vernix in the uterus, s/he would emerge looking like a prune. The vernix also acts as a lubricant as the baby passes through the birth canal. Some babies are born with dry-looking, scaly skin; this happens most frequently if the baby is postmature. The baby may have some fine, downy hairs, called lanugo, on various parts of the body. The lanugo is usually concentrated around the shoulder area and on the ears. The younger the fetus, the more of this hair will be present. It will fall out during the baby's first few weeks of life.

It is not unusual for a baby to be born with a spot that resembles a bruise mark on its back or bottom. This is called a Mongolian spot, and it has nothing to do with the form of mental retardation known as Mongolism. This spot is most often present in babies of dark-skinned or Asian races, however Caucasian babies sometimes have it. In babies of color, the spot will blend into skin tone, and in white babies it will disappear.

A few days after birth the baby's skin starts to peel, and for several days it may look something like a peeling sunburn. It's best if this skin comes off at its own rate, and that parents not add lotions or creams, nor pull it off.

The newborn's head is large in proportion to its body. The head comprises approximately ¼ of the total body length. The baby's head is composed of five large bony plates that slip together and overlap to adapt to the shape of the mother's pelvis. This molding is normal, and essential to the birth process, but it does cause some babies to have rather misshapen heads for the first few days. The bones involved do return to a normal position, and the baby will probably have a nice round little head by the end of the first month or so. This natural molding does not cause brain damage to the baby. In the case of a birth where the head is not the presenting part (such as a breech presentation) the head is not molded, but is round from the start. During the molding process, the plates close over the fontanels (the soft spots) in the baby's head. When the skull returns to normal, the soft spots are evident. The posterior fontanel is small and usually closes within several months. The larger anterior fontanel doesn't close for 18 to 24 months.

Because it is so large, and because neck muscles are not well-developed, the baby's head wobbles and must be supported for the first few months. Most babies have enough strength quite soon after birth to turn the head from one side to the other while lying down, but cannot hold it straight up. The newborn's neck is short.

Some babies are virtually bald and others have a full head of hair. The amount of hair the baby has at birth is not at all correlated with the amount of hair the child will have later. Much of this first hair, often darker than later hair color, may fall out before permanent hair comes in anyway.

The newborn baby's eyes are usually blue or a slate gray color. Permanent eye color is achieved sometime during the first six months to a year. The baby can see, but s/he has trouble with focus. Many babies appear to be cross-eyed for the first few days or weeks because muscle development is not yet balanced. As the first days go by, and as the baby becomes more interested in the outside world, s/he will try very hard to focus. With practice, hard work and muscle development on the part of the baby, soon s/he'll be able to focus well. The baby has no functioning tear glands and won't for several weeks. That doesn't mean s/he can't cry, it just means that the crying is tearless.[5]

Either at birth or shortly after the baby may develop what looks like acne. **These spots are called milia and look like little whiteheads.** They're mostly concentrated across the nose, on the chin and the forehead. They are immature oil glands and should not be tampered with; they will eventually disappear with no treatment. Trying to squeeze them can result in infection.

The baby may look like s/he has a receding chin when first born. This facilitates nursing, and will become a normal-looking chin in due time.

At birth the baby may have very long nails, and may even have scratches on the face that were self-inflicted while still in the womb. The nails reach the end of the fingertips sometime during the eighth month in utero. The baby's nails are very soft and pliable and easy to trim. Some mothers who are nervous about using scissors find it easier to just make a very small cut on the side of the nail and then peel the rest of the nail off by hand. Some mothers prefer to trim the baby's nails while the baby is sleeping.

The baby's liver is large because it has had special functions dealing with the production of blood cells. The size of the liver and other abdominal organs, coupled with weak muscles, cause the abdomen to be round and large.

Shortly after birth the umbilical cord is clamped in two places, and cut between the two clamps. The double clamping is a precaution against hemorrhage. A short length of the cord is left attached to the baby, and within 7 to 10 days this cord stump will dry up and fall off if it is kept clean and dry. The umbilical cord itself is usually approximately two feet long, but can range from very short (6 inches) to very long (70+ inches). Some doctors cut the cord as soon as the baby is born, and others wait for it to stop pulsing in the belief that the infant receives more placental blood if such a course is followed.

The external genital organs of both male and female babies are often swollen at birth because of maternal hormones of pregnancy that have passed to the baby. The swelling will disappear quite soon after birth. Little boys often have very large scrotum, and some are born with testes that have not yet descended. If this problem does not correct itself eventually, surgery can. The little boy's penis may look either larger or smaller than parents expect it to. Things will change during the first few months, so what he's got at birth is not necessarily what he'll have later!

A girl baby's clitoris may be so swollen that it looks as if she has a little penis. The swelling will recede gradually. She may have a little vaginal bleeding. This is a menstrual flow of sorts caused by estrogenic hormones from the mother's body. It is no problem, and will disappear within a very short time. Large amounts of blood from the vagina, or any blood from the rectum should be reported to the doctor.

It's not uncommon for both boys and girls to have milk in their breasts for several days after birth. This milk is caused by the same hormones that have prepared the mother's breasts for lactation. Sometimes a little of the milk may drip from the breasts, but the milk disappears within a few days and is nothing to be concerned about. In days gone by, this secretion of milk was called "witches' milk."

As with most other things, it takes time for the baby to establish regular digestion patterns, and early digestion is irregular and unpredictable. During the first couple of days, the baby excretes meconium. This is a tarry, black substance that is the waste material that the baby builds up during the pregnancy. Some of the fetal waste products are removed through the umbilical card and placenta; the meconium is what remains in the large intestine of the fetus. The newborn passes this before s/he has normal bowel movements. If the baby is cared for in the central nursery, and the mother and baby do not leave the hospital until 2 or 3 days after the birth, the parents may never see the meconium. A breastfed baby's stools will eventually be loose and yellowish. The stool contains small curds and is fairly odorless. A formula-fed baby has a firmer, darker stool that has a much stronger odor. A baby, like an adult, has a unique pattern of regularity. Some babies have very frequent stools (as often as with each feeding) while others may go as long as a week between bowel movements. Constipation is judged by the hard consistency of the stool and the difficulty with which it is passed.

Approximately 50% of all babies develop a condition within the first 24 to 36 hours called physiological jaundice. This condition is characterized by a yellowish cast to the skin and the whites of the eyes. The baby is born with an immature liver, and it takes several days for the liver to develop the capacity to handle the excretion of the red blood cells as they are destroyed. As the old red blood cells are destroyed, the red hemoglobin is changed to yellow bilirubin. In older children and adults, this bilirubin is excreted by the liver into the intestine and from there it is carried out of the body. Before the baby's liver begins processing this bilirubin adequately, it is left in the blood and causes the yellow color. If the jaundice is particularly severe, the doctor may perform tests to ascertain the exact concentration of the bilirubin in the blood. If necessary, placing the baby under bright lights ("bilities") destroys the bilirubin and helps to eliminate the jaundice.

The newborn has many natural reflexes. Medical personnel can judge the baby's normalcy by carefully observing the baby's response to certain stimuli. Some of the reflexes are to aid in feeding, and others are defense mechanisms against outside intrusions.

The baby will make sucking movements whenever anything brushes its lips. The baby sometimes starts practicing sucking as early as the seventh month of pregnancy. Some babies are born with callouses on their thumbs from sucking them in utero. This sucking reflex is what causes a newborn baby to suck on anything that comes within range.

The rooting reflex causes the baby to turn its head toward anything that touches its cheek. Later on, the lips protrude as the head turns. This is how the baby finds food. All the mother need do is brush the baby's cheek with her nipple; the baby will automatically turn its head in the appropriate direction. The rooting reflex is why it is very important not to touch both of the baby's cheeks at the same time. Don't grab the baby by both cheeks to try to guide its head toward the nipple. The poor baby just ends up confused and frustrated if handled this way.

The presence of the Moro (or startle) reflex indicates awareness of equilibrium on the part of the

infant. Any sudden stimulus, such as a loud noise or a sudden change in position, will cause the infant to draw up its legs and throw the arms out with the hands open and then draw the arms toward the body in an embracing motion. Crying is sometimes elicited. These movements are symmetrical and the Moro reflex is harder to elicit after two months of age.

The tonic neck reflex describes the position the infant takes when lying on its back. The head rotates to one side and the arm and leg on the side the baby is facing are either partially or completely extended. The limbs on the other side are flexed. This reflex is a representation of the immaturity of the newborn infant's nervous system. This reflex, also called the fencing reflex, disappears sometime between the ages of three and six months.

The Galant's (or salamander) reflex causes the trunk of the baby to curve when it is stimulated between the ribs and the hip. This reflex disappears after the second month and reappears later. This reflex exists in the adult.

If a newborn baby is held upright with its feet touching a surface, s/he will make stepping or dancing movements. This is called the stepping (or dancing) reflex and it disappears soon after birth, usually by about 6 weeks. This reflex should not be mistaken for attempts to walk and the baby should not be allowed to try to support its weight on the legs at this early age.

The grasp reflex causes the infant to grasp any object placed in its hands. The baby will grasp with such strength that s/he can support his/her own weight. The baby's foot acts the same way, and when the sole of the foot is stroked, the toes will turn down. The foot has the same strength that the hand has; it just doesn't curl enough to actually grab something. After the age of approximately two months, the baby's toes will turn upward and spread apart when the sole of the foot is stroked. This is called the Babinsky reflex. The Babinsky reflex disappears when the child is about

2 years old. An adult's toes will curl downward when the sole of the foot is stroked.

For the first few days the baby will exhibit the doll's eye reflex which causes the baby's eyes to lag behind when the head is rotated rapidly.

The baby has a gag reflex that causes the infant to gag if s/he takes more into his/her mouth than s/he can swallow.

Both the sneeze and the cough reflexes help to clear the respiratory passages of mucus and any other irritation. The baby will sneeze in response to irritation of its nose, or even in response to bright lights.

The baby will blink when s/he's subjected to bright lights. Stimulation of the eyelids, whether the baby is asleep or awake, will also cause blinking.

CIRCUMCISION

If the baby is a boy, the parents will have to decide whether to have him circumcised. Circumcision is an emotional issue and doctors who advocate circumcision advocate it vehemently and doctors who discourage circumcision discourage it with equal conviction. The doctor can provide the parents with facts supporting both sides of the argument, but the responsibility for the decision properly rests with the parents.

Circumcision is widely thought to be a simple, relatively painless operation when it is performed on the newborn. In truth the operation requires experience and meticulous technique, and the newborn certainly does not consider it painless. The circumcision area must be cared for conscientiously until the area heals. Unfortunately, serious complications resulting from circumcision are not rare. However, precise technique and comprehensive care of the area can effectively reduce the risks involved. To make the operation as safe as possible, circumcision should be delayed until at least 12 hours after birth. This period of time allows for stabilization of the infant's body temperature and thorough examination of the external genital organs in order to rule out conditions which would contraindicate circumcision. The waiting period also allows the parents time to make an informed decision if they have not considered the question previously. Many physicians perform circumcision on the second or third day of the infant's life.

It is often argued that the boy who is not circumcised at birth will undoubtedly have to be circumcised later in life when the operation is more traumatic to the individual, but it has been established that most men can avoid circumcision later in life by practicing good personal hygiene. While it is true that in terms of memory the operation makes less of an impact on a newborn than on an older male, it is not necessarily true that the procedure is less painful for the infant. In any case, studies have indicated that unless circumcision is mandatory, it should not be performed on a boy during the period of time that he is learning to identify himself as a male; generally this development takes place between the ages of 4 and 7 years.

It has been established that circumcision of the newborn is definitely linked to prevention of carcinoma of the penis. It is also true that good personal hygiene prevents carcinoma of the penis. And, in any case, penile carcinoma is not common in the United States.

Though early studies indicated that circumcision prevented cervical cancer in the female partner, continuing studies have not confirmed the earlier studies. Researchers now believe the early link may have been more related to factors such as heredity, promiscuity, and poor nutrition, for example, than to the circumcision factor of the male.

It has been claimed that circumcision prevents prostatic carcinoma; however, it is now believed that the variations in mortality from this cause between the gentile and the Jewish populations are genetic rather than directly related to circumcision.

According to urologists in the military service, circumcision appears to have some protective value in regard to venereal diseases. However, good personal hygiene may do as much to protect against problems caused by venereal disease as circumcision does.

It appears that one of the most important factors to consider when deciding whether or not to circumcise an infant is whether the father or a sibling is circumcised. Sexual identification with family members, involving "looking the same," seems to be important to psychosexual development of the child. This close identification with the male parent and siblings seems to be more important to the developing child than any peer group reaction to the appearance of the genital area.

Unless it is medically contraindicated, the infant should be circumcised if the family's religion and tradition dictate circumcision.

Those who discourage circumcision claim that circumcised men are deprived of complete sexual pleasure. This claim is unsubstantiated. Those who promote circumcision claim that circumcised men are able to maintain an erection for a longer period of time than uncircumcised men. This claim is unsubstantiated.

All in all, circumcision is not a clear-cut issue. Experts do not recommend circumcision across the board as they did a few years ago. A family tradition of good personal hygiene seems to minimize the problems associated with uncircumcised men, but it is easier for a male to keep the penis clean when he is circumcised. Parents must consider both the risks and benefits of circumcision and decide what they think is best for their son.

ACCEPTING YOUR BABY

A newborn baby has never been a baby before. S/he doesn't know what s/he is supposed to look like, how s/he's supposed to act, nor what time s/he's supposed to eat or sleep. If new parents consciously realize all of this, it will be much easier to adjust their lives to being parents. The parents' acceptance of the physical appearance of their newborn is important for the development of close parent-child bonds. Sometimes this is difficult because we live in such an appearance-conscious society and because most people expect a newborn to look like an older baby. Great changes in the baby's appearance will take place during the first few months. So even if your baby is not "cute," accept the infant without reservation and realize that s/he will change considerably by the end of the first year. Seeing many pictures and films of newborns before actually giving birth yourself can make your expectations of your baby's appearance more realistic and probably reduce any disappointment you may feel when you see the infant for the first time. The baby's first requirement is unqualified acceptance and love. The love will come after the acceptance.

Breastfeeding

In addition to choosing how to conduct the birth experience, couples can choose how to feed the baby. The method of infant feeding should be chosen with the same care and serious thought that accompanies the other intelligent decisions. The choice between the breast and the bottle should not be made lightly. Nor should it be made blindly; education is highly recommended.

Because most babies in America are bottle-fed, few women know very much about breastfeeding. Many women bottle-feed simply because their mothers, friends and neighbors bottle-feed. Breast milk, obviously the most perfect food for the human baby, is often overlooked in favor of the latest formula with the biggest advertising campaign. The formula manufacturers openly admit the superiority of breast milk with advertising slogans that tout individual products as being "closest to mother's milk." And bottle manufacturers admit the ultimate suitability of the human nipple when they design "natural-shaped" nipples. A considerable amount of money is tied up in trying to duplicate the equipment and product that human mothers already have. If the choice of breastfeeding or bottle-feeding were made entirely on economic considerations, every woman who cared about the family budget would breastfeed. All that breastfeeding requires financially is that the mother eats a nutritious diet, and she should be doing that anyway.

But the whole question is not, and cannot, be based on financial considerations. Many, many cultural and societal forces come into play. In our modern society the female breast is regarded as the ultimate representation of sexuality. It is very difficult for many people to relate the breast, a blatant symbol of sexual desire and attractiveness, to the innocence that a baby represents. It is simply a contrast in terms. Fortunately for the generations of human beings born before artificial methods of infant feeding were invented, this way of regarding the breast is a recent phenomenon. This view, and the accompanying modesty about displaying the breast, are probably the two most common objections to breastfeeding that people have (either consciously or subconsciously). Because of the sexual concept of the breast, many men do not want anyone, including the baby, to have visual or physical access to their woman's breast. These men seem to feel they have a proprietory claim to the breast that they won't relinquish even to the baby.

Again, as with childbirth, it is unfair to blame the men and women who feel this way. It is only fair to educate them. The same society that produced the Ostrich Approach to childbirth produced the decline of breastfeeding. For years little boys and girls, and some big ones, have been snickering over pictures in National Geographic of women with exposed breasts. And one certainly does not think of breastfeeding and small babies when looking at pin-up pictures. All of this is to point out where some of our culture's attitudes have led us.

Breastfeeding advocates are certainly not recommending that we remove the breast from the arena of sexuality. What they are recommending is that the original function of the breast be considered valid and accepted in the mainstream of society.

Human milk is perfectly suited to baby humans. Cow's milk is perfectly suited to baby cows. Cow's milk has large tough curds which are well-handled by the animal's multi-stomached digestive system. A human baby comes with only one stomach, and it is hard for the baby to digest the curds properly, even after the milk is diluted and heated. For the convenience of the parents, the child's difficulty in digesting the cow's milk formula may be welcomed because the large curds remain in the baby's stomach longer, and produce a feeling of fullness for the baby. This means the baby can go longer between feedings.

On the other hand, human milk is easily digested by the newborn's immature stomach, therefore it does not remain in the stomach as long. The human milk is utilized more efficiently by the baby; its contents are almost completely used in supplying the baby with the necessary nutrients. Once the milk supply is established, the communication that the frequent nursings allow the mother and baby is satisfying to both.

Another factor that is closely related to the content of each kind of milk is that of allergy. Some babies are simply allergic to cow's milk; these babies must be fed either breast milk or expensive formulas containing goat's milk or milkless formulas made with soybeans. Some babies can tolerate only human milk. Human babies are simply not allergic to human milk.

Breastfed babies usually do not need any additional source of nutrition until they are 4-6 months old. This delayed introduction of solids lessens the chance of allergic reactions to individual foods. The younger a baby is when a particular food in introduced, the more likely that s/he will exhibit some sort of allergic reaction. Delayed introduction of solid foods is a very good way to minimize allergies. Breastfeeding and late solids are especially recommended if allergies are common in the baby's family.

This first substance in the breast, colostrum, appears to be extremely important to the newborn baby. Colostrum develops in the breasts during pregnancy and remains for a day or so after the birth. It is a thick, yellowish liquid. The colostrum carries viral disease antibodies which will protect the infant from specific diseases until s/he is six months old. This immunization continues through the first six months whether or not breastfeeding is maintained past the first days of life. It is thought that colostrum may clear the infant's gastro-intestinal tract of infectious organisms. It is important to note that the baby does not receive either the immunization or the cleasing power through the placenta. The colostrum is the only source.[1]

The mother's breasts do not start producing actual milk until 24 to 72 hours after the birth. A supposed advantage of formula-feeding is that parents can rest secure in the knowledge that the baby is getting enough to eat during these early hours before the milk comes in. What they don't realize is that the baby doesn't need the milk during this period of time; s/he does very well drinking the colostrum which precedes the actual milk.

Babies who are breastfed are less likely to have diaper rash and other skin disorders than babies who are bottle-fed. Breastfed babies are also less prone to getting serious respiratory infections such as bronchitis and pneumonia.

The active sucking required of the breastfed baby promotes good facial development. Adults who were bottle-fed during the early months of life are more apt to have poorly-developed facial structures than are those who were breastfed.

One perceived advantage of bottle-feeding is that the mother can save time because she can prop the bottle up on a pillow, and let the baby eat while she goes about her household chores. So she can do two jobs at once. This advantage for the parent is a serious disadvantage for the infant. Aside from the rather obvious physical dangers of leaving the baby and the bottle alone together (particularly if the bottle is glass), there are developmental hazards. Study after study has shown that the physical, touching part of nurturing is as important to the developing human as the nourishment is. Even at its best, bottle-feeding does not provide the extensive skin-to-skin contact that breastfeeding does. At its worst (a propped bottle) it provides nothing but an improperly-placed, improperly-formed nipple filled with milk. The cuddling that a baby gets when s/he is being breastfed helps to give the infant a feeling of security. When a baby is bottle-fed, s/he should be held very close and provided with the contact that is unavoidable in breastfeeding. Bottle-feeding mothers should offer the bottle on both sides. If the mother always holds the baby in her left arm and the bottle in her right hand, the baby's eye coordination can suffer.

Now, in contrast to the above statements, it can also be established that breastfeeding can leave a mother freer to do other things during the feedings than can properly-done bottle-feeding. A breastfeeding baby can easily be held in one arm to be nursed. The baby still gets the necessary contact and cuddling, and the mother's other hand is free to hold a book, write a letter or dial the telephone. Bottle-feeding takes two hands; breastfeeding doesn't.

An apparent disadvantage to breastfeeding is that the mother is the only one who can feed her baby. During the early days this can be a bit of a burden. As the mother and baby develop a nursing relationship, and as the mother's milk supply becomes established, it becomes a natural and satisfying fact of life.

The fact that the mother is the only one who can feed the infant can be important to developing an appropriate mother-child relationship. Grandmothers and other women love to help with the new baby. These helping individuals are often much more experienced with baby care than is the new mother. It is possible for a new, inexperienced mother to feel so inadequate in caring for her own baby that she completely withdraws and allows others to assume full responsibility for the infant for as long as possible. In her eagerness to help, the helping individual gladly accepts full care of the infant. She doesn't realize that she may be actually damaging the new mother's perception of herself as a mother instead of helping her. Some helping individuals actually try to wrest the responsibility away from the mother whether she wishes to relinquish it or not.

The breastfeeding mother has a distinct advantage over bottle-feeding mothers in these sorts of situations; she is the only one who can feed the baby. Someone else can change the baby's diapers, someone else can hold the baby when s/he cries, and someone else can change the baby's clothes. Even if the more experienced people find fault (naturally in a "helpful" way) with most of the mother's caretaking skills, still the breastfeeding mother retains the sole ability to feed the child. It can be a terrific ego-builder.

It is true that the mother will probably have to contend with skepticism about breastfeeding, particularly if the helping individuals are confirmed bottle-feeders, or "didn't have enough milk" for their babies. About the only thing the new mother can do to combat the arguments supporting bottle-feeding is to continue nursing the baby and show everyone just how alert, healthy and bright-eyed the infant is. If the baby happens to be a fussy baby, it is good to point out to the helpers that the fussiness is not necessarily due to hunger. The baby may have wet pants, s/he may be cold, the blanket may be wrapped too loosely, the blanket may be wrapped too tightly, or s/he may want to be held. If the baby has frequent wet diapers, s/he is getting enough to eat. If friends and relatives get too troublesome, it is a good idea to give them a good book on breastfeeding and tell them you will continue the conversation after they've read it. It usually does the trick; and if it doesn't swing them to your side, at least it has given you a week or so to further establish your milk supply and nursing relationship with the baby. By the time the baby is 4 to 6 weeks old it will be obvious that s/he is thriving on breast milk alone, and it's very possible that the people close to you will change their attitudes about breastfeeding. And by that time your confidence will probably be built up to the point that it doesn't matter whether they hassle you or not.

The father obviously can't do the middle-of-the-night feedings for the mother (and many fathers think that this is a definite advantage to having a breastfed baby). This can seem like a disadvantage for the recovering mother, but it really needn't be. The breastfeeding mother can get up, go get the baby and pop back in bed with it. Once she's back in bed, all she has to do is help the little one find the nipple. Then the mother and the baby can snuggle up together in the cozy warmth of the blankets. If the mother is concerned about falling asleep, she can sit up in bed and lean against pillows.

This is certainly an easier, more relaxed way of feeding the baby in the middle of the night than stumbling to the kitchen and heating a bottle while the baby lets the whole world know that s/he's hungry. Babies just don't understand that it takes time to heat a bottle; and they aren't very patient creatures. Breast milk doesn't have to be heated; it is always just the right temperature for the baby's sensitive mouth.

If the mother is particularly tired, or recovering slowly from a difficult birth, the father can do the actual carrying of the baby from the cradle to the parents' bed and back again. This situation can be even more restful to the mother than listening to the baby cry while the father is heating the bottle.

Another advantage of having the milk ready at all times is that it is so easy to travel with the baby. Traveling with a bottle-fed baby can be a harrowing experience. Formula must be kept cold. Bottles must be sterilized (or at least kept spotlessly clean). Formula must be heated before the baby is fed. Unused formula must be discarded. A long car trip can entail stopping at many roadside dinners to have the bottle heated. Traveling with a breastfed baby is much easier. Whenever the baby seems hungry, all the mother need do is put him/her to breast. That's it. There's no need to stop the car. There's no need to carry a large cooler for the formula. There's no need to wonder how the bottles are going to get cleaned (or what to do if you run out of plastic liners for the other kind of bottles in the middle of the night).

On the other hand, it is difficult to go very far without the breastfed baby. A mother who is bottle-feeding can easily leave the baby with someone else while she takes short or long jaunts away from home. It is easy for her to take a day-long shopping trip and leave the baby at home. All she has to do is leave the appropriate amount of formula with the babysitter. The breastfeeding mother must make some advance preparations if she plans to leave for more than a couple of hours. She can either express breast milk and leave it in bottles for the baby, or she can have the babysitter give the baby prepared formula in her absence. Because breast milk is produced strictly on a supply and demand basis, formula should not be substituted for breast milk until the milk supply is well-established. Feeding the baby a large number of supplemental bottles would mean that the infant would eat less breast milk, consequently the breasts would produce less milk. And too long an absence would prove to be uncomfortable for the mother. Her breasts would swell with milk, and begin hurting if the baby went too many hours between feedings. With a little planning, the mother can easily arrange to make short outings. If she must make longer outings, it is easy to take the breastfed baby with her. This doesn't prove to be too inconvenient for most new mothers because many are quite reluctant to trust anyone else with the baby during the early weeks anyway.

Even if you lead a very active lifestyle, it is not necessary to rule out the possibility of breastfeeding. The human body is a marvelously adaptable mechanism. Once the milk supply is well-established, after the first couple of months, many mothers have found it possible to go back to work full time and continue to breastfeed their babies. Some of these mothers leave bottles of breast milk for the baby to drink during the day; others prefer to leave formula. Even if the mother works full-time, it is possible that the baby will not need solid foods until s/he is 4 to 6 months old.

Breastfeeding is particularly nice for these working mothers because they are able to spend their time at home feeding the baby and taking care of other things rather than preparing bottles and bottles of formula. Preparing a day's worth of formula can be time-consuming and boring, especially if the baby's doctor recommends sterilizing the bottles. A breastfeeding mother can spend this substantial amount of time enjoying the baby instead of preparing formula. Breastfeeding also gets a mother off of her feet and gives her a built-in chance to rest.

An advantage to breastfeeding that everyone can appreciate is that as long as the baby is totally breast-fed, its stools are soft and have a relatively mild odor. Breastfed babies do not get constipated. Bottle-fed babies sometimes have extremely uncomfortable, hard stools. A bottle-fed baby's bowel movement smells much more unpleasant than does a breastfed baby's. The breastfed baby's stool is often yellowish and thin. Some breastfed babies have bowel movements several times a day; some go several days between bowel movements. Both situations are entirely normal, but they may cause concern to people who have never breastfed a baby. Just remember that a breastfed baby does not get constipated.

A frequently-cited shortcoming of breastfeeding is that the mother cannot see how many ounces of milk the baby is getting. It's true that short of weighing the baby immediately before and immediately after a feeding, on a very accurate set of scales, it is impossible to determine just how much the baby has eaten. Whereas it's easy to see just how much a bottle-fed baby drinks at each feeding because the ounce markings are printed right on the side of the bottle. It's important to determine just whom this information is important to. The baby certainly doesn't care how many ounces of milk s/he drinks; all s/he cares about is whether s/he gets enough to eat. The baby's body does a great job of answering that question. However, the parents care how many ounces of milk the baby drinks. Somehow they think they can determine whether the baby is getting enough to eat by measuring formula and keeping track of how much s/he drinks at each feeding. Actually about all they can determine is whether the baby has had 8 ounces of formula, or 3 ounces or 2 ounces.

People who are overly hung-up on ounces are extremely concerned if the baby quits drinking after s/he has had only 6 ounces instead of the "goal" of 8 ounces. These parents tend to force the baby to eat the last 2 ounces whether or not s/he wants it or needs it. This can lead to overfeeding and patterns of obesity early in life. Bottle-fed babies are often heavier than are breastfed babies. On the other side of the coin, the baby could still be hungry when its ration is gone; overdependence on measuring and ounces does not allow the individuality that each baby has a right to.

Of course, it is important that the baby gets enough to eat. But the baby is the best judge of that. A breastfed baby eats until s/he is satisfied. Then s/he quits. As the baby's appetite increases, so does the milk supply. As long as the baby has frequent wet diapers and is alert and healthy-looking, the baby is getting enough to eat. This may be a hard point to get across to bottle-feeders.

Some women fear that breastfeeding will ruin the shape of their breasts. This is simply not true. The changes that take place in the breasts during pregnancy, not during lactation, are the ones that can cause sagging breasts. Good breast support, especially during the last part of pregnancy and the immediate postpartum period, can lessen the damage that pregnancy can do to the breasts. Other women are concerned that the amounts of food necessary during lactation will make them fat. Actually, most women lose weight faster when they are breastfeeding. It takes approximately 1,000 calories a day to produce the breast milk for the baby. Another advantage to the figure that breastfeeding offers is more efficient involution of the uterus. When the baby sucks at the breast, the mother's body releases oxytocin. This hormone causes the uterus to contract and return to its normal size more quickly.

Do not believe the claims that you will not get pregnant as long as you continue breastfeeding. It is true that ovulation (and menstruation) is usually suppressed as long as a woman is totally breastfeeding her baby, but don't depend on it. Even if ovulation is suppressed that long, when supplemental bottles of formula and solid foods are added to the baby's diet, ovulation will probably begin again. However, unless you really don't care if you get pregnant again, you should use some method of contraception. It is possible that you can ovulate before you have your first menstrual period; it is possible that you could get pregnant with that ovulation. Most doctors recommend not using birth control pills during lactation; it is not known what effects the hormones in the pills have on the nursing baby. And in most cases the pills inhibit the production of milk.

Some mothers (and fathers) are very concerned about how the mother can feed the baby in public. Nursing can be done very discreetly, and it is not uncommon for a mother to be nursing the baby and have people just a few feet from her unaware that the baby is eating. The choice of appropriate clothes makes it very easy to nurse discreetly. Three-piece pant suits are especially good. The mother can pull up the shell top and hold the baby over her exposed skin. The jacket or sweater helps to hide the baby and what s/he's doing. Breastfeeding is usually less obvious if the mother unbuttons her blouse from the bottom rather than from the top. Women who sew have come up with very clever darts and tucks which allow the baby easy, and hidden, access to lunch. Some patterns are available commercially for clothes that have concealed openings. A little bit of practice in front of a mirror and a couple of attempts in a secluded public place will produce a feeling of confidence that everyone really doesn't know what you are doing. This is one of those things that must be accepted on faith until you try it yourself. In most public places you will be able to find a rather quiet corner that is well-suited to a private nursing.

It is fairly easy to plan outings with the baby so s/he won't have to eat during the time you are in busy public places. It's also easy to plan appropriate places to go. Taking a nursing baby to the movies is extremely simple. It's dark in the theatre, and if the baby wants to, s/he can nurse for the whole length of the movie; the people sitting next to you probably won't have any idea what you are doing, but they will more than likely be highly impressed with what a good baby you have. Taking a bottle-fed baby to the movies could be a much less pleasant experience.

IF YOU CHOOSE TO BREASTFEED

If your doctor, hospital and pediatrician approve, you can first attempt nursing your baby on the delivery table. If you are too tired, or have been heavily medicated, you won't feel like it. If the baby is too sleepy or has too much mucus, s/he won't feel like it. However, if both of you are in good shape, it's fun to try. This early stimulation of the nipples does help the placenta detach and reduces blood loss. In addition, the colostrum that the baby gets starts a laxative action that helps to clean the meconium out of the baby's bowel tract.

If the hospital allows rooming-in, you should take advantage of the option. Demand feeding is the best way to establish a good milk supply. If the baby is rooming with you, you will be able to pick it up and nurse him/her whenever s/he seems hungry. If you cannot have rooming-in for some reason, try to get the nursery to bring you the baby for demand feedings. If that doesn't work, see whether they will let you have the baby every 3 hours instead of the customary 4 hours. The frequent nursing is important to both you and the baby. Some hospitals will defer to the pediatrician's written orders requesting a demand schedule or a 3-hour schedule; some will not. It's good to know ahead of time what the situation will be.

In any case, be sure the hospital nursery doesn't give the baby any supplementary feedings of formula. If the baby eats in the nursery, s/he won't be hungry enough to eat when you try to nurse him/her. Supplementing with formula is the most effective way to make early breastfeeding difficult. If the baby can only be brought to you every four hours, it is appropriate to let the nursery staff give the baby a little glucose water if the baby gets too upset between feedings. Of course, it is more reasonable for them to bring the baby to you and let you nurse it, but some hospitals are very inflexible.

The PKU test is done somewhere between the second and fourth day of the infant's life; it must be given after a high protein feeding. It is not necessary to give the baby formula for the PKU test—colostrum provides enough protein for the test to be accurate.[2]

If the nursing staff on the postpartum floor, or in the nursery seem unsupportive of breastfeeding, try to ignore them. It is nice to have their support and help, but not essential to breastfeeding success. To keep up your morale, take a breastfeeding book to the hospital and keep reading. It is also helpful to have personal or telephone contact with friends who have successfully breastfed. If you don't know anyone in this category, call the local chapter of La Leche League. La Leche League is an international group of breastfeeding mothers who offer information and support to each other. You need not be a member, nor know anyone in LLL to get help. An LLL mother will be happy to spend time answering your questions and offering suggestions to help in your breastfeeding efforts.

When you are first helping the baby to find the nipple, remember the rooting reflex that newborns have. Don't grab the baby by both sides of the head and try to guide its mouth to the nipple. Brush the baby's cheek lightly with the nipple and the baby will automatically turn its head in that direction. A little guidance from you will put the nipple in the appropriate place. Premature babies will probably need more help in finding the nipple.

It's important not to be discouraged if your roommate is breastfeeding her baby with great success and you seem to be getting nowhere with yours. Don't give up. It just takes some babies longer to decide to nurse. Some are eager from the start; others are not.

If you have been given pills or shots to dry up your milk supply by mistake, don't worry. Of course, it's best not to have received such medication, but it is still possible for you to go ahead with your plans to nurse. Frequent nursings will bring the milk in. By the same token, if you change your mind after you receive such medication, you can nurse successfully.

One of the best things you can do to influence success in breastfeeding is choose a pediatrician who is supportive. The pediatrician who suggests supplementing with formula, or putting the baby on a strict formula diet as soon as a problem appears is not supportive. Nor is the pediatrician who recommends the early introduction of solids. Adding formula and solid foods to the baby's diet will decrease the baby's need for your milk. That will decrease your supply of milk. Remember that most healthy, full term infants have no need of additional food until they are between 4 and 6 months old. It's hard enough for a breastfeeding mother to argue the point with bottle-feeding relatives and friends without having to fight her pediatrician, too.

The dark area around the nipple, the areola, as well as the nipple must be in the baby's mouth when s/he is nursing. If s/he just has the nipple, s/he won't get any milk. Sometimes mothers have to work with the baby a little before s/he will take the whole area into the mouth. However, do not just shove the nipple and areola into the baby's mouth. That is likely to scare the poor little thing. With practice the baby will become highly proficient.

Even though the real milk does not come in for a

while after the birth (normally between 24 and 72 hours, but sometimes as long as a week), it is important not to supplement with formula before it comes in. The milk will come in as the baby sucks out the colostrum. Supplementing will just delay your milk from coming in and necessitate further supplementation. And don't try to keep the baby on a strict schedule. It will simply frustrate both of you and probably send the whole household into an uproar. Frequent nursings is the key. Remember that the baby has a built in weight reserve of 10% to tide it over until your milk comes in.

The let-down reflex is the reflex in the mother's body that allows the milk to be released when the baby sucks. A relaxed atmosphere promotes a good let-down reflex. Tension, distraction and embarrassment all serve to inhibit the let-down reflex. During the first few weeks you should make every attempt to have things quiet and peaceful when you sit down to nurse. If you prefer to be alone, then be alone. It's common to get quite thirsty soon after the baby starts nursing, so it is a good idea to have a glass of juice, water or beer close at hand.

It doesn't matter what position you choose for nursing. Some women prefer to lie down, some prefer to sit on the sofa and some prefer to sit in a rocking chair. The important thing is that you and the baby are comfortable. As you and the baby become more proficient, the environment and position will become less and less important.

The first time that the phone rings while you are nursing and you quickly pull the baby away from the nipple, you will learn how not to detach the baby from the breast. The correct way is to insert your finger in the side of the baby's mouth to break the suction; then you can remove the nipple from the baby's mouth easily.

In order to establish and keep up your milk supply, it is important that you get an adequate amount of rest. If you can afford it, or if you have a mother or mother-in-law available, it's nice to have help the first few days after you and the baby come home from the hospital. But remember to remind the help that she is there to do the dishes, sweep the floor and dust the living room furniture. She is there to cook dinner and answer the telephone. You are there to take care of the new baby. Take advantage of the help; it is soon enough that you will again have all of these responsibilities in addition to caring for the baby. If there is no one to help you during the first couple of weeks, it is important for you to realize that the baby is more important than doing the dishes. The housekeeping will keep until the baby is a little older. To be sure that you get enough rest, you should nap when the baby does.

Because of the opposition (sometimes violent) that you may encounter from family and friends, it is a good idea to let people know ahead of time that you plan to breastfeed the baby. You may be able to get some of the problems hashed out before the baby is born that way. One drawback that this plan entails is that you may become so discouraged before you start that you doom yourself for failure. However, if you can take negative reactions as a challenge, and use them to your advantage, you'll get an extra boost. Telling people ahead of time also allows you to sort of test the waters. If it looks like you will get hassled a lot, call La Leche and get some early advice about what to say to opponents of breastfeeding.

Besides offering support to new nursing mothers, the LLL chapters in each area sponsor a series of four monthly meetings open to anyone who is interested. LLL recommends that mothers attend the meetings before the baby is born.

If the father, the grandmothers, and other interested individuals feel left out because they can't help feed the baby, let them offer the infant water in a bottle. It's a good idea to let the baby experience an artificial nipple occasionally, after the first 3 or 4 weeks, just in case an emergency arises wherein the baby must be fed from an artificial nipple. If s/he's experienced one before, s/he is more likely to take it with less trouble if it becomes necessary.

Be prepared ahead of time for the appearance of breast milk. Sometimes the early milk is mixed with colostrum and looks quite creamy, but the milk by itself is thin, bluish and watery. Bottle-feeders are prone to telling breastfeeding mothers that the breast milk is "no good" and that it isn't substantial enough to nourish the baby properly. Even mothers who have very little high quality food produce milk that is adequate to feed the baby. Mothers who have good food available (as we in America do) produce milk that is extremely nourishing. It is supposed to look thin, bluish and watery.

If things have been going along just fine and then the baby develops a rash or gas, it may be caused by something you ate. Examine your recent diet and see whether you can discover a particular spicy food. If you can discover what the food was, remove it from your diet; the gas or rash will probably go away. Wait a few weeks and try the food again to see whether it still produces the same reaction. There's no need to avoid any particular food unless it seems to bother the baby. Different foods will bother different babies. Many babies aren't bothered by any foods at all.

It is possible to freeze breast milk for up to several months in a 0° freezer. All you need do is hand express the milk into a sterile container and freeze it. To thaw it, you can hold it under warm water. La Leche League, or any book on breastfeeding, can give you more detailed information on the storage of breast milk.

If it is necessary for you to wean the baby before s/he has shown a desire to be weaned, do it as slowly as possible. It is hard on the baby to take the breast away suddenly. Mealtimes are a real source of security, especially to the breastfed baby. Give up the early morning nursing and the bedtime nursing last. If the baby is old enough, you may be able to wean directly to the cup, and avoid bottles altogether.

Leaking

Leaking breasts are fairly common, especially for the first 4 to 6 weeks while the milk supply is being established. Usually the problem can be nicely handled by inserting nursing pads in your bra. Disposable pads are available, but if you'd rather not go to that expense, you can cut 4-inch circles out of old fabric and sew several thicknesses together to make your own. Do not use plastic bra liners; they can easily cause sore, cracked nipples. If there's a possibility that a little of the milk may leak through to your outside clothing, it is a good idea to wear print fabrics or colors that won't show the wet spot. Normally if you have a nursing pad, or even a handkerchief, in your bra there's no problem.

At first many mothers experience leaking from the opposite breast when the baby starts to nurse; it's just because both breasts are letting-down at the same time. As the let-down reflex becomes more and more efficient, it's very common to let-down automatically whenever you hear a baby cry. Any baby, not just your own. A baby crying on a television show will probably do it, as will a baby crying in the supermarket. When you feel the tingling that signals the beginning of the let-down reflex, try folding your arms across your chest and pressing on the breasts. That usually takes care of it. Another time that you may leak is when you are out shopping, for instance, and you suddenly wonder whether the baby is hungry. The response your body has to verbal and thought stimuli is amazing.

Leaking does not go on forever, and some women don't experience any at all. During the early weeks it is a good idea to take a thick towel to bed with you to put under your breasts; that way you won't get the whole bed wet if you leak during the night. Leaking sounds like a worse problem than it really is; it just takes a little adjusting to.

Sore Nipples

Some women experience sore nipples, especially during the first few days of breastfeeding. Sore nipples aren't really serious, just painful. To avoid irritating the nipples do not use soap, alcohol, tincture of benzoin or petroleum jelly; use only mild preparations such as pure lanolin, Vitamin A & D cream and Masse breast cream. The nipples should be kept dry as much as possible. If you use nursing pads, either commercial or homemade, be sure to change them often. Plastic bra liners will protect your outer clothing, but they keep the nipples wet almost constantly. Expose the nipples to air and sunlight as much as you can (but take care not to get the breasts sunburned). You can use a sunlamp if you're very careful about the amount of time you expose your breasts to the lamp.

Continue to nurse the baby frequently. If you must, limit sucking time to between 8 and 10 minutes on the sore side, but try not to limit it any more than that. At each nursing, offer the baby the breast that is the least sore first. That way the baby won't suck as hard on the sore side because s/he will have at least partially satisfied the hunger pangs while nursing from the first breast. Don't let the baby play around with the nipple. Chewing is definitely out. Be sure s/he has the entire areola inside of his/her mouth.

It is helpful if you change nursing positions at each feeding. Holding the baby at different angles and sitting or lying in different positions means that pressure is not applied at the same place on the breast each time.

To ease the discomfort as the baby nurses, take an aspirin, drink a glass of wine or have a bottle of beer about 15 minutes before each feeding. These things can all help relax you and can ease the let-down reflex. Sometimes it helps if you hand-express some milk before the baby starts nursing; s/he will not have to suck so hard if you're already produced the let-down reflex. If you are having real difficulty with the let-down, talk to your doctor about prescribing some oxytocin to help you.

Engorgement

In contrast to nipple soreness, engorgement is a condition that affects the total breast. It is characterized by swollen breasts that feel very hard and are extremely tender. A common time for engorgement to take place is between 3 and 5 days after birth. The engorgement is caused by increased circulation of blood in the breast, swelling of the breast tissues and the pressure of the milk. Application of either ice packs or heat usually helps lessen the discomfort. Some women prefer the ice and some women prefer the heat. Some women find it most effective to alternate the two. Frequently a warm shower will help a great deal.

To help the baby, and make the first few pulls on the breast less painful for you, you can express some milk manually before each feeding. This relieves some of the pressure in the breast and makes it easier for the baby to get the nipple and areola in its mouth.

With engorgement, as with sore nipples, an aspirin, glass of wine or perhaps a bottle of beer a few minutes before the feeding can take the edge off of any pain and relax the mother. Be sure your bra is supportive and well-fitting; it should not be too tight.

Women who are able to demand-feed the baby from the time the baby is born are less likely to suffer from engorgement. If engorgement does occur, frequent nursings are also helpful.

Mastitis

Mastitis is a breast infection which may be produced by a clogged milk duct or possibly a staphylococcal infection. The condition should be suspected if the mother feels generally lousy, and has a fever, a headache, and engorged breasts that feel warm to the touch. If you believe you have mastitis, you should contact your doctor immediately. If caught at the beginning, the condition will not become serious. Perhaps the doctor will prescribe an antibiotic. Get off your feet as much as possible. Apply heat to the breasts with wet washcloths. Wear a supportive bra that is not too tight.

It is important to continue nursing from the affected breast. Doctors used to order women who had mastitis to discontinue nursing immediately. Now it has become evident that the breast heals more quickly and with less chance of complication if the mother continues to nurse the baby. The baby will not get sick from nursing the infected breast. If your doctor advises you to quit nursing if you get mastitis, call La Leche League and get the references for the latest articles regarding breast infection and whether or not the mother should stop nursing during the infection. Continued nursing will help clear any clogged ducts and get the milk flowing again. Offer the sore breast to the baby first at each feeding. If you do that, there is a better chance of the breast being completely emptied. As the breast is completely emptied, the clogged duct will be unclogged.

Breast Preparation

Some people feel that preparation of the breasts during late pregnancy will lessen the chances of sore nipples when nursing starts. Several things can be done to toughen the nipples. Don't use soap or anything else that tends to dry out the nipples. A simple procedure that can be especially helpful if your nipples don't protrude very far is nipple-rolling. To do it, pull the nipple out a little way with your thumb and forefinger. Then roll the nipple gently between your fingers for a couple of minutes. You can do this two or three times a day for the last few weeks of pregnancy. After your bath or shower, rub the nipples gently with a rough washcloth or towel; the cloth can be wet or dry.

Expose your nipples to air and sunlight as much as possible without sunburning them. It's a good idea to go braless occasionally to let the nipples rub against your outer clothing.

Following these hints on toughening the nipples does not guarantee that you will have no nipple soreness when you start nursing, but many women have found them to be helpful. Some women never experience any tenderness at all, even if they have not prepared the nipples ahead of time.

TO BREASTFEED SUCCESSFULLY

Determination and self-confidence are probably the two most important factors to successful breastfeeding. If you've got those two things, chances are that you and the baby can work out any minor problems you may encounter. It is very common for the self-confidence to run low in the face of criticism from bottle-feeding friends and a crying baby. Either call a breastfeeding friend or La Leche League. Very few women who really want to succeed at breastfeeding are unsuccessful.

If you don't know whether you would like breastfeeding or not, try it. It is much easier to change from breast to bottle than from bottle to breast. Even after bottle-feeding for months, it is possible to begin breastfeeding, but it is a long, hard, tedious process which takes a great deal of patience on the part of both mother and baby. So, if you are undecided about breastfeeding, go ahead and try it. You may like it, and you may not, but at least you will have tried. That will give you the basis for an educated decision.

The Postpartum Challenge

Whatever you expect life to be like after the baby is born, it probably won't be that way at all. It's fairly safe to say that no matter how well-prepared you are for the adjustments that a new baby brings, there will be additional changes that you hadn't even considered. Babies are little people, little people whose capacity for making demands is phenomenal. They demand food, love, attention, security and clean diapers. The really hard thing about meeting these demands is that they are made on a 24-hour a day basis.

Many expectant parents have heard that newborn babies sleep more than 20 hours a day. It certainly doesn't sound difficult to devote about four hours of each day to the baby that you've waited so long to have. Even if the baby does sleep that much (and that doesn't always happen) you must remember that it is the baby, not the parents, who chooses which four hours of the day will be devoted to caring for the baby. S/he really doesn't care if mother is right in the middle of fixing dinner or if it is 3 o'clock in the morning. In addition to the poor timing that babies are notorious for, sometimes they can't communicate their specific needs very well. So devoting those four hours may not be so easy as it sounds.

Postpartum is the period of time following the birth; literally it means "after the separation." For the sake of convenience, the postpartum period is often said to last until the six-week check-up. But the end of the postpartum time cannot really be so rigidly defined. In a sense, postpartum never ends because parents are constantly adjusting to new situations as their child grows older. It is true that the adjustments made during the early postpartum period are more drastic and total than those made at any other time during the child's life.

Some aspects of the postpartum experience are related directly to the physical process of childbirth and others are based more in emotional reactions to the new life situation. The physical and emotional aspects are intertwined and affect each other a great deal.

During the postpartum hospital stay, it is common for new mothers to concentrate more on the physical aspects of recovery; the emotional aspects frequently do not play a big part while the mother is still in the relatively protected environment of the hospital. Unless she has 24-hour a day rooming-in, the mother does not have to deal with the infant on such a total basis as she does at home.

Following the delivery of the placental materials, new mothers have a flow of blood called lochia. The lochia is a discharge of blood, mucus and tissue from the uterus. It is very much like a menstrual flow at first, then it gradually gets browner, then tends toward a pinkish-brown and is finally a yellowish-white or colorless discharge. The flow of lochia commonly lasts from one to six weeks following the birth. At first some rather large clots may be passed. This is fairly common, but is something you should mention to your doctor. If the lochia has begun to turn brownish, then suddenly is a bright red, you should notify your doctor.

Chances are that you have been doing too much, and s/he will suggest that you get more rest. Lochia can really be profuse, and it is a good idea to have an adequate supply of sanitary napkins waiting for you at home. Your hospital might charge you per pad for its sanitary napkins, so you may want to take some in your suitcase. Most doctors advise their patients to use napkins, rather than tampons, until the six-week checkup. Breastfeeding tends to reduce the bleeding more rapidly.

Bowel movements and urination may be difficult and/or painful for the first few days. That is not unusual. If a woman has had an episiotomy, she may be afraid of straining at stool for fear of rupturing her stitches. The doctor can prescribe a stool-softener to help get things going; if that doesn't work, a laxative will.

No matter what sort of medication is offered in the hospital, be sure that you ask what it is. Don't let the nurses get away with telling you it is "stitch medicine" or whatever; ask what the purpose of the medication is and what the name of it is. This is especially important if you are allergic to any medications. In any case, it is your legal right to know what you are being given. If you are planning to nurse, be sure that none of the pills or shots will affect your milk supply; some mothers have been given "dry up" drugs by mistake. Even if you did receive this kind of medicine, it is still possible to nurse, but it will take more work. If you are Rh−, talk with the doctor about getting your RhoGAM injection. This must be given within 72 hours of delivery. If the father of the baby or the baby is Rh−, this injection will not be necessary. Due to specific blood characteristics, some women cannot receive the RhoGAM. But if you are Rh−, and no one has said anything to you about the shot, be sure to find out why. It is too good a protection for future babies to be "forgotten."

Walking, sitting, and even turning over may be painful for the first few days. Most of this discomfort will probably be from the episiotomy stitches. If there is a great deal of swelling in the perineal area, an ice pack application may help bring it down. If the pain still persists, there are a number of things that you can do to help yourself. The hospital will have a heat lamp available that may be helpful. This same lamp can also be used very briefly on your breasts as a relief for sore nipples. The hospital will also have a sitzbath available. This is a chair with water circulating in it. You just sit down in the water and it circulates all over your perineal area and the "sitting" portion of your body. Even if you aren't having trouble with your stitches, it's a good idea to try the sitzbath as long as you have one available. It is a very soothing, relaxing experience. Warm showers and warm, shallow tub baths are good, too, in relieving discomfort from the stitches.

Some over-the-counter drugs may help, too. Perineal pads such as Tucks are placed between the sanitary napkin and your stitches and afford some relief. Local anesthetic creams and sprays are also sold over the counter and can be particularly helpful if you find that you are having trouble with urination and bowel movements. It's less expensive to have someone pick these things up at the drug store for you than to have the doctor prescribe them and they come from the hospital pharmacy.

In addition to those aids mentioned above, the doctor and nurses may be able to suggest more. Don't suffer silently. If you are hurting, let someone know. It's usually helpful to put a pillow on hard chairs; if there's not an extra pillow in your hospital room, ask the nurse for one. Once you get home, you can carry your pillow from chair to chair with you. Don't be embarrassed about it; be comfortable. If a particular chair is most comfortable for you, let other people know that you would like to sit there.

You may be given an irrigation bottle in the hospital. The nurses will have you fill it with either water or some sort of dilute antiseptic solution and irrigate the perineum every time you urinate, have a bowel movement or change your sanitary napkin. Another aspect of "peri care" is wiping from the front to the back and dropping the tissue without bringing it forward again. This prevents material from the anus from entering the vagina and urethra and causing infection.

It's common to perspire quite profusely during the first few days and nights after delivery. This is especially noticeable at night. Don't be worried about it, and don't think that you will continue to perspire that much for an indefinite period of time. Your body is merely ridding itself of excess fluids accumulated during pregnancy. You will be able to wash yourself daily at the hospital. At first the nurse may bring a basin of water for you to use in giving yourself a sponge bath; she will help you wash the hard-to-reach places. Most hospitals and doctors encourage early ambulation for maternity patients, so on the day after delivery, or maybe the second day after delivery, you will probably be allowed to walk to the shower and bathe yourself completely. If you feel like taking a bath or shower earlier than the nurses offer you the opportunity, ask someone if you can. Prepared mothers are typically more eager to get back on their feet after childbirth than the Ostrich. Hospital routines are often geared to the Ostrich patient, so let the staff know just how you feel.

The postpartum period starts in earnest when you leave the hospital. For a woman in very good condition this may be just a few hours after delivery. For a woman who had a difficult vaginal delivery or a Cesarean delivery this may be a week or more after the birth. The average hospital stay for new mothers is somewhere between 2 and 4 days after delivery. Let your doctor know how you feel and what your wishes are regarding the hospital stay. As long as you are feeling okay and you are healing well, you should be able to leave the hospital as soon as you want to. By the same token, if you don't feel like going home on the third day, let your doctor know that you would like to stay longer. Some women, particularly those who normally go to bed late and sleep late, find it very difficult to get any real rest in the hospital. Others find the stay to be very restful and wish to prolong it. Communicate with your doctor.

In order to make the most of the hospital stay, find out early about the routines and what time meals are served, etc. It can help you to adjust your own schedule to the hospital schedule.

During the hospital stay, the nurses will check the involution of the uterus quite frequently. After delivery the uterus is normally at the level of the navel. From this position it descends a little each day until it returns to its approximate prepregnant size and location. Contractions, sometimes quite strong, can be felt during this involution period. The nurses will knead your uterus to help the involution process and may show you how to knead it, too. If you go home from the hospital shortly after delivery, it is very important that you know how to determine whether the uterus is remaining hard and that everything is progressing normally. Postpartum hemorrhage is extremely dangerous.

Many mothers tend to jump back into a normal routine as soon as they get home. After a few days (or hours) they find that it is physically and emotionally impossible to live the sort of non-pregnant life they were used to just a few months before. Wearing a robe and slippers home from the hospital and not getting dressed until the baby is two or three weeks old helps to combat the tendency to overdo.

Remember that you and your body have been through a lot. It takes time and rest for you to completely recover from childbirth. This problem is compounded by the fact that the baby makes it so difficult to get the necessary rest. In this new life as parents, things must be adjusted, at least to some degree, around the demands of the baby.

Care of the baby goes on for 24 hours a day. This is really a rude awakening for some mothers. It is a fact of life for all new mothers; even if this total involvement with the baby has been foreseen by the mother, the magnitude of it doesn't really become apparent until the mother and baby leave the hospital. Few mothers are prepared for the feeling of total exhaustion that is common during the first weeks at home with the baby.

As hard as it may be to get, rest is essential for the proper recovery of the mother's physical and emotional self. A good, healthy diet, including a lot of fluids is important, particularly for the nursing mother. Plenty of roughage and fluids can help relieve possible constipation. Hemorrhoids may be a problem, particularly if they developed during pregnancy. The doctor will be able to prescribe an appropriate laxative and some sort of medicine for relief of the discomfort. A cardinal rule of the postpartum period is to nap when the baby naps. Don't use this important time to pick up the house or cook. This is an almost impossible rule to follow if you have other children, but you can use the time for some quiet activity with the older children; reading, playing guessing games or watching television are all things that the children might enjoy doing with you. Engaging in one of these quiet activities will allow you to rest as well as spend time with the children (who might be feeling left out with the arrival of a new baby).

If there's any way you can arrange it, it is a good idea to have help at home for the first few days. If there's no relative or friend available, you can hire a high school girl or boy as a "mother's helper" for very little. It is money well spent. No matter who helps you, whether it is the baby's grandmother, a friend of yours, a relative, the father or a hired mother's helper, be sure that the helper takes care of the cooking, cleaning, and household chores instead of taking care of the baby. The baby is your job. It is important to get to know the baby and how to care for it during these early days. Let the helper take charge of the older children. The prime responsibility of the helper is to give you adequate rest and adequate time to care for your new baby. If you are the sort of person who finds it hard to accept help from others, force yourself. It will be better for both you and the baby in the long run. However, if you are breastfeeding and the only helper you can find is hostile to breastfeeding, or if the only helper you can find makes you feel inadequate, the help is not worth the personal hassles involved.

If you do not have help at home, don't worry about how the house looks. The same house and dishes will be there for years; the baby will only be a baby for a very short time. It can be very difficult to close your eyes to the mess, but it's better to do that than to do too much, hemorrhage and end up back in the hospital for a few days. Some women have found delivery service for dairy products and bread to be very helpful during the early weeks.

Be selective about who visits. If you do not feel like having company, tell people that the doctor (either yours or the baby's) has ordered no visitors for the first week or two. If you do receive guests, don't try to be Super Hostess; it is just too tiring.

If you are nursing, select your clothes with that in mind. Things that open down the front or that are two-piece make nursing very easy. Positioning may be a bit of a problem for the first two or three weeks, but by the time the baby is about a month old you will probably both be fairly comfortable with each other and know which positions work best.

If you feel like there is something wrong with your physical recovery, call your doctor. Loss of appetite for an extended period of time, or a sudden increase in bleeding, passing large clots in the lochia, or a sudden bright red color in the lochia can all indicate that there may be a problem. Do not wait until your six-week check-up if you think there may be something wrong before that.

The emotional adjustments are partially due to hormonal imbalances during the postpartum period, and to the physical sensations of the body. The postpartum adjustments must be made in an intense, highly-charged atmosphere.

It's not at all uncommon for parents to have a preconceived idea of what the baby will look like and be like. If the baby does not "measure up" to these expectations, the parents can be upset about it. If the baby is the "wrong" sex, this feeling can be intensified. The parents may even feel as if the baby is not really their baby—that some mistake must have been made at the hospital because the baby they have is so different from the baby that they had expected. This is a real advantage of prepared childbirth; both parents are able to see and identify the baby from the moment of birth. This is not the case when a woman has given birth under the effects of general anesthesia. It is common for a woman who has been completely anesthetized to ask about the sex, size and condition of the baby again and again in the recovery room. The prepared woman knows about the sex, size and condition of the baby. And she knows what the baby looks like; she doesn't have to wait several hours to meet her new infant.

Despite all the talk about the "maternal instinct," love does not automatically appear at the moment of birth. After the initial excitement about the birth wears off, a mother is frequently upset about her feelings. If she does not love the baby with an overwhelming, total love she wonders what is wrong with her. There is absolutely nothing wrong with her. Love takes time to grow and develop. As the parents get to know this new little creature, they will come to love it. It is extremely important to understand this. Love is always a growing, changing process. It is not suddenly complete. This is particularly important to remember if the baby is one which has been desperately wanted. Parents who plan and hope for a baby for years are sometimes extremely upset when "parenthood" and their attitudes toward the baby do not measure up to what they had expected. As the baby grows and starts to develop a personality of its own, the love will come. When the baby is able to respond positively to the parents, s/he seems like more of a little person capable of love.

It is very common for a new mother to feel resentment toward her baby. In fact it has been said that every mother feels resentment toward her baby at one time or another; if she says she doesn't, she is lying, to herself or others. The resentment is natural and normal. The baby takes up a tremendous amount of the mother's time and energy. She no longer has time for all of the things that she did before the baby was born.

A new mother is frequently upset by her lack of expertise in caring for the baby. In the past, women learned baby care skills early in life because of the extended family living arrangements. Now it is likely that a woman's contact with her own baby is the first contact she has ever had with a small baby. The responsibility of caring for a new baby can be overwhelming, especially if the mother feels as if she doesn't know how to do things "right." Baby care is like anything else that must be learned; it just takes time and practice. The baby isn't going to be any worse off if the diaper isn't on exactly right. What really matters is the cuddling and the attention that you give the baby. By the end of the first couple of months you will have changed so many diapers and fed the baby so many times that you will probably be quite self-assured. Don't let people who are more experienced with babies than you are intimidate you. If their suggestions sound reasonable, try them, but maintain your own integrity in the situation. It is your baby.

One of the hardest things about caring for a new baby comes at the time that the baby is fed, dry, burped and still crying. It is very hard for even experienced parents to know just why the infant is crying and upset. Try everything you can think of to comfort the baby; if nothing works, realize that maybe the baby just needs to cry.

Remember that the baby's "stages" don't last very long. If the baby cries every night from 7 to 9 for no apparent reason, don't think that s/he will still be crying every night when s/he is a year old. Some parents enjoy second babies more than first babies because the parents realize consciously that each of the second baby's stages will come to an end; the first child is proof of that.

Many new mothers find that dinner time is the most

frustrating time of the day. Other adult members of the household are usually used to having dinner at a fairly consistent time. But the mother has probably had a very busy day with the baby; and the baby cares nothing about schedules and such. It does not take just good planning, it takes the planning of a genius to have dinner on the table at the "right" time every day if that time is a specific time such as 5:30 p.m. Many babies choose this time of the day to be particularly fussy. Meals that are prepared ahead of time and frozen can be a big help, but probably the biggest help is having the other people who depend on the mother be patient and helpful.

It is easy for a new mother to feel that her own validity as a person is being judged by the ability she is showing as a homemaker and mother. It is important for her to realize that she is still very important as an individual and that she has an identity apart from that of the baby and her partner. Contact with other adults can help her to maintain her own identity, and can help her grow in her new role. Adult, intelligent conversation that does not revolve entirely around the baby is important. It is important to get out and away from the house or apartment, with or without the baby, as soon as you feel like it. It's easy to take the baby, particularly the breastfed baby, in a back or front carrier and go shopping or visiting. All it takes is a little getting used to. This getting out can help you get over the feeling of being confined to the house.

It's good to get used to using babysitters early in the baby's life. It's good for both you and the baby. Your presence is important to the baby, and rightly so, but the baby should be used to being cared for by other adults as well. If some emergency calls you away for a period of time, it is less traumatic for the baby if s/he has had some experience away from you beforehand. It's understandable that you will be very concerned about leaving your baby with someone else, particularly the first few times. If you can't leave the child with someone you know well, ask friends for the names of sitters. You can also call the counselors in local high schools and you may be given the names of several students to contact.

Before you actually leave the baby with the sitter, it is a good idea to invite the sitter over for a visit. That way you can meet the sitter and watch the sitter with the baby. If you use the sitter as a mother's helper, and let him/her care for the baby some, too, you will be able to judge the person's competency in baby care. Make your first outing short; the next time you will feel more comfortable. Eventually you will find a sitter with whom you are very comfortable and in whom you have the utmost confidence.

It's also good to look into the possibility of joining (or starting) a babysitting co-op in your area. This method of child care proves to be very satisfactory for many mothers. Families exchange baby-sitting and pay one another with points or coupons rather than with money. Co-ops can be an ideal arrangement for people who don't mind caring for someone else's children occasionally. This gives you a pool of several sitters, most of whom are quite experienced with small children.

Remember that your own needs, both physical and emotional, are still important. You have a right to make demands, too. When you feel ready to venture out by yourself, do so. But don't feel pressured to do more than you really want to. Examine your own feelings and try to figure out just how you feel and what you need.

Be aware that you are not the only one who is adjusting. Everyone in the family is affected by the arrival of a new baby. The arrival necessitates the development of entirely new relationships. In addition to the original relationship between the two adults, there is now a father-child relationship and a mother-child relationship. To make things even more complicated, the father-mother relationship is probably different from the original relationship between the two adults.

Part of this change in the relationship is probably due to the sexual adjustments necessary during the postpartum period. Many, many conflicts are apparent in the early postpartum sexual relationship. It's common for the woman to be afraid of intercourse because of pain. This fear is prevalent among most women during the first few weeks, but particularly among those who have had stitches. The first time intercourse is attempted, the experience may serve to confirm the fears about pain. It is probable that the woman's vagina will not lubricate as much or as easily as before the birth. Many couples who have never had any problem with lubrication are completely taken aback by this turn of events. This lack of adequate lubrication is particularly evident in women who are nursing. It involves both postpartum hormonal balances and the trauma to the genitals that has taken place during childbirth. KY Lubricant, available over the counter, or a cream recommended by your doctor, can help the problem. The important thing is to be prepared to deal with the problem in a forthright and honest manner. The father's understanding, consideration and gentleness are exceedingly important in allaying fears.

Communication is very important for the reestablishment of the sexual relationship. The woman is sometimes very sure that the man is ready (and anxious) to resume having intercourse before she feels ready either physically or emotionally. If she goes ahead just to please the man, sex is likely to result in some problems that could have been avoided if she had discussed her feelings fully and honestly. Sometimes the father is concerned about resuming the relationship; he may be concerned about hurting the mother, or he may wonder how sex could possibly feel the same after her vagina stretched enough for the baby to get out.

Some new parents have the feeling, either consciously or subconsciously, that mothers shouldn't do "that sort of thing" and have a difficult time reestablishing the sexual relationship because of that feeling. Some new mothers (and fathers, too) associate the mother's body more closely with the baby than with the father.

Another problem that new parents have to get used to is the fear that the baby will wake up and start crying right in the middle of things. The whole sexual re-adjustment is a difficult one to make at best, and if the mother is physically exhausted, it is even more difficult. Rest and communication are important.

The father may not realize exactly why you are so tired. When he's gone all day, it is hard for him to realize just how much time and attention the baby demands of you almost constantly. Arrange to take a Saturday "off" and leave him with the baby. It will be a real eye-opener for him, and may give you a whole new lease on life. Even if you don't leave for a full day, it is important to share the baby care responsibilities with the father. The best way for a good relationship to develop between the father and the baby is for them to do things together. Don't hover while he is caring for the baby. Mothers tend to stand very close and offer a constant stream of advice as the father attempts to relate to the baby. Certainly the mother has found which things seem to work best when she is caring for the child, but unless the father asks for her advice, she's better off staying out of it. That way the father can develop his own ways of interacting with the baby. And it's quite possible that he may find some even better ways to do things!

The father is going through a lot of the same postpartum adjustments that you are. His adjustments are usually to a lesser degree, but still they are there. The father may also feel neglected and think that you are paying too much attention to the baby and not enough to him. Leaving the baby with a sitter and going out to dinner or a movie together can be really good for both of you. Do the things together that you enjoyed before the baby was born. The birth of your baby shouldn't be the end of your "together" relationship.

Many of the postpartum experiences are common to all new mothers and fathers. It is important for you both to realize this. It somehow makes things seem better when you realize that you are not the only ones experiencing the difficulty in making the adjustment from couple to family.

Many mothers find postpartum discussion groups to be helpful. Your childbirth education instructor may be able to direct you to one. If not, and if you can't find one through a nearby community college or public health facility, consider starting one yourself with the other mothers (and fathers, too, if you like) in your childbirth education class. Discussion of problems can lead to creative solutions and a feeling of support for each other.

Women who are especially concerned with weight problems may have added stress during the postpartum period. Most women lose between 10 and 20 pounds during the birth and the immediate postpartum period. That means that most women have more weight to lose after the first three or four days. For some women the rest of the weight comes off very easily; for some women the rest of the weight doesn't want to come off at all. A mother should take care to maintain an adequate, nutritious diet while her body is recovering from the stress of pregnancy and childbirth. A good program of postpartum exercise can help.

Women who are determined not to accept any medication during labor and birth are also apt to have special problems during postpartum. If such a woman does accept medication (medically-indicated or not), she may be very disappointed in herself when she looks back on the birth experience. The choice to accept medication is a personal one, and should be made surely and with no regret. If the mother does accept medication, she must realize that she cannot go back in time and make that decision over again. It does no good to fret about it after the baby is born. The best way to avoid such a dilemma during the postpartum time is to enter the labor period with an open mind. It is not reasonable to decide ahead of time that you will absolutely refuse all medications. Accept that there is no "failure" in childbirth.

Cesarean mothers sometimes have special feelings to cope with after the baby is born. It has been found that many Cesarean mothers (and fathers) are frustrated and angry that things didn't go "like they were supposed to." A mother usually feel this more intensely than the father because she may feel that the Cesarean was somehow her "fault." She may have strong feelings of failure, guilt, and disappointment. She may feel as though she is a failure as a woman because she couldn't push her baby out on her own.

The Cesarean mother may have difficulty in accepting the baby as hers. This is a fairly common feeling among all women (even those who deliver vaginally), but is especially prevalent among Cesarean mothers. The Cesarean mother has not had the feeling of "completing" the birth process. Women who were under general anesthesia at the time the operation was performed may have the most difficult time relating to their babies.

It is also quite common for a Cesarean mother to feel jealous of women who are able to deliver vaginally. Hearing about a woman's happy, satisfying, normal vaginal birth may send the Cesarean mother into a real state of depression.

Many, many Cesarean mothers feel guilty about all of the negative feelings they may be having. People tell the Cesarean mother that what is important is that she has a healthy baby. They point out that the baby is the important thing, and that it doesn't matter how the baby was born. That attitude on the part of friends and relatives can be very damaging to the Cesarean mother's self-esteem and emotional outlook.

Contact with other Cesarean mothers seems to be very effective in sorting through thoughts and bringing things into focus. Cesarean birth support groups are listed in Appendix C.

THE POSTPARTUM CHALLENGE

The postpartum period is very difficult for some and only slightly difficult for others. Everyone must make adjustments and changes when the baby comes. How easily these changes come about has to do, in part, with how well-prepared you are for the challenge of postpartum as a whole.

The tremendous isolation I feel at times makes me almost desperate. I don't know how other women feel, but I feel I must not be the only one.

I feel both childbirth and parenting are so important, not only to me personally, but to society, that we must humanize and communicate with our children.

I know a great deal is happening to my son even now psychologically, but I don't know just what is happening. I so much do not want to imprint him with something that may affect him negatively for the rest of his life. Yet at the same time I feel like I'm nothing but a caretaker, that day after day we do the same things; that there is no immediate feedback as to whether what I do is right or wrong.

I live on an emotional see-saw. I love him more than I ever loved anyone. But I hate him intensely for taking away my freedom. Sometimes I feel I have lost myself in the shuffle of trying to do the best thing for him.

Birth Day Stories

The following birth stories were written by parents. They were originally written as reports to childbirth education instructors. Even though the facts surrounding each birth are quite different, all of the reports are similar. Each of the couples seems to consider childbirth a positive, creative event that the father and mother should experience together.

A large percentage of the stories are about unusual birth situations (breech, multiple birth, Cesarean birth, etc.) because it is important for expectant couples to know that prepared childbirth techniques are useful for all labors, not just the so-called textbook labors.

RICHARD EDWARD

Born: March 11 at 3:49 a.m.
Due: March 7

Weight: 7 pounds 1 ounce
Length: 19 inches
Pregnancy #2

Our first childbirth experience is very sketchy as I was in a fog much of the time. Labor was induced with Pitocin in a glucose drip. Contractions came fast and furious. I had a block for delivery. It was nice, but I knew there must be something better.

Richard was the one that introduced the idea of "natural" childbirth. I was interested because I had heard that at our hospital fathers were not allowed to participate if they had not had any training. And we so wanted to share this experience.

Even during classes I wasn't quite sure I would be able to go through with it. March 11 at 12:45 a.m. I woke to use the bathroom. Lost mucus plug. Felt a strange excitement, sort of a disbelief. As I got back into bed, chills came. I couldn't get warm so I woke Richard at 1:10 a.m. and asked him to hold me. As soon as he touched my stomach, contractions began. They came much stronger than I expected. Deep chest breathing was all I needed to keep on top. They were 4 minutes apart and getting stronger.

At 2 a.m. I took a warm shower to relax and warm up. At 2:15 we called the neighbor to take our 3-year-old daughter. Richard called the hospital to let them know we were on our way. At 2:30 a.m. Richard took Mindia next door and I was blowing like crazy. Contractions were 60 seconds long and 3 to 4 minutes apart.

Richard came back to finish getting our things together. He was running around fixing coffee, getting dressed and checking on me all at the same time. I think he was very nervous. He told me that our labor coach guide wasn't with the goody bag. Our daughter loves to put things away and it was nowhere to be found, so I told him to forget it; if we didn't know it by now, it was too late. Besides that, I needed to get on the road.

At 2:40 a.m. we left for the hospital. Contractions were still 3 to 4 minutes apart. Blowing to control and between contractions deep breathing into my hands because my fingers were tingling. Richard drove as fast as he dared. I was wishing he'd go 200 miles an hour. Bucket seats aren't exactly the most comfortable place to have contractions.

At 3 a.m. we arrived at the hospital. The orderly that helped me in hit every corner and bump in the corridor; he must have been nervous. I signed in and rushed to the third floor. Richard disappeared to park the car. I didn't see him for what seemed an eternity.

The nurses were super and I was impossible. I felt I needed some help; the nurse said "sorry." Then I got nasty and she told me I was dilated to 7 centimeters, but that didn't even register with me. The nurse told me to use what I had learned. My doctor checked me and said I had 10 minutes. I felt a bit better knowing I only had a few more contractions to work with.

Transition made me very confused and being alone without Richard didn't make me very happy. I'm sure he would have calmed me. And made me aware of what phase I was to work with. Two nurses went to work quickly between contractions. Prepped me and gave me a glucose drip; of course, the first attempt to find a vein failed. So they worked frantically always giving me a kind reassuring word or glance. Rectal pressure was great; felt as if I were going to burst.

Took me to delivery. I didn't see Richard (he was in the Fathers' Waiting Room). I needed him. The nurse didn't know if he would be allowed in delivery. But I insisted and the next thing I knew, there he was comforting me. We were both so excited.

Then the urge to push was so overpowering, the doctor said to go ahead and I forgot how to push. I arched my back and lifted my chin. But Richard put me straight and with the following contractions I felt the baby move down. The doctor explained each step he was taking. Gave me an injection for the episiotomy.

With each push I felt more excited and was thankful that I knew how to hold air and push with my diaphragm because I was able to hold the block without even thinking about it.

On the second to last push the doctor said, "Stop" then Richard yelled, "Stop!" That was the hardest part of the whole labor and delivery. The cord was around the baby's neck. I blew like mad; it was easier after he explained the situation. Then with the next contraction the doctor said to push and there was our beautiful son. Time: 3:49 a.m. I remember Richard and I looking at each other, then together we said "Praise the Lord" and he kissed me. A warm glow of relief and exhaustion came over me.

The placenta was delivered at 3:55 a.m. The doctor was so informative. We discussed all that we had done and he told us how he enjoyed working with Lamaze parents and thanked me for being so quick. Richard was busy taking pictures of our son while the nurses were busy helping him get going. He was full of mucus so it took him a minute or two to get going strong. The doctor gave him an APGAR score of 7 at one minute and 8 at five minutes.

At 4:10 a.m. the nurse brought the baby to us. He is beautiful. The doctor congratulated us, then they took me to recovery all wrapped in warm blankets and Daddy went to the telephone.

I had a dish of gelatin and soda crackers to relieve my heartburn—had it all during pregnancy, labor and delivery but it's gone now. The nurse sat down to visit with me about Lamaze. Relaxation techniques taught in class helped when the nurse had to knead my stomach.

I felt upset for the lady groaning with pain in the labor room. I could hear her tighten up with each contraction. I wanted to help her but all I could do was pray for her.

On the way to my room Richard told me all about his conversations with our folks. I could see and feel his pride in what we had just done and in our wonderful son.

I didn't get much sleep because the IV made me uncomfortable. The nurse told me I couldn't get up for 6 hours. I asked her why. She said it was because of the medication that I had received. When I told her I had had nothing, she looked at me in disbelief.

At 8 a.m. a nurse came in to help me to the bathroom. I had to drag that IV stand along. I felt faint and barely made it back to bed. At 9:45 a.m. another nurse came to help me back to the bathroom. I was still unable to empty my bladder. The doctor decided I needed a catheter. My temperature was somewhat elevated. Catheterization wasn't bad and I felt like a new person. Soon after, my temperature came down. Richard came that afternoon and went to the nursery. I didn't go because I was still weak and tired.

Tuesday morning I woke tired and weak because I had had a bad night. They had given me two Darvon for my stitches and a sleeping pill. The room spun all night. I woke up with a hung-over feeling. But I felt so good that afternoon that I walked to the nursery twice before Richard came and once with him.

I woke at 1 a.m. Wednesday unable to sleep. I was so homesick. The nurse gave me a cup of hot cocoa. We talked about prepared childbirth and I went off to sleep. I woke again at 5 a.m. Got cleaned up, went to the sitzbath and could have spent the entire day there because it felt so good. The doctor came into my room at 9 a.m. and asked if I'd like to go home. Of course I wanted to. Our son hadn't been circumcised, so I had to wait. By the time Richard got to the hospital it was 1 p.m. The baby was ready and waiting.

I had worried needlessly about Mindia's reaction to her brother. When we walked in she was laughing and crying with excitement to see her "baby brother." She gave me a kiss and asked to hold "MY brother."

Our childbirth experience was so wonderful that it is easy for us to share it with others. A friend asked if I had stitches. She couldn't believe it because I was sitting tailor-style on the floor 5 days after delivery. She couldn't sit down for 2 weeks. Those 150 Kegel exercises each day made the difference for me. Our son is nursing to his heart's content, gaining weight, getting strong and is very alert. I feel wonderful and am enjoying both of my children and my husband. I know I wouldn't feel this good had I had medication. I was longer getting back after my first, medicated, birth.

My mother says she thinks this method of childbirth makes for better mothers and babies. I feel this experience has given me a self-satisfaction and confidence I would never have gained without it.

Richard, thanks for all your time, patience and love. I could never have gone through it without you. We thank our childbirth education instructor for all of the time and information she gave us.

EMILY ATHERTON

Born: July 7 at 4 a.m.	Weight: 6 pounds 14 ounces
Due: July 9	Length: 19½ inches
	Pregnancy #1

In November, when Rick and I found out that I was pregnant, the pro-Lamaze letters started coming from my older sister Molly. She had had a Lamaze baby the previous summer. All winter long the letters kept coming; Lamaze this and Lamaze that. By May 1, when it was time for our classes to begin, I'd almost been Lamazed to death. I'd had it up to my neck. Luckily my head still told me to give it a try, for we couldn't lose anything by going to the first class. If we didn't like it, we wouldn't have to continue. The instructor immediately made class fun, interesting and informative. I was very leary of an unmedicated birth, but she put my mind at ease by saying that Lamaze was to prepare one for labor and delivery even if a woman chose to have some sort of medication. I guess I just wasn't sure that Lamaze could really work. After our first class, Rick and I looked forward to Mondays when we could learn more about what was happening and what was to happen. Our due date wasn't until July 9, but on June 27 at my doctor's appointment I was two centimeters dilated; zero per cent effaced, but I was excited because those two centimeters had gone by completely unnoticed. The story of Emily had begun. I had some rather heavy spotting for a few hours, but nothing else happened.

On June 28 at 6:30 p.m. my mucus plug came out. Seems to me that they've really misnamed it; mine was a 3-4 inch long vein-looking, string-like particle. Luckily the instructor had told us about it or I really would have been frightened thinking that it was something essential to the baby. I was at a friend's home and called Rick and told him to put the suitcases in the car. His reaction was priceless. Being a bit nervous he said, "Why, are you having convulsions?" No, no convulsions, and seven days passed without anything else to report.

On my appointment on July 5, I was still 2 centimeters dilated, but was now 50% effaced. The doctor gave me some castor oil to take July 9 (my due date) in case nothing had happened before then. Yikes, I had only four days left. That evening the doctor's nurse called to say that he'd changed his mind. I was to drink that awful stuff on the 8th. Three days! Were we really prepared? Had we practiced enough?

Saturday, July 6 I was so sluggish that I felt like a turtle turned over on its shell. I rested all day. My stomach kept getting really hard on top. I thought that Emily was just stretching so I thought nothing of it. I did mention it to a friend and she said that I was having contractions of a sort. I wasn't feeling any of the back pressure or menstrual cramps, so I wasn't quite sure that I believed her. Connie got out the stopwatch to time my so-called contractions. All was quite discouraging because they were highly irregular and I really couldn't say for sure when I was having one.

About 10:30 on July 6 I started having the menstrual cramp feeling with a few of the contractions. We crawled into bed about 11. As soon as we went to bed, Rick fell asleep. I was too excited to sleep, so concentrated on my contractions. I couldn't believe it but they seemed to be quite regular and felt like contractions. The doctor had told us to go to the hospital when the contractions had been 5 minutes apart for one hour. I timed the contractions and they were almost exactly 5 minutes apart. At 12:20 a.m. on July 7 I realized that it had been at least 45 minutes of regular contractions at 5 minutes apart, so I woke Rick.

He woke immediately, ready to go. While he dressed, I made him a thermos of coffee. Then he drank one cup and I put on some eye-liner and polished my rings. I guess those two things were important to me. It's funny what becomes important at such an hour.

The ride to the hospital was very pleasant. My contractions were still walking-talking ones. I continued to apologize to Rick, saying that I hoped this wasn't a false alarm. He reassured me by saying that it wouldn't matter if it were false and that if I wanted to get checked at the hospital, that was fine. Occasionally I'd use slow deep chest breathing, but mostly to practice with a real-live contraction.

We got to the hospital at 1:05 a.m. I was wheeled down to the maternity ward even though I could have walked easily. The head nurse checked me. I was 4 centimeters dilated and 50% effaced, so she sent Rick to admitting. She prepped me and gave me an enema. By 1:30 a.m. Rick was back and with me in the labor room. The nurse, seeing that we were Lamaze students, said that she'd leave us alone, and to buzz if we needed anything. Another nurse popped her head in the door to ask if I was going to want a caudal. I said only if I found out later that I needed or wanted it. My contractions were 3, 4 and 5 minutes apart. I used early breathing techniques and some effleurage. Rick placed my focal points, pictures of our friends' child, Brandon, around the room. All seemed to be going quite well.

At 2:04 a.m. I experienced a popping sensation in my stomach. I gasped with excitement, told Rick and he called the nurse. Yes, my water had broken and at 2:17 a.m. I was 5 centimeters dilated and 100% effaced. My doctor was not on duty that weekend so I asked the nurse if he would be coming. She said yes, that he had asked to be called if I came into the hospital in labor. I really do think that because we were using Lamaze, that he was interested and wanted to help us do the whole thing successfully. Either that or he's always that nice to first-time mothers. I like to think that it was because of the Lamaze preparation.

At 2:30 a.m. I had to go to the bathroom. I didn't have to use a bedpan even though my water had broken because it was leaking slowly. Right after I went to the bathroom, my contractions got harder and closer. They were coming 1½ to 3½ minutes apart and were lasting about 2 minutes. I moved up to more advanced breathing and stopped the effleurage so I could concentrate totally on the breathing. By 3:10 a.m. I was in hard labor, working labor. My contractions were peaking at the beginning now so were difficult to control. I was doing very rapid breathing and my hands started tingling. I was hyperventilating and got scared. Luckily, Rick recognized this and was able to calm me right away. I got worried because I was already using the highest level of breathing and it seemed that we'd been there for a short time. So Rick called the nurse to have her check me. She said that I was 8 to 10 centimeters dilated and could push if I wanted to. I hadn't even realized that I'd wanted to push, but with that suggestion I gave it a try. I wasn't very successful, mostly because I wanted the doctor to get there before trying too hard.

The doctor finally came into the labor room at 3:30 a.m. I lifted my head and said, "Oh, you're such a beautiful sight to see." He said that I could push in the labor room or we could go right into the delivery room. I thought that the delivery room was a beautiful idea. Sounded quite good actually. Rick said that he felt that the doctor was giving us both a good looking-over to see how we were doing, to see if it was going to be all right for Rick to come into the delivery room. Apparently we were doing okay, because the doctor told Rick to follow him.

While Rick changed, they took me into the delivery room and prepared the stirrups. Having my left leg raised like that felt so good that I kept trying to put my right leg up even though they weren't ready with the right stirrup. Finally the doctor and Rick came into the room. We really had trouble with the delivery table. First it wasn't the right height for the doctor so adjustments had to be made. Then they slid a slippery plastic cloth under me and said to push with the next contraction. In pushing you are supposed to roll your pelvis forward. I'd do this and slip forward on that nasty plastic paper. I kept feeling as though I were going to slide right off the table into the doctor's lap. After a couple of attempts, I told them the problem and was allowed to scoot back on the table. Finally all was ready.

We were ready, but my mind wasn't. I had forgotten how to push. I couldn't remember at all and blurted out, "I can't remembeer how!" Thank God for a cool, well-prepared coach. Rick re-taught me, slowly and patiently. I finally got back into it and had some good pushes. The next thing I knew, Emily's head was born. I'd missed the crowning because I was concentrating on pushing correctly. We both oohed and aahed about the head and with one more good push, Emily was born. Our daughter was here. She cried immediately. After tickling her feet, the doctor announced that she got an APGAR of 9. She was beautiful; no head molding, no forcep markings. Since we were able to use the Lamaze techniques without medication, the forceps were unnecessary. The nurses cleaned her up so that the doctor could hold her up for us to get a good look at the baby we had created. A beauty, our Emily!

I'd been given an injection for the episiotomy, so the stitching didn't hurt. Rick left the room as the stitching started. It seemed to take forever because I got the shakes. The poor doctor. I was shaking so much that I was sure that he was going to sew my legs together just to keep them still. It wasn't until later that I thought that I could have been doing some breathing exercise to force myelf to relax. On the way to the recovery room, Rick met me, all smiles. We got to have Emily for about 15 minutes. I was still shaking so I could hardly hang on to her.

I've rattled on much too long now, but I get such a high whenever I tell Emily's story that I don't want to omit anything. It is definitely the most exciting experience that Rick and I have ever shared; it was total togetherness. And now we have a beautiful, healthy daughter. Two people couldn't be happier. Thanks to Molly who pestered me into giving Lamaze a try, thanks to Lamaze, but mostly, thanks to our childbirth instructor, Paula.

MARGARET KATHRYN "MEG"

Born: August 9 at 1:27 p.m.	Weight: 8 pounds 11 ounces
Due: August 3	Length: 20½"
No Regular Contractions	Pregnancy #1

From a father's point of view:

Since I called the doctor to find out the results of the pregnancy test, I was able to tell Betsy that we were going to have a baby! Looking back, I realize that I had little understanding of what it would involve. At the time I felt very happy and close to Betsy; I also thought it was fun to announce having a baby and looked forward to telling everyone. I knew from the start we were going to have a girl, and by our calculations she would be born on August 3. It didn't take long to realize I wasn't going to just sit back and wait. We decided at the beginning to have a prepared childbirth with me present through both labor and delivery. Betsy wasn't working and used her time to read many books on the subject. This allowed her to screen the books and then I could read those which were most informative. We had fun discussing our baby's development and looking at pictures as the pregnancy progressed. During the seventh month when I saw our baby moving, the prospect of being a father became suddenly real. In the meantime the never-ending game of picking a name continued with Betsy proposing and me disposing until we agreed on Margaret Kathryn.

In June we started our Lamaze classes which continued for six weeks. By this time I felt fairly confident about my knowledge of childbirth but soon found out my education had just begun. The classes met once a week and we practiced faithfully five or six days a week. Practice included a morning session of prenatal exercises before I left for work (which we both did to keep Betsy inspired) and an evening session of breathing and relaxation. At first it was a chore keeping on schedule; however, after we learned these techniques, we came to enjoy the practice sessions. They gave us a feeling of working together and of confidence in each other's ability and attitude. The six weeks went by quickly but things slowed down during the month between the classes and the baby's birth. Betsy just seemed to get rounder and rounder and our activities became more and more restricted. We went on two hospital tours and were pre-registered at the one we chose. Then August 3 came and went. Betsy had no signs that the baby's birth was imminent. The week that followed lasted forever.

On August 8 Betsy started having mild contractions in the morning. We went about our normal activities. That afternoon Betsy had a doctor's appointment but there was no indication of when the baby might come. By the time we went to bed that night the contractions were close enough together to start timing them. We called the doctor about 1 a.m.; he told us that even though the contractions were irregular, they were under 10 minutes apart, so we could go to the hospital. It was exciting that the baby was finally on the way and that the waiting had ended. After gathering the suitcase and Lamaze bag together and talking for a while, we left for the hospital. I was keeping a record of when the contractions occurred, but unlike normal labor, the contractions remained irregular throughout the entire labor. During the next few hours the contractions were easy to control with deep chest breathing. In our class we had been told to take a bag full of lollipops, cards and other items to help pass the time. However, since the contractions were irregular, we had no idea of when the next one would occur and never opened the bag. We spent most of the morning talking and began wondering if it were a false alarm. The contractions seemed to be coming less frequently, but when the nurse came in to check Betsy, we found that dilatation was continuing.

By 10 a.m. it seemed as if the contractions had almost stopped. Transition began suddenly at 11 a.m. At this stage, Betsy had a great deal of trouble controlling her breathing; I worked very hard to keep her concentrating on her focal point. At this point I realized the importance of those many weeks of practicing breathing and relaxation. Betsy did rapid breathing through the intense contractions without thinking out her actions. She followed my coaching to look at the focal point and relaxed as much as possible between contractions. The nurses were very helpful and spent time with us to keep both Betsy and me calm. Around noon the doctor arrived and examined Betsy. He found that the baby's heart rate had dropped. Betsy was moved to the delivery room so that she could have oxygen and the use of the fetal heart monitor.

While she was being cared for by the doctor and nurses, I was told to wait in the corridor outside the delivery room. The transition period had left me feeling exhausted and the rapid-fire pace with which everything was moving made me feel a little lost. Finally, a nurse told me to wash and put on the delivery room outfit. In the delivery room I found Betsy up on the table pushing when the doctor told her to do so. I was given the job of wiping off her forehead with a wet cloth. This task made me feel very useful and a part of the team. By this time Betsy had been pushing for half an hour but was making little progress in getting the baby out. The baby was turned so that the face was up, and the doctor couldn't turn it around. He decided to do a forceps delivery.

Betsy had an episiotomy and the first medicine she received since entering the hospital, a local anesthetic shot on each side of the cervix (paracervical). I remember beginning to worry when I saw the forceps.

But the next thing I knew, the baby was out! I had my little girl. She was born at 1:27 p.m. Even though the labor and delivery were a little more hectic than we had planned, we were thankful to have shared this most wonderful of experiences—the birth of our child.

ALISA VICTORIA

Born: June 2 at 7:18 a.m. **Weight: 6 pounds 10 ounces**
Due: May 21 Length: 20¼ inches
Breech Birth Pregnancy #1

On May 1 the doctor said I was "carrying the baby very well" and that the head was down in good position. On May 9 the baby was at station −1. On May 15 the baby was at station +2 and the doctor said the cervix had "changed dramatically" since May 9 and that I should deliver within a week. On May 22 the baby moved back up to station 0 and on May 30 the baby had gone all the way back up to station −2. Understandably I was getting a little discouraged. It seemed like the baby had decided to crawl back up inside and not come out at all! Later we found out that what she had done is gone back up and turned around to come down in a breech position. But we didn't know that until I was in labor.

Between May 26 and June 1 I had some very mild contractions, with no pain at all, just a tightening of the uterus. Many I would not have even been aware of had I not had my hand on my stomach. There was no regularity at all. Even though they were Braxton Hicks contractions, they were something.

During the afternoon of June 1 I began having stronger contractions, but I didn't bother timing them; they weren't very strong and they were too far apart. By 7 p.m. they were getting closer together and somewhat more regular. Between 9 p.m. and 11:30 p.m. they were 4 to 5 minutes apart and they lasted about 45 seconds. They still weren't painful and I wasn't using any breathing.

Between 11:30 p.m. and 1 a.m., I didn't time them; I was trying to go to sleep, but was too excited. Finally I dozed off about 1 a.m. and slept until 3. I woke up at 3 a.m. quite hungry so I ate some cottage cheese with taco sauce (this is not recommended as an early labor meal, but it is something I enjoy pregnant or unpregnant). Then I was too awake and the contractions were too strong to go back to sleep. From 3 a.m. until 4:30 a.m. the contractions were 5 to 7 minutes apart and quite strong; about 45 seconds in length. At about 4 a.m. I started using some slow chest breathing. At 4:30 a.m. I woke Philip because the contractions were getting too hard for me to control by myself. At first he told me to get back in bed and try to sleep so I would be rested when labor really started. Finally I convinced him that labor had started and he woke up to help me.

I was feeling very discouraged at this point and lost control of some of the contractions because I felt I couldn't be too far along in labor, and if it were this hard now, what would it be like toward the end? Philip encouraged me to use a more advanced breathing technique. I did and it helped. By 5:30 a.m. the contractions were 2 to 3 minutes apart but were only about 30 seconds long. They were short, but very hard. At 5:30 a.m. my membranes ruptured with great force. I had Philip call the doctor and he said to come right in. With each contraction after the membranes ruptured, I felt a rush of warm fluid coming out of the vagina. I assumed it was amniotic fluid, but when I got up to get dressed to go to the hospital, I discovered that it was a tarry black substance. I assumed that I had lost control of my bowel function and was very embarrassed. There was so much that I had to put a washcloth in my underwear for the ride to the hospital. On the way to the hospital I started using some transition breathing.

We arrived at the hospital a little after 6 a.m. Philip stayed for a few minutes to make sure I got settled, then had to go back home for some papers. It's part of the hassle of being in the service and having a baby at a civilian hospital. Luckily it was only a 20-minute round trip. It seemed like much longer to me.

The nurses who prepped me were not helpful in the least. They kept asking questions during contractions and were not happy about waiting for answers until the contraction was over. Then another nurse took over and said to forget the urine specimen and the enema. She filled in my chart and asked as many questions between contractions as she could. She also offered encouragement during the contractions. She was very helpful. When she asked me what I had last eaten and when, I told her about the cottage cheese, but I was afraid to admit that I had had the taco sauce on it.

After she completed my chart, she checked me. I was amazed when she told me I was almost fully dilated and at a station +2. It was very pleasant news. But she also had some unpleasant news; she said the baby was in breech position. The black, tarry substance was meconium from the baby. I felt a lot better when I learned that it was the baby's mess instead of mine!

I told her I thought I wasn't doing too well and she said I was doing beautifully, especially considering the baby's position. Until Philip returned about 6:30 a.m., she fed me ice chips and helped with pillows. When Philip got back he took over the ice chips and pillows, but the nurse stayed in the room. Philip was very patient and calm with me throughout labor, but was especially helpful at this stage. I kept saying that I just wanted to go to sleep. Earlier Philip had tapped my shoulder to help me keep my breathing rhythms on, but during transition, I didn't want him touching me at all. It was a very strange feeling. I entered transition about the time we got to the hospital, and had to handle most of it without Philip's help. I'm thankful that I had such a supportive nurse. It could have been a terrible experience if the nurses who prepped me had remained with me throughout labor.

About 6:45 the nurse told me I could push if I wanted. I still hadn't seen the doctor. I didn't particularly feel like pushing, but with each contraction I felt a warm sensation throughout my lower abdomen. After several more very hard contractions, I decided to push even though I didn't feel the urge to do so. It felt better than just using transition breathing, so from then on I pushed with each contraction. The nurse let Philip go around to the foot of the bed and see the baby when I pushed.

I was on my side the entire time in the labor room except during a couple of exams. Most of the time she checked me while I was on my side; I really appreciated it.

About 7 a.m. the doctor finally came in to check me and then they took me to the delivery room. I heard the doctor saying he wanted to talk to Philip and when I got into the delivery room they put me on my side instead of in the stirrups so I was pretty sure the doctor was going to insist upon medication even though I didn't feel the need for any. Philip told me later that he and the doctor had argued a little about who would tell me about the saddle block that the doctor wanted to give. Philip won; it was decided that he would be the one to tell me because he felt I would accept the news better from him. Just after he told me that the doctor was going to insist upon a saddle block because the baby was breech and would require some maneuvering, I had a very strong pushing contraction. No one had told me not to push so I did. Hard. I was still on my side on the delivery table, so naturally my legs weren't in the stirrups, nor my wrists in the straps. I was not draped. The doctor wasn't even at the foot of the table; my supportive nurse was, though. After the contraction I looked in the mirror and the baby's body was mostly out. The nurse was holding her and calling for the doctor. Finally the doctor got there. He gave me an episiotomy and delivered the baby's head at 7:18 a.m., just a little more than an hour after we got to the hospital.

The only medication I had had at all throughout the entire labor and delivery was the Xylocaine for the episiotomy and the stitches. Philip and I were both ecstatic. We had a brand new healthy daughter and had avoided the saddle block. She had an APGAR of 8 at 1 minute and 9 at 5 minutes.

The recovery room period was strange because I felt so terrific and the other women who came in while I was there looked and sounded miserable. I was in the recovery room for almost 5 hours because there was no room on the postpartum floor. It was a frustrating experience. When I did get to my room at about 1 p.m., I told the nurse that I wanted to go to the bathroom. She said she would get a bedpan; I said I would prefer to walk to the bathroom. But she insisted that I must stay in bed because I had had the baby less than 6 hours before then. I thought that was a little silly, particularly when the other woman in the room asked for a bedpan and the nurse told her she would not bring her a bedpan because she had delivered three days before and it was time for her to get up and walk to the bathroom. The idiocy of the whole thing astounded me. When the nurse left to get me my bedpan, I got up and went to the bathroom. When she got back with it I told her I didn't have to go to the bathroom anymore. It was difficult feeling so good in the hospital and having the nurses treat me as if I were sick. Nurses kept telling me that I was supposed to take it easy because of "the medication I had received." It upset me because it seemed to me that they could have looked at my chart and found out that I hadn't had any medication.

It was all a fantastic experience. We're so glad we were able to share it.

GABRIEL

Born: November 11 at 9:23 p.m.
Due: October 28
Cesarean Birth

Weight: 7 pounds 11 ounces
Length: 20 inches
Pregnancy # 1

It's now more than two months since my Cesarean section, and the birth of our son, Gabriel. I waited to write because I had hoped that in time my mind would become able to accept it, and I could write more clearly. But, instead, all of my memories have become clouded subconscious feelings; instead of being obsessed with the Cesarean, I am now haunted by it.

I'd like to go back to the very beginning of my basic feelings about childbirth and where they came from. But I have never been able to find the beginning. Perhaps they begin at my own birth. I vaguely remember speaking to my mother about childbirth, and being somewhat frightened of this strange pain that no one could explain. But by the time I was in college, a few of my friends were having their children "naturally" and the more I learned the less fearful I became. By the end of my pregnancy, there was nothing I wanted more than a "natural" home delivery with Philip and our friends. I wanted to be surrounded in labor and delivery by those people I love and who I know love me. But Phil constantly reminded me of the "chance" I would be taking, and refused to agree to a home delivery. So I put my heart into making my hospital delivery as natural and sensitive as possible. I read everything I could, and spent many hours talking to and pleading with doctors, nurses and even the Board of Health.

In general, my entire childbirth experience was very intense. My excitement was phenomenal! I had a part of my ego at stake, too. I knew childbirth would be painful and I also knew I had a notoriously low pain threshold. Before and even during our childbirth classes, Phil would remind me of this great contradiction. I became more and more intense about having a "drugless" delivery (for the health of the baby, but also for my own ego). I needed to prove to myself that if others could do it, so could I.

I also had this strange assumption of normalcy. Even when meconium was found in the amniotic fluid, and they put me on the fetal heart monitor, somehow a Cesarean section never crossed my mind. My only fear was of stillbirth, which now seems somewhat significant to me. Perhaps without the Cesarean section, a stillbirth might very well have been the result. So in a sense the Cesarean was certainly a blessing.

Actually, once my water was broken, labor progressed quite well, and I was surprised to see (feel) how well the techniques that we had practiced so diligently actually worked. Simple relaxation with no breathing took me quite a way, and I remember the nurses saying what a good job I was doing with my relaxing. It seemed that the need for the breathing crept up on me. I never decided consciously to start the breathing; when I needed it, it just happened. I stayed with the early breathing techniques well into the accelerated phase of labor.

Then signs of fetal stress showed that the baby needed more oxygen than he was getting. They gave me a mask and had me turn on my side. The pain increased and became almost unbearable; it forced me into using more advanced breathing techniques. Although Phil had been very important all along, it was at this point that his presence became truly significant. I was losing touch with reality; time, people, nothing around me had any significance except Phil. I couldn't bear him to leave me. He was worth more than all the drugs anyone could ever have given me. He held me. He talked to me. He took all the emotional stress from me.

Then the urge to push came and almost startled me. I thought it was too soon. So I began using the techniques to avoid pushing. I was amazed by the strength of the urge. But it seemed a very short time had passed when my doctor examined me and just said, "Okay." I didn't understand. Did that mean to go ahead and push? Yes!! I was so happy. Not only did it feel good to be able to push instead of fighting such an intense urge, but I knew it wouldn't be long; soon I'd be in the delivery room watching myself deliver my baby into the world. I would see its head, hear it cry, and feel it move out of my body. And I would hold it, and nurse it. And the three of us would be together.

After a while the happiness turned to concentration

on getting the most out of every push. I pushed unbelievably hard, and I was glad I was in such good shape. I had exercised a great deal during my pregnancy. Even the doctor said I was pushing well. It wasn't too long before I began to feel an intense rectal pressure which made it difficult to tell when contractions were beginning and ending. It caused me to grunt and groan involuntarily. I remember apologizing to the nurses for the noise I was making.

Soon there was a crowd of people around me watching for any change. With every push they would watch, and I would ask if they had seen anything. After a while I asked how much longer this would take. They reassured me that things were normal, and that it just takes a long time sometimes. But somewhere in the back of my mind, I began to feel that this wasn't the way everyone described the expulsion stage; it just didn't feel right. It felt like something was stuck. Then the pressure grew stronger and stronger. Philip would hold me between contractions. It was becoming difficult to stay in control because of the constant pressure; there were no rest periods.

The doctor checked me again, and said he might have to do a Cesarean, but since I was doing so well at pushing, he would let me go another hour. I screamed, "Another hour!" I wonder now if I had tried a squatting position, if gravity might have helped. At the time the idea of the Cesarean didn't bother me. It meant only the end in my mind; and anything to get this over was okay with me.

What happened to my dreams of birth? I look back and somehow I feel I failed. I chickened out at the end. After no drugs for all that time, I quit in the end. I had no will to go on. I only wanted the pain to go away. I couldn't understand why, if they were going to do a Cesarean, they didn't put me out, then and there. From the time the decision was definite, until I got the spinal in the operating room, it seemed like an eternity of pressure and pain. I was aware of very little that was happening, even Phil was almost nonexistent in my mind.

I do remember them taking blood, shaving me and changing my clothes, and, at Phil's insistence, pinning my cross to my hospital gown. Never have I heard Phil so insistent, so emotional; he wanted anything, but not an operation. He was afraid for my life. He didn't care about the baby. All he cared about was me. I know he wanted me to deny permission for the operation; when I did sign the papers, I could hardly control the pen. But I was gone, and totally out of control.

The worst was when Phil was gone. I felt all alone. I kept asking them to put me out, and I remember squeezing a nurse's hand during a contraction and realizing it wasn't Phil's. I never felt such relief as I did when they gave me the spinal. Usually the sight of a needle makes me cringe, but I didn't even feel it. I fell sound asleep. The doctor said I was the only patient he'd ever had that snored on the operating table. I awoke to the cry of my baby. "It's a boy! 9:23." I thought, "My, it really was a big baby. No wonder I couldn't deliver him." Somehow 23 ounces didn't sound at all right, but I couldn't figure out why. I fell asleep thinking about it. Then they brought the baby for me to see. He was red and wrinkled, and I wanted to touch him, hold him. But I couldn't. I hadn't the energy to fight, so I fell back to sleep.

The next thing I knew, I was being moved, and it hurt. But Phil was there. He said the baby was fine. He had been with the pediatrician when he did the APGAR scores of 8 at one minute and 9 at five minutes. Phil said he weighed 7 pounds 11 ounces. I was surprised and a little disappointed to find out that 9:23 was the time of day, not the baby's weight. The fact that he wasn't such a big baby made me feel all the more inadequate.

I wanted Phil to stay with me that night. It's difficult to explain why it should be so important, but I had missed his presence so greatly, that I didn't want him to leave again. He had to call the head nurse, and she refused to let him stay. She even refused to see him face to face to discuss the matter. I feel very strongly that this was total insensitivity on the part of the hospital staff.

That night was painful and lonely, filled with strangers with hypodermics loaded with Demerol forcing me to move when all I wanted was to lie flat and open a window. I was so hot I thought I would die. I'd spent 12 hours of labor in the hospital and 24 hours before that.

The next day was painful, but Phil was there early in the morning. He helped me to take my first steps. I felt like either a baby or an old lady; I'm not sure which. But certainly not like the active new mother I had dreamed of being. Soon they brought Gabriel to me to nurse. It was the most beautiful time I have ever spent! A spiritual experience beyond belief. Finally the three of us were together. Holding him was glorious. He made everything else a drop in the bucket. For two or three days I was high on my son. Phil spent every moment he could with us. Since I originally had requested 24-hour rooming-in, they brought Gabriel whenever Phil was there. Phil amazed me. He seemed so at ease with Gabriel; not at all like all the other fathers I've heard about who are afraid to hold their babies. I attribute that attitude to our being together; we were in labor, we had our baby.

Then it hit me. I had failed. I'd had a Cesarean, and more important, I'd lost control. I had become the screaming idiot I'd tried so hard to avoid being. My "drugless delivery" had become a nightmare. And worse, I would never have a chance to prove I could do it. I kept thinking, "Once a Cesarean, always a Cesarean." My ego was crushed. I felt it was my own fault. If I hadn't given up, I might have had him naturally.

I became embarrassed with the doctor. It was the most important event of my life and most of it I can't even remember. My conscious mind was no longer censoring what I shared. My greatest secrets, blurted out, involuntarily, revealing my very essence. My soul reaching out in vain, so totally vulnerable, so very alone. And the people there witnessed it all! It frightens me to know they know more about me at the birth of my child than I do. I have lost that "something" deep in the recesses of my mind and I must retrieve it in order to accept what has happened. I need to be able to talk to the doctor and the nurses. I need them to tell me what I cannot remember. But we are not close. We are not friends. To them I was just another patient. How I wish they could be my friends! If they could understand the spirituality of a birth and could respond on the same level, I feel they could be the friends I had hoped for. Maybe next time our souls will touch.

The hospital was a strange, callous place. It wore on me like sandpaper from the inside out. I ached for my freedom. I would gaze outside and cry. Visitors were my only connection with "real life." Finally, after a spinal headache and an infection in my incision, I was released from what seemed to be jail, eight days later.

Home never seemed so beautiful. The trees and the animals had never been so special. I longed to be able to hike and run through the woods again. It seemed it would never happen. Gabriel exhausted me. Phil stayed home a week and a half with me. I don't know how I could have possibly made it, if it weren't for him. He did everything for me. And I loved him for it. But every night I would cry; cry about the Cesarean. I was emotionally obsessed with my failure. I would talk to my friends about it, but they seemed to feel that I shouldn't be so upset. Intellectually I agreed. I had a healthy, beautiful, unbelievably good baby and what did it matter how he came out?

But somehow it mattered a great deal. And still does. But now, instead of obsession it's a kind of haunting. I can be doing anything, anything at all, when suddenly my mind slips back to that day, recalling things that are neatly tucked away most of the time. I have not told it all. I can't. The memories are like the misty bog; never clear, seen only in eerie patches. And still I wonder, will the haunting ever be gone? Will I ever be free enough for my heart to agree with my head about the events and their consequences of that birth day of my son, November 11? It seems now he was not delivered or borne by his mother; but taken by a stranger; a kind, good stranger, but still a stranger.

I keep hoping that the next time will be different. That somehow I'll find someone who will let me try again. And that even if I need a Cesarean, that I won't lose control, that Phil will still be there, and ideally be the one to take the baby from me.

Gabriel is awakening now, so I must stop. He brings me out of the past, back from the future, and into the present, which is always the healthiest place to be. Thank you, God, for Gabriel!

CHRISTOPHER ROBERT

Born: June 3 at 9:47 p.m.
Due: June 11
Cesarean Birth

Weight: 6 pounds 7½ ounces
Length: 18 inches
Pregnancy #2

The day began normally although I felt less energetic than usual. About 3:30 p.m. I started feeling just awful so I lay on the rug with a pillow. When David came home I told him I thought I'd be in labor soon, but had had no contractions yet. I was developing the most terrible pain in my right side and I couldn't find any comfortable position. I wondered if I were having an appendicitis attack and worried about what that might do to the baby. A few minutes later, at 4:50 p.m., I was aware of what I thought might be a contraction.

By 5:30 p.m. I was pretty sure they were real labor contractions (2 and 3 minutes apart, but very weak) so I bathed and we alerted the babysitter, then tried to call the doctor. His line was busy and we tried for an hour and a half to get him. I wasn't really too worried about such weak contractions. I put on make-up so I could be pretty for the baby. At 7:20 p.m. we called the operator to break in on his line and ended up leaving a message at a restaurant.

David insisted we leave, so I checked into the hospital at 7:40 p.m. My nurse wheeled me to my room (I couldn't walk because of the pain in my side) and helped me undress. I was annoyed with myself for feeling so bad and explained to her that I felt no pain with the contractions, but I had this ghastly pain and lump in my side that I couldn't understand. She checked me and found I was at 3 centimeters. Then we timed my contractions. They were 60 seconds long and 10 seconds from the end of one until the start of the next one. I thought it was great and anticipated a short labor. She called the doctor for instructions, and then came in with an external fetal heart monitor. David was there by then and was rubbing my back, trying to make me more comfortable.

No kind of breathing or position helped so finally I sat up tailor style and could tolerate it. The contractions began to register as pain even with deep breathing, so I tried a more advanced breathing technique. Nothing helped. The nurse checked me again at 9 p.m. and I was still at 3 centimeters. I was horrified. All that inexplicable pain for nothing. She had me lie down; it was agonizing and I lost some control of my face with every contraction although they still felt really weak. It was because I was so tired from the constant pain in my side.

At 9:05 p.m. I felt a burst of fluid and said, "There went my waters." The pain in my side immediately stopped and I said, "Oh, what a relief!" I peeked under the covers so David and I could joke about the mess I'd made and I said, "That's funny. I don't remember all that blood when my waters broke with Shane." The nurse gave a casual look and went out. I assumed she was routinely calling the doctor to warn him of quick progress.

At 9:10 a.m. the doctor walked in and I told him how nice it was for him to come while I was still at such an early stage. He smiled cheerfully and said he was on his way through to see another patient, checked me, said I was still at 3 centimeters and left. The nurse closed the door and I felt the first twinge of uneasiness. She gave me a lame excuse for doing it, and I decided to collar the doctor about it when he returned.

I didn't have to. He came back and sat down by my bed, took my hand and said, "That's not a good sign." I said, "What?" (It still hadn't registered.) He said, "All that blood." He explained that I was hemorrhaging, my membranes hadn't ruptured and that it might be a placenta previa. He hadn't detected it before because the placenta was not completely over the cervical os, it was attached to the right rim. I was surprised to find that the liquid gushing out was blood, but it didn't occur to me to be afraid.

At 9:15 p.m. the specialist that my doctor had called walked in. He sent David out while he checked me and confirmed the diagnosis of placenta previa. In an effort to speed my labor he ruptured the bag of waters. He was trying to avoid a Cesarean section. Then he put the baby on the internal heart monitor. The heartbeat jumped from 116 to 176 beats per minute during my contractions. I said, "That's bad!" He turned around and yelled to the staff, "It's a section. Get them rolling!" Then he turned to me and actually apologized for not being able to bring the baby vaginally. I told him to never mind, to just get the baby.

The next five minutes was a flurry of calm activity. An IV, a quick discussion with the anesthesiologist and a transfer to a cart. They insisted I must have sodium pentothal although I wanted to see the birth. I knew they were thinking of me, so I didn't object. I said goodbye to David and told him not to worry about me. I wondered why they were racing me down the hall. I waited outside the operating room while they asked me what I had eaten, and I signed the necessary papers. I was getting pretty dreamy in the operating room while they prepped me and took fingerprints, but I noted how quick and efficient everyone was and how concerned for me they all seemed. Someone told me they would drape me now and the sheets would feel heavy, but I only remember how warm they felt and then I passed out.

Christopher was born at 9:47 p.m. The next thing I knew, it was 3 a.m. and a nurse was saying, "Let us help you." I was vaguely aware that I had been struggling against the anesthetic. I told her I was okay and asked what kind of baby we had. They said a boy. I asked how David had taken that because I knew he'd wanted a girl; they said just fine. A hesitation. I asked if he had any defects. They said no, but that he was having trouble breathing. I thanked them for telling me, then they gave me a pain shot and I slept until 8 a.m. when David came. He told me they hadn't expected the baby to live through the night, but by some miracle, he had and now he had a 50/50 chance of living. David said that if Christopher lived, he probably would be brain-damaged, extending anywhere from being a complete vegetable to a slow learner. He had run completely out of oxygen and they didn't know how long he had been out. The specialist had started suction and mouth-to-mouth on him before he even got him to the baby table. They took twenty minutes before they could get him to breathe. He had tried to breathe inside of me and had aspirated a considerable amount of mucus, blood and amniotic fluid. He had seizures and stopped breathing every two or three minutes.

I was shocked, but knew that worrying would not help him. I felt he was getting the best care possible and that I must get strong enough to cope with whatever lay ahead.

The first day I just laid there kind of drugged from the pain shots and had my transfusions and IV. I had a nurse in attendance almost constantly. They all seemed so concerned.

The second day I was up and around. My nurses all helped me very much physically and emotionally. They were cheerful and we joked at my ability to urinate immediately after having a surgical catheter. They thought my prenatal exercises had a lot to do with it. I began to feel like a human again and felt pleasantly surprised that my incision didn't hurt nearly as badly as I thought it would.

I didn't see Christopher until the third day. I wasn't in a lot of pain, but was just too weak to walk to the nursery. When I did see him, I was blacking out and got an impression of a pale little baby that looked bald. I was more determined than ever to breastfeed him. I felt he needed every advantage he could get even though the doctors had decided I would be too weak. I guess they thought I would be strong enough to stand for hours fixing formula and sterilizing bottles. Besides, Christopher was allergic to cow's milk (he still is at 9 months) and wasn't doing well with soy formula.

The only nurse I had trouble with was the nursery nurse. She thought he would do just fine on formula because her babies did. I was weak, but found strength enough to get very firm with her. My nurse came every three hours all night to help me pump my milk for him. They called all over town to get a Nuk pacifier to retrain Christopher's sucking reflex for breastfeeding. They stayed right by me, holding his head, using the pacifier, encouraging me not to be disappointed until we taught him to nurse. When I was released from the hospital, the nurses gave me many helpful hints as to solving future trouble with breastfeeding, what to do about it if he had seizures and how soon I should expect my strength to return for housework, different activities, etc.

The only postpartum blues I had were during the first week I was home. I developed a massive abdominal infection. Never having had surgery before, I thought it was normal to have a swollen, red abdomen and take twenty minutes to turn over in bed. Four days after I went home, a stitch gave and the infection poured out. The relief was immeasurable. I saw my doctor the next day. He removed a tension stitch, prescribed massive doses of iron and gave me lots of encouragement about how well I was healing. The night after he removed the stitch, I was able to stand up straight and it was the most wonderful feeling. I didn't worry too much about Christopher, just calmly planned what to do for any level of retardation, from institutions to home care. I must say here, however, that when the doctor pronounced him normal at his one-month check-up, our floods of relief and joy can't be expressed. All of a sudden the world became sunny.

What really impressed me, on thinking back, was the total calm of my labor nurse. I remembered, with a start, that she hadn't even shaved me. She must have detected something wrong because of the lump in my side when she checked me. And I couldn't get over how quick they were—42 minutes from the start of hemorrhaging to Christopher's birth.

I was actually pleased about the abdominal infection because it proved to me that they had respected my wish to have Christopher attended to first. I did wonder why they had insisted on general anesthesia. My doctor explained that I was in physical shock at the time and if I hadn't passed out I stood a good chance of dying of the additional shock of seeing the baby's condition and all of the emergency work over him. He explained every question I had, even how much blood I lost. I look at Christopher now, developing normally, and think of those few minutes packed with quick action. I remember that even during all the drama, they talked to me, smiled at me and explained things to me. I feel even now that they were intent on saving two human beings rather than just preventing two undesirable statistics.

JOSEPH DONALD

Born: February 22
Due: February 5
Cesarean Birth

Weight: 8 pounds 12 ounces
Length: 20 inches
Pregnancy #1

Our first birth experience was the culmination of four years of trying to have a child. When I finally became pregnant, the joy was indescribable. I was convinced that being pregnant was the epitome of all that was good and beautiful. Consequently, my birth expectations were very high; I truly looked forward to giving birth and actually welcomed every aspect of the process of birth. In joyful anticipation of our baby's birth, Joe and I attended childbirth education classes and listened intently, enjoying each moment and learning as much as we could about pregnancy, birth and postpartum adjustment. Neither of us was apprehensive; we just knew that we could look forward to our desperately wanted baby. We knew there would be no complication to mar this beautiful experience.

When I was 2½ weeks overdue, I finally felt my first real labor contraction at 8:30 p.m. We were thrilled; here was the moment. Now was the time for us to finally share the most precious of all gifts—giving birth to a child. As the first stage of labor progressed, we prepared to go to the hospital. Joe timed my contractions, I did my breathing. When the contractions were 5 to 6 minutes apart, I called my doctor. Time to go! I walked into the nursery, looked around, and thought about how wonderful it would be to watch our child grow and what a beautiful family we would be.

As labor progressed, I reminisced about the four years of waiting. Four years of not ever really believing I'd have a child. Now we were eagerly anticipating our baby's birth, thanking God for this generous opportunity.

All during the night we were together—laboring, breathing, concentrating on this enormous "job" of birth. Joe was my needed strength. He encouraged me when I couldn't seem to breathe just right, coached me when the strength of a contraction overpowered me, supported me every second, helped me as no one else could.

At 6:30 a.m. my doctor came; this was really it! With the next contraction I could push! I pushed and pushed and pushed with every ounce of strength.

Two hours later, I was still there, in that labor room, pushing. We began to realize that something was wrong. Why hadn't the baby's head come down? After x-rays, we were told that the baby was too big for my pelvis, and that a Cesarean delivery must be done.

The shock of that moment (three years ago) has never gone away. Joe and I were crushed. Why? What was going to happen? What is a Cesarean? As I laid there, trying to gather strength, trying to take this in, I desperately tried to remember what had been said about Cesarean birth at our childbirth class. Suddenly I realized that nothing had been said. No information had been given. We had received absolutely no preparation. If we ever needed some knowledge, it was now and none was available. How could this happen, how could a childbirth education class ignore what was inevitable for us—a Cesarean birth? Consequently we felt alone, totally ignorant and completely frustrated. I desperately wanted the contractions to go away now; I suddenly realized the fruitlessness of my trying to cope.

Joe was told he could not go into the operating room, but at that moment his main concern was for me. He looked terrified for me; he wanted my pain to go away; he just wanted it over with. I turned toward him and I will never forget the look of absolute helplessness on his face. He looked beaten; what we wanted to share so much was so abruptly taken away, and we could not do one thing to change it. How sad we felt to be separated when we both most needed to be together. The coldness of that few minutes was so cruel. If I had to have a Cesarean, if the baby was in trouble, or if I was in trouble, then we both needed Joe and he needed us. Joe and I conceived this child and we should have shared in our baby's birth.

We had a beautiful 8 pound, 12 ounce boy. We were both thrilled, very happy, and thankful that all had gone well. Finally we had the child we had wanted so much; what a precious gift we had.

Since then I have had another, planned, Cesarean birth—and we have another boy. Joe and I were separated for the birth, but at least I was more prepared the second time. I knew what would be happening and consequently it was a better experience, but still not completely positive. I look forward to the next time because I know it will be a shared birth. Joe will be there. He felt alone, and not a part of his children's births. He shouldn't have to wait outside in the Fathers' Waiting Room if he wants to be with me. Cesarean couples need each other.

ETHAN PAUL and ANNE MARIE

Born: December 1
Due: November 25
Multiple Birth
Pregnancy #3

Ethan Paul	Anne Marie
Weight: 7 pounds 15 ounces	Weight: 7 pounds 1 ounce
Length: 21 inches	Length: 20 inches

I became interested in prepared childbirth classes because learning to relax and breathe properly seemed to me to be the important necessities I lacked during my two previous labors.

My first pregnancy ended with a rather short (5 working hours), but hard, labor. It was not a prepared birth and I really felt scared, I received a caudal 45 minutes prior to the delivery of our first beautiful, healthy baby boy. He was 7 pounds 11 ounces.

My second pregnancy ended with even a shorter labor (4 hours). I received an epidural 30 minutes after being admitted to the hospital and had quite a comfortable delivery and our second beautiful, healthy baby boy was born. He was 8 pounds 8 ounces.

On December 1 at 5:30 a.m., after a solid night of comfortable sleep, I awoke to go to the bathroom and discovered my amniotic fluid was leaking. I had no pains, but thought it best to tell my husband and prepare ourselves for the trip to the hospital due to my rather short labors of the past.

By 6:30 a.m. I had established labor with contractions less than 5 minutes apart and began deep chest breathing which seemed to help. We were on our 11-mile trip to the hospital and the contractions began coming every two minutes and were approximately 45 seconds long. During the drive to the hospital I was using a more advanced breathing technique which helped somewhat even though I was beginning to find difficulty concentrating and staying in control.

By 7:15 a.m. I was in the labor room and they began to prep me and upon examination the doctor learned I was 8 centimeters dilated. Terry was waiting to be permitted in the labor room to assist me. At this time the contractions were very strong and close, and I'm afraid I wasn't timing them. When they were through prepping me at 7:30 a.m., I was fully dilated and on my way to the delivery room. At this point I felt out of control, tense, but breathing every technique that came to mind. I asked the nurse for medication, but she encouraged me to go on and I did. I pushed three times and our baby boy's head was born. One more push and he was completely born. I had the feeling of elation I never experienced with my other two births and I find it difficult to describe the emotions that I had at that time.

Then the news—the doctor began examining my uterus and stated, "I think there is something else there—I think it's a leg!" He called for another doctor and they agreed that there was another baby to be born. The baby was very high in my uterus, lying in a transverse presentation. The amniotic sac had not been broken. The doctors said they would have to put me to sleep They turned the baby and our beautiful baby girl was born head first at 8:04 a.m.

All this time Terry was unaware of what was going on and was still waiting to assist me in labor. They wheeled me from the delivery room with our babies in my arms and I awoke with my husband looking down in a state of shock!

I am very pleased that we took the childbirth education classes, even though the labor and births were so quick and strong. I feel it would take quite an exceptionally prepared woman to have maintained control throughout this kind of a birth. I was very disappointed that Terry was not with me because his words of encouragement on the drive to the hospital were very reassuring. He was very skeptical of the Lamaze approach, but from the beginning, until I left him for the labor room, I was amazed at his encouragement and recall of the methods to assist me.

I do recommend that all women should be prepared for the birth of her children. I am sure, especially with the first child, that it can be a less painful and more rewarding method of birth.

SHELLY

Born: October 14 at 8:42 p.m.
Due: October 15
Induced Labor

Weight: 6 pounds 14 ounces
Length: 19½ inches
Pregnancy #1

We became interested in childbirth preparation classes through experiences of friends of ours. We decided to take the classes for our own knowledge and then to use whatever portion was appropriate to our situation at the time of our baby's birth.

The pre-labor stage started sometime on Saturday in a very mild way. At the time I didn't recognize it as that; it merely felt to me like I had sore muscles in and around the pelvic floor (similar to sore muscles from exercises or a new sport). In looking back, I realize this slightly achy feeling was the beginning of the dilatation process. This feeling was not really uncomfortable, and we went about all our regular activities on Saturday and Sunday. I had felt no contractions, but I did pack my suitcase on Sunday because the due date was Tuesday.

On Monday morning, I had the same feeling of "sore muscles," and doing pelvic rock now and then relieved it somewhat. Tom went off to school as usual; I did some vacuuming and house cleaning and washed some baby things.

At 2:30 p.m. I went to the doctor's office for my regular prenatal visit. The doctor asked if I'd been having any contractions. I replied that I'd only noticed the irregular Braxton Hicks contractions, but that I'd been having a rather strange feeling in the lower abdomen and pelvic floor.

The doctor gave me a pelvic examination and then announced that I was 3 centimeters dilated. He explained that it is rather unusual with a first pregnancy to reach that stage without experiencing any contractions.

He gave me two tablets of buccal pitocin to see if these would establish contractions. I sat in the examining room sucking on the tablets for about a half an hour. Now and then the doctor would come in and check for contractions. He said that the tablets were getting the contractions started. They seemed very vague to me, and I couldn't tell very well when I was actually having one.

My doctor explained that the baby was in the proper position for labor and everything else was fine. He felt I would probably start having regular contractions late that night or the next morning if left on my own. He said he planned to induce labor for another patient that evening, and if I wanted to go ahead, he would do the same for me. We had impatiently been waiting for the baby's arrival, so I agreed to go ahead. He told me to be at the hospital by 5 p.m. and that we could expect our baby to arrive by 11 p.m.

I drove home from the doctor's office and began packing the Lamaze goody bag that I had been sure we wouldn't need for another week. When Tom got home from school at about 4:15, I asked him, "Are you ready to go have a baby?" It was very exciting to think that the long-awaited time had finally come.

At about 5 p.m. we got to the hospital. I was taken to the maternity wing while Tom parked the car and went to the admitting office. In the labor room, I was given a partial prep and an enema; the enema felt like a 20-minute attack of flu, but after that I felt fine. The nurse checked me and said I was about 3 centimeters dilated. She said I was carrying the baby very low and would probably have to resist the urge to push later. Next the nurse hooked up a regular IV bottle and another IV bottle of a solution containing pitocin—that was referred to as "the drip." She very painlessly inserted the two needles on the back side of my wrist and taped them in place; this set-up fortunately didn't interfere with any of the techniques to be used. The pit drip started at 5:40 p.m., and then Tom was allowed in the labor room.

Within 10 minutes, I began to feel contractions. I felt the contraction very low in the pelvic floor and toward the back; then gradually and lightly I felt it across the upper abdomen. Tom started to time them, but I was still barely able to tell when one started and stopped. They were somewhat irregular at first, but by 6:30 p.m. they were coming about every 2 minutes and lasting about 30 seconds. Tom kept checking me for relaxation. I didn't need to use any of the breathing techniques yet.

At 6:40 p.m. the doctor checked me. I was still at about 3 centimeters, but he said the contractions were coming along fine. After an hour in the labor room, Tom and I felt almost funny that everything was still so easy. I think we were expecting it to be harder by then. The contractions continued at 2-minute intervals lasting 30 seconds; I felt very comfortable with them and still only needed to relax. I was beginning to experience some discomfort in my back, but changing positions seemed to help.

At 7:20 p.m. the nurse checked me and announced that I was 4 centimeters dilated which didn't seem to us like very much progress after about 1½ hours. Then the doctor came in and asked if any of my contractions had been "toe-curlers." When I said no, he laughed and indicated that things would probably change fast now because he felt at this point it would be advisable to rupture the membranes.

At 7:30 p.m. he ruptured the membranes. This procedure was not uncomfortable, but I found it helpful to relax and use slow breathing while it was being done. Within 5 minutes the contractions began to lengthen out to 45 seconds or 50 seconds. By 7:40 p.m. the intensity of the contractions had increased to the point that I felt it was really necessary to start using the breathing techniques.

At 7:45 p.m. I switched to more advanced breathing for the peaks of the contractions. They were coming every 2 minutes and lasting about 50 seconds. I concentrated very hard on the focal point picture, but the back labor which had started about an hour before was getting to be quite uncomfortable. I tried using effleurage, but soon quit because the baby had moved so far down that effleurage felt very strange.

I was starting to get worried because the contractions were getting so much stronger so quickly; and the peaks were coming at the beginning of each and that made them seem more intense. I wondered how much harder they would be to handle soon. The saying, "take one contraction at a time" was especially in my mind at this time, and that helped a great deal.

At 7:50 p.m. the back pain was getting to be extremely strong, so we started to use counter-pressure. I was on my side and just as a contraction was about to start, I would signal Tom to start the counter-pressure. We would keep that going good and hard for the length of the contraction and that made me feel a lot better. It was only the counter-pressure that made the back pain manageable. I think this must have been transition.

It was about 8:05 p.m. when the feeling of the contractions suddenly changed, and I suppose that this change must have been the urge to push. I had the feeling that the baby was coming at any second and told Tom; he went to call the nurse. Tom had been able to feel the baby's head "like a baseball banging against the spine" while he had been doing the counter-pressure; he said it felt exactly like it was described in class. We knew that things were happening fast even though we expected transition to last much longer. It was important here to remember to believe what you feel; evidently the induced labor had shortened and concentrated the various stages.

At 8:07 p.m. the nurse checked me and announced with surprise that I was fully dilated and could start to push. I began to do labor-room pushing then, and it really felt good to work with the urge. I worked with pushing for about 5 minutes in the labor room. Meanwhile I heard the doctor telling Tom to gown for delivery. I was surprised to hear Tom say okay, because we had discussed this, and Tom had decided he would prefer to be in the labor room only.

About 8:15 p.m. I was taken into the delivery room. It was quite surprising to find that the strange position in the stirrups was very comfortable. The doctor administered a local anesthetic, and I couldn't really tell when he did the episiotomy because I avoided looking in the mirror.

The nurse showed Tom how to lift me to help push during contractions. We had not yet covered delivery-room pushing techniques in our classes, so we had to just go ahead as with labor-room pushing which we had learned about 5 days earlier. The pushing was not uncomfortable; it was hard work, but gave me the feeling of doing something very active.

During each contraction, there was time for about 3 pushes. I kept asking, "Is it almost there?" Tom kept reassuring me and saying that everything was fine and that we were almost there. It wasn't that I was uncomfortable; I was just so excited at this point. In the mirror I could begin to see the baby's head.

I felt somewhat clumsy about the pushing efforts, but after about 8 or 10 contractions as I was lifted forward pushing, I suddenly saw her little head emerge. The doctor suctioned out her nose and mouth; then her little body just seemed to slide out into the doctor's hands without any more pushing, and we heard her begin to scream lustily at 8:42 p.m.

Tom and I laughed and shouted as we looked at that amazing little creature. We could hardly believe things had gone so well and she was here. Shelly was checked over, put in the little cart, was wheeled off to the nursery after they had let me touch her.

I was not able to tell when the placenta was expelled. Next the doctor started to do the stitching; this took longer than expected because the baby's head had bruised some internal structures during delivery. It probably would have been more comfortable if I had remembered to relax during the repair, but I was still so excited.

When Shelly was about an hour old, they brought her to us in the recovery room, and we got to hold her and look at her and she nursed for the first time.

Tom's being with me and helping me the whole time meant something to me that I can never begin to explain; I wouldn't want to do it any other way. We both feel that this kind of shared experience and immediate close contact with the baby gives parenthood an especially warm and meaningful start.

AMI MICHELE

Born: July 14 at 7:55 p.m.
Due: July 23
Precipitous Birth

Weight: 7 pounds 10 ounces
Length: 21 inches
Pregnancy #2

On July 2 my doctor told me I was dilated to 3 centimeters and that delivery would "undoubtedly" be within a week. Ha. A week later I was dilated to 4 centimeters and the doctor recommended an induction because he said when the baby came it could come fast and that it would be more comfortable for me if I were in the hospital when I went into transition instead of in the car on the way to the hospital. We set up the induction for July 12, but on July 11 we cancelled the induction because we felt the child would come when it was supposed to come. The doctor agreed with us fully, and reiterated that it was only for my own comfort that he had recommended the procedure in the first place.

During the 12 days between the time the doctor told me I was at 3 centimeters and the time I delivered, I had painless Braxton Hicks contractions that would come and go. Finally two days before delivery there was a tiny bit of cramping with the tightening of the uterus, but no pain.

Sunday, July 14 was a lovely sunny day. We took a 3-mile walk. We got home about 4 p.m. and I took a nap. A little after 7 p.m. I got up and went to the bathroom. While I was urinating I heard a quiet little sound that sounded like someone rubbing their finger on an inner-tube. When I went back to the bedroom, I told Philip that I thought my water had broken, but that I really wasn't sure. I sat down on the bed on a towel and waited for a couple of minutes. Philip kept telling me to lie down. Finally I did. That position change allowed the amniotic fluid to escape (apparently the baby's head had been preventing it from running out previously).

Philip wanted to call the doctor, but I said to at least wait until I had a contraction or two. About 7:10 I had the first contraction (I hadn't even had any Braxton Hicks contractions during the preceding 2 days). At 7:14 I had another mild one and at 7:18 I had one so strong that I couldn't stand up. So I decided the doctor might like to know about it. I talked to him at 7:20 p.m. He said he'd notify the hospital. I said I'd be there in about a half hour and he said I'd best be there sooner than that!

We left the house at 7:30, got to the hospital rather quickly and we checked into the hospital at 7:41 p.m. The nurse checked me and said I was 7-8 centimeters dilated and that I would be going into transition shortly. Philip was getting dressed in his delivery room clothes. I had two contractions in the labor room and then I informed the nurse that I had an urge to push. She checked me again and she said I was fully dilated, so she wheeled me off to the delivery room. By this time Philip was ready and he was with me.

The doctor still had not arrived and the nurses left me on the labor room bed even after we got into the delivery room. I think they thought that maybe I would feel less like delivering if I stayed on that bed than if I were on the delivery table. The two nurses and Philip had me control the urge to push through two very strong pushing contractions. Then I asked if the doctor was in the hospital yet. They told me no and I said I was sorry, but that he wasn't going to be there for the birth. They must have believed me, because they put me on the delivery table and said go ahead.

At 7:55 p.m. the nurse delivered Ami Michele. It wasn't necessary for me to push with even a fraction of the power that I wanted to push with. During the delivery Philip had been bouncing all over the delivery room recording the whole thing on film. He also kept up steady verbal coaching.

At 8 p.m. the doctor, still in street clothes, stuck his head in the delivery room door and looked at Philip, looked at me, and looked at Ami over in the corner and said, "Well, did you get your pictures?" Then he got changed and scrubbed and came in and put my legs in the stirrups, draped me, etc. (kind of after the fact it seemed to me) and delivered the placenta. Then he put in one stitch and it was all over.

I thought it was all kind of exciting that only an hour before that I hadn't had any contractions and I hadn't even been sure that my membranes had ruptured and now I had a 7 pound 10 ounce little lady!

I spent about 20 minutes in the recovery room and the doctor told me I could go home then if I wanted to, but that he preferred that I stay overnight. I felt great and really wanted to go home, but Ami had a possible blood complication (I am O– and Philip is AB+) and I wanted her in the nursery overnight. And I couldn't go home without her! So I stayed until the next morning at 11.

Philip smuggled me ice cream and stayed at the hospital with me until a little after midnight. He came to get us the next morning and we were home by 11:30. Ami was about 15½ hours old. Philip and I have enjoyed both of our children's births very much. We wouldn't consider being apart during childbirth. I think childbirth is great fun.

Hints, Leftovers and Miscellany

This chapter is a short collection of suggestions that some new and expectant parents have found to be helpful in dealing with pregnancy, birth and infant care. What appears here is by no means all-inclusive, nor will every suggestion be appropriate for every parent. Don't feel that you must carry out each suggestion mentioned here any more than you should follow every suggestion given in books of baby care. You, as a parent, must make choices that are appropriate to your own lifestyle, personal beliefs and sense of what is "right" for your own child.

It is important to remember that the baby, indeed, is yours. S/he does not belong to your mother, your mother-in-law, neighbor or friend. The responsibility is yours to develop your own philosophy of child-rearing. It's undoubtedly one of the most important things you will ever do, but remember that it can be fun, too.

Read through the following collection of hints and suggestions, and choose what is right for you and your baby.

Before the Baby is Born

Don't make pregnancy a contest. Some women tend to make it a contest to see who can be the sickest. Some women tend to make it a contest to see who can lead the most "normal" life until the day the baby is born. Move with the pregnancy. Do what your body tells you is right. If you are tired, rest. Some women truly are sick through much of the pregnancy; if you are, accept it and do what makes you feel better. Some women make themselves sicker by trying to lead a completely normal life and not making provision for the fact that they are physically upset. Don't work up until the day of delivery just to prove that you can do it. If you honestly feel strong enough and energetic enough, and if your doctor agrees that there's nothing in your physical condition to contraindicate your continuing to work, it's fine to work. But don't do it just to prove something to someone.

By the same token, labor and birth should not be a contest. Ostriches often seem to compete for the most painful ordeal possible. Prepared women sometimes tend to minimize any pain and discomfort in an attempt to have experienced the most pain-free labor. It's important to communicate honestly with your childbirth education instructor and with expectant parents in order to be helpful to each. Being honest with your childbirth education instructor can help her to develop the most effective teaching strategies and to concentrate on those techniques that most of her sudents find most helpful. Being honest with expectant parents enables them to best prepare for the birth experience.

Take handwork or reading material to your prenatal appointments. Sometimes the wait can be quite long, especially if you go to a clinic.

To remember your early-morning urine specimen, put a small bottle on the closed toilet lid the night before your appointment.

Take a list of questions with you on your prenatal visits. As questions occur to you between appointments, jot them down on a piece of paper that you leave in your purse or coat pocket.

Take your coach to at least one of your prenatal appointments. It is good if the coach meets the doctor (and vice versa) before you enter the hospital in labor.

Wear simple clothes to your prenatal appointments. Getting dressed and undressed in a doctor's office is no fun at best, but simple clothes can make the task simpler.

Be honest with your medical care-takers. If you want to know what your blood pressure is, ask. Let them know if they are doing something that you don't like.

Some doctors will make a photocopy of your prenatal records for you to carry with you during the last weeks of your pregnancy. This assures that if you go into labor before the hospital has received your chart from your doctor, you will have the pertinent information for the nurses when you arrive. It is also a good safeguard if you go into labor while you are a long way from home and find it necessary to enter a hospital other than your own.

Find maternity clothes that you really like, and really feel comfortable in. Three or four outfits that make you feel stylish and attractive are more helpful to your frame of mind than ten outfits that do nothing but cover up your body.

Accept offers of loaned maternity clothes. If someone has four or five things she is offering to loan you, you just may like at least one or two of them. It's not necessary to wear every piece of clothing that you are loaned. After your pregnancy, remember to loan your clothes to others.

After the Baby is Born

Remember that is is your baby.

Remember that the baby came to live at your house. The baby will adjust to your schedule and lifestyle if you are reasonable in your expectations. There's no need to schedule everything for the baby's benefit. After the first few months, the baby's sleep schedule will settle down, and you can train him/her to sleep when it is most convenient for you. For instance, it is not a Universal Rule that all babies and toddlers must go to bed at 7 p.m. and wake up at 6 a.m. Some children go to bed at 11 p.m. and get up at 10 a.m. It's all in what fits your lifestyle and the way you train the child. Admittedly, if you are shopping at 10 p.m. with the baby tucked under your arm, you may get some strange and disapproving looks from some people. Remember that it is your baby.

Some babies like to be wrapped very tightly in a blanket. Apparently they like the security.

Some babies like to be on the floor on a blanket from the very first days. Apparently they like the freedom to kick and move about.

Even when babies are very young, they love to look at things. If you don't have a mobile to hang over the baby's crib or cradle, try hanging a piece of aluminum foil on a string. The baby will be delighted with the way the light is reflected as air currents move the foil. The aluminum foil works just as well, perhaps better, than expensive mobiles available from the stores.

If the baby spits up, try sponging the spot with a teaspoon of soda or vinegar mixed in a glass of water. The sour smell will go away without changing the baby's whole outfit.

If the telephone is a problem at your house, perhaps it would be a good idea to have a phone jack installed that allows you to disconnect the phone when you don't want to be interrupted. The phone company gets very irate when people leave the phone off the hook.

Don't use oils and powders on the baby's skin. They are unnecessary, and are not good for the baby's skin. If you particularly like the smell of baby powder, sprinkle a little onto the baby's clothes after s/he is dressed.

Leave the cord stump exposed to air, clean it with alcohol at every diaper change, don't clip it and don't get it wet. It will fall off within a week or ten days.

It is not necessary to bathe the baby daily. Every three or four days is often enough for a full bath. The only part of the baby that gets really dirty gets washed with every diaper change anyway. A word of warning: it may be very hard for grandmothers to accept the idea that the baby does not have to be bathed every day exactly at 10 a.m. (or 2 p.m. or whenever). Remember that it is your baby.

Some parents, particularly those who are uncomfortable handling a slippery, wet baby, find it easier to take the baby into the bathtub when the parent bathes. If you do this, it is a good idea to have someone around that can take the baby from you when you are ready to get out of the tub. The baby may get chilled while you are drying off if there is nobody to help dress and dry the baby.

Let the baby get used to normal household noises. Don't turn off the stereo and ask everyone to whisper when the baby is sleeping. The baby will learn to sleep through a fair amount of noise. If strict silence is maintained when the baby is sleeping, it will have to be maintained when the toddler and young child is sleeping.

Instead of buying commercially prepared baby foods, consider making your own. Table foods can be put through either a blender or a baby food grinder before the baby is old enough to handle regular food.

As the baby is learning to feed himself/herself, put either a large plastic sheet, or newspapers under the high chair to make cleaning up after the meal easier.

If you have unexpected twins, both babies can sleep in the same crib for the first few months.

If you have twins, do the same thing for each baby at the same time. Change both at the same time, feed both at the same time, bathe both at the same time.

Place a folded cloth diaper under the baby's head when s/he is sleeping. If s/he spits up, the whole sheet won't have to be changed to get rid of the sour smell.

Disposable diapers are very convenient for traveling. Use of disposables eliminates the need for carrying the wet and soiled diapers home in plastic bags.

Appendix A: Glossary

ABDOMEN: The part of the body between the lower ribs and the pubic bone.

ABORTION: Termination of pregnancy before the baby is able to survive outside of the uterus. An abortion may happen spontaneously or be induced by chemical or surgical means.

AFTERBIRTH: The material expelled from the uterus after the baby is born; includes placenta, umbilical cord and membranes.

AFTER-PAINS: Lower abdominal cramps sometimes felt after the baby is born; caused by the uterus as it returns to its original size. The greater the number of children a woman has borne, the greater the discomfort is likely to be.

ALBUMIN: A protein substance; its presence in the urine may be an indication of a medical problem. A pregnant woman's urine is checked frequently for albumin.

ALVEOLI: Small, hollow air sacs in the lungs that the baby must inflate with its first breaths.

AMNESIC: A drug which causes temporary memory loss.

AMNIOCENTESIS: Process of withdrawing amniotic fluid through the abdominal and uterine walls; the fluid can be studied to find out much about the developing fetus. Amniocentesis carries little risk to the fetus, but the safety of the fetus dictates that the procedure be done only if there is some special cause for concern about the fetus.

AMNION: The innermost membrane holding the amniotic fluid and the fetus in utero.

AMNIOTIC: Having to do with the amnion.

AMNIOTIC FLUID: The liquid the fetus floats in in the uterus.

AMNIOTIC SAC: The sac containing the amniotic fluid; bag of waters.

AMNIOTOMY: Artificial rupture of the membranes.

ANALGESIA: Lack of sensibility to pain while still conscious.

ANALGESIC: A drug used to relieve pain and produce analgesia.

ANESTHESIA: Loss of sensation or feeling.

ANESTHESIOLOGIST: Doctor who has specialized training in the administration of anesthetics.

ANESTHETIC: A drug used to cause loss of sensation in a specific region of the body or to produce unconsciousness.

ANESTHETIST: Registered Nurse who has specialized training in the administration of anesthetics.

ANTERIOR PRESENTATION: When the top of the baby's head leads the way down the birth canal with the baby facing toward the mother's back; this is the most common presentation.

ANTIGEN: Protein substance found in blood.

ANTISEPTIC: An agent which destroys microorganisms that can cause disease and infection.

ANUS: The outlet of the bowel.

APGAR SCORE: A method of rating the physical condition of the newborn baby. The infant is rated at one minute after birth and at five minutes after birth. Either 0, 1 or 2 points is given for each of the following: heart rate, respiratory effort, muscle tone, reflexes and color. A score of 7-10 is good, 4-6 is fair, 0-3 is very poor.

AREOLA: The dark ring around the nipple.

BABY BLUES: A term used for postpartum depression.

BACK LABOR: A term applied to labor which is felt in the back; often caused by a posterior or breech presentation.

BAG OF WATERS: Amniotic sac.

BARBITURATE: Analgesic used to induce sleep.

BILILITES: Lights used to help destroy bilirubin in a severely jaundiced infant.

BILIRUBIN: Yellowish substance that is a waste product produced as red blood cells are broken down.

BIRTH CANAL: The vagina.

BLADDER: Pouch which receives urine from the kidneys.

BLOOD TYPE: The classification of blood into one of a number of groups; blood can be A, B, AB or O as well as being Rh+ or Rh−.

BLOODY SHOW: Mucus tinged with blood; this may be one sign that labor is about to begin. Sometimes blood-tinged mucus appears after a vaginal examination.

BRAXTON HICKS CONTRACTIONS: Uterine contractions which occur periodically throughout pregnancy as the uterus enlarges to accommodate the growing fetus; more noticeable in late pregnancy; false labor contractions.

BREECH: Buttocks; a breech presentation is one in which the fetus emerges from the vagina buttocks or feet first.

BROW PRESENTATION: When the baby's brow leads the way down the birth canal; brow presentation is very rare.

BUCCAL: Having to do with the cheek; a buccal "pit" is a method of inducing labor which consists of placing oxytocic tablets in the woman's mouth and letting them dissolve.

CALIPERS: An instrument the doctor uses to measure externally the fundal height.

CAPUT: The head; used to refer to the swelling on the presenting part of the fetal head.

CATHETERIZATION: Insertion of a small tube through the urethra to empty the bladder.

CAUDAL: Anesthetic injected into the caudal space at the base of the spine.

CENTIMETER: Measurement used to indicate the dilatation of the cervix; one inch is equal to 2.5 centimeters.

CEPHALO-PELVIC DISPROPORTION: When the baby's

head is too large to pass through the mother's pelvic structure; CPD.

CERVICAL OS: The opening of the cervix which effaces and dilates during labor.

CERVIX: The narrow, "neck" of the uterus which opens into the vagina.

CESAREAN DELIVERY: Birth of the baby through incisions in the abdominal and uterine walls, Cesarean Section; C-section.

CHLOASMA: Mask of pregnancy; dark pigmentation which may appear on pregnant woman's face.

CIRCUMCISION: Surgical removal of all or part of the foreskin of the penis.

CLITORIS: Small erectile organ of the female genitalia located at the anterior of the vulva.

COCCYX: The tailbone; small bone at the end of the spine.

COLOSTRUM: The yellowish substance which precedes breast milk.

CONCEPTION: Union of the male sperm and the female ovum.

CONFINEMENT: Term applied to childbirth.

CONTRACEPTION: Prevention of conception.

CONTRACTION: Shortening and tightening of the uterine muscle and fiber during labor; labor "pains."

CPD: Cephalo-pelvic disproportion.

CROWNING: When the baby's presenting part stretches open the perineum; as the baby crowns the perineum bulges.

DEFECATION: Evacuation of the bowels.

DELIVERY: The birth of the baby; properly used it refers to a birth in which the mother is assisted with forceps, etc.

DELIVERY ROOM: The room where the baby is born; in American hospitals the delivery room is usually separate from the labor room.

DIAPHRAGM: The muscular partition between the chest and the abdomen.

DILATATION: Opening of the cervix during labor; 10 centimeters is full dilatation.

DILATION: Dilatation.

DIURETICS: Drugs which increase the discharge of urine.

DORSAL POSITION: Delivery position in which the

mother lies on her back with her knees flexed and her feet flat on the delivery table; opposed to the lithotomy position in which her legs are elevated into stirrups.

DUE DATE: The projected date of the baby's birth.

ECLAMPSIA: Toxemia.

ECTOPIC PREGNANCY: When the fertilized egg grows somewhere outside of the uterus, such as in the fallopian tube.

EDEMA: Swelling of body tissues caused by excessive fluid retention.

EFFACEMENT: The thinning of the cervix during labor; effacement may occur before or during dilatation; it is measured in percentages; 100% effacement indicates the cervix is fully effaced.

EFFLEURAGE: Fingertip massage of the abdomen performed by either the mother or the coach; tends to relieve tense muscles and provide a distraction for the mother.

EMBRYO: The product of conception in the uterus from about the third week after conception to about the fifth week after conception.

EMESIS: Vomiting.

ENDOMETRIUM: Mucous membrane which lines the uterus; is shed during menstruation, and remains in the uterus during pregnancy.

ENEMA: Injection of a solution into the rectum and colon to cause the lower intestine to empty.

ENGAGEMENT: When the presenting part of the fetus has settled into the upper part of the pelvic canal; lightening.

ENGORGEMENT: Excessive fullness of the breasts, often present when the milk comes in.

EPIDURAL: Anesthetic injected above the caudal space; does not enter the spinal fluid.

EPISIOTOMY: A surgical incision of the perineum done just prior to the birth of the baby in order to widen the opening and prevent tears.

ESTROGEN: Hormone secreted by the ovaries and the placenta; responsible in large part for feminine body characteristics and for the changes that take place in the uterus during pregnancy and menstruation; the female hormone.

FALLOPIAN TUBES: The ducts that connect the ovaries with the uterus; fertilization of the egg by the sperm usually takes place within one of the fallopian tubes.

FALSE LABOR: Contractions that resemble true labor contractions, but cause little or no dilatation and effacement of the cervix.

FAMILY-CENTERED MATERNITY CARE: Maternity care that focuses on, and fulfills the needs of, the laboring couple and the new family.

FEAR-TENSION-PAIN SYNDROME: The theory that fear causes tension and that this tension can cause and heighten the amount of pain felt; this increased pain causes more fear and the cycle continues.

FERTILITY: The ability to reproduce.

FERTILIZATION: Conception; the beginning of pregnancy; the fusion of the sperm and the ovum.

FETAL DISTRESS: Condition whereby the fetus is under too much physical stress; fetal distress is detected by excessive slowing or speeding of the fetal heart tones, or by the presence of meconium in the amniotic fluid.

FETAL HEART TONES: The baby's heartbeat in utero; ranges between 120 and 160 beats per minute.

FETAL MONITOR: An electronic machine designed to detect and record the fetal heart tones during labor; both internal and external monitors are in use today.

FETOSCOPE: A modified stethoscope used to listen to the baby's heartbeat during pregnancy and labor.

FETUS: The baby in utero from about the end of the fifth week of pregnancy until birth.

FHT: Retal heart tones.

FIRST STAGE OF LABOR: The part of labor during which the cervix effaces and dilates.

FLOW: Lochia.

FOCAL POINT: A picture or object that the mother uses during labor as a point of visual concentration; use of the focal point is a method of distraction for the mother.

FONTANELS: The two "soft spots" on the baby's head that allow for the molding of the baby's head during passage through the birth canal.

FOOTLING BREECH: Baby whose feet lead the way down the birth canal.

FORCEPS: Obstetrical instruments used to help pull and ease the baby out of the birth canal in difficult deliveries.

FORESKIN: The fold of skin which covers the glans penis; prepuce.

FRANK BREECH: Presentation in which the buttocks of the fetus lead the way down the birth canal; the feet are up near the face of the fetus when the baby is in this position in utero.

FUNDAL HEIGHT: The distance, measured in centimeters, from the pubic bone to the top of the uterus.

FUNDUS: The upper rounded portion of the uterus; the top of the uterus.

GENE: An hereditary factor in the chromosomes which carries on hereditary traits.

GENERAL ANESTHESIA: Anesthetic which removes consciousness.

GENITAL: Pertaining to the reproductive organs.

GENITALIA: The reproductive organs.

GESTATION: The condition of pregnancy.

GONADS: Term referring to the male sex glands (testicles) or the female sex glands (ovaries).

GRAVID: Pregnant

GRAVIDA: Pregnant woman

GYNECOLOGIST: Physician who specializes in diseases peculiar to women and their reproductive organs.

GYNECOLOGY: Branch of medicine dealing with diseases peculiar to women and their reproductive organs.

HEMORRHOIDS: Varicose veins of the anus.

HORMONE: Chemical substance produced in any organ; carried to an associated organ by the blood stream a hormone influences in the latter organ a functional activity.

HYMEN: A membranous fold of tissue which partially or wholly occludes the external vaginal opening.

HYPERVENTILATION: An imbalance of the oxygen-carbon dioxide levels in the blood caused by exhaling too much carbon dioxide; hyperventilation is characterized by dizziness and a tingling or numbness in the limbs.

IMPLANTATION: The embedding of the fertilized ovum in the lining of the uterus; if implantation occurs outside of the uterus, the result is an ectopic pregnancy.

IMPREGNATION: Fertilization of an ovum by a sperm.

INDUCED LABOR: A labor started by physical or chemical means by the physician.

INDUCTION: The starting of a labor by physical or chemical means.

INERTIA: Inactivity; uterine inertia is the state whereby the uterus produces inefficient contractions.

INFERTILITY: Inability to reproduce.

INTRAVENOUS: Injected into the body through a blood vein.

INVOLUTION: The return of the uterus to normal size after the birth of a baby; involution takes approximately six weeks; during involution the uterus contracts and gets smaller until it reaches its normal size.

IV: Intravenous; a procedure whereby a needle is inserted into the back of a patient's hand, taped in place, and attached to a rubber tube; glucose water with, or without, medications can be given via this tubing.

JAUNDICE: Condition characterized by a yellowish tinge in the baby's skin; caused because the baby's immature liver is unable to excrete red blood cells as fast as they are destroyed, and as the red blood cells are destroyed, the hemoglobin is changed to yellow bilirubin.

KEGEL MUSCLE: The pubococcygeus muscle; a muscle of the pelvic floor that surrounds and contracts the vagina and the urethra.

KEGEL MUSCLE EXERCISE: Exercises devised by Arnold Kegel, M.D. to strengthen the pelvic floor muscles; contractions of the vagina.

LABIA: The outer lips of the vagina.

LABOR: The process by which the products of conception are expelled from the mother's body.

LABOR 'PAIN': Uterine contraction during labor.

LABOR ROOM: The hospital room in which a mother spends the dilatation and effacement part of her labor; some pushing may also be done in the labor room.

LACERATION: A tear.

LACTATION: The process of making milk in the breasts; the period of time during which the baby is being nourished by breast milk.

LANUGO: The fine, downy hair on the body of the fetus and newborn.

LET-DOWN REFLEX: The reflex which allows the baby to receive milk from the mother's breasts.

LIGHTENING: Engagement of the fetal presenting part.
LINEA NIGRA: Dark line that may develop on the pregnant woman's abdomen between the umbilicus and the bottom of the abdomen.
LITHOTOMY POSITION: A position whereby the mother lies on her back with her legs raised and spread apart by stirrups; this is the most commonly used delivery position in America.
LOCAL ANESTHESIA: An anesthetic which affects only a limited part of the body.
LOCHIA: A discharge of blood, mucus and tissue from the uterus for the first days or weeks after delivery.
LUNAR MONTH: A month of 28 days.
MASTITIS: A breast infection.
MECONIUM: The tarry dark green or black substance found in the large intestine of the fetus or newborn; substance that the baby passes before having bowel movements.
MEMBRANES: The sac which contains the baby and the amniotic fluid; the amniotic sac; the bag of waters.
MENOPAUSE: The time in a woman's life when menstruation ceases; the 'change of life.'
MENSTRUATION: The cyclic uterine bleeding which occurs throughout a woman's childbearing years, except when she is pregnant.
MIDWIFE: A person trained in the management of normal labor and birth.
MILIA: The small white bumps on the nose and forehead of the newborn.
MISCARRIAGE: A spontaneous abortion.
MOLDING: The shaping of the baby's head so it will adjust itself to the size and shape of the birth canal; during molding the bony plates of the baby's head slide together and overlap.
MUCUS PLUG: Heavy mucus inside of the cervix that protects the contents of the uterus from contamination.
MULTIPARA: A woman who has given birth before.
MULTIPLE BIRTH: When two or more children are born to one mother at the same time.
NEVUS: Birthmark.
NULLIPARA: Woman who has never given birth.
OBSTETRICIAN: Physician who specializes in the care of pregnant women.

OBSTETRICS: The branch of medicine concerned with pregnancy and childbirth.

OS: The opening of the cervix.

OVA: Plural of ovum.

OVARY: Sexual gland of the female in which ova develop; ovaries also produce female hormones.

OVULATION Cyclic release of ova from the ovaries.

OXYTOCIC: Drug which stimulates uterine contractions.

OXYTOCIN: Pituitary hormone which causes the uterus to contract.

PAIN THRESHOLD: The amount of sensation that one can experience without perceiving the sensation as pain.

PAP SMEAR: Papanicolaou test; examination of cervical secretions to detect possibly cancerous cells.

PARACERVICAL: Anesthetic injected into the cervical rim.

PATHOLOGICAL: Referring to the scientific study of disease.

PEAK: The most intense part of the contraction; some contractions have more than one peak.

PEDIATRICIAN: Physician who specializes in caring for infants and children.

PEDIATRICS: The branch of medicine devoted to the care of infants and children.

PELVIC EXAM: A vaginal or rectal examination done to identify the placement of internal organs, or the position of the baby; also done to determine the progress of labor.

PELVIC FLOOR: Pubococcygeus muscle group; trough-shaped group of muscles that forms the support for the rectum, urethra, bladder and the internal reproductive organs.

PELVIMETER: Instrument used for measuring the size and shape of the pelvis.

PELVIMETRY: Determination of the exact measurements and shape of the pelvis.

PELVIS: The basin-shaped bony structure that rests on the lower limbs and supports the spinal column.

PENIS: Male organ of copulation.

PERINEAL: Pertaining to the perineum.

PERINEUM: Area between the vagina and the rectum.

PERISTALSIS: Wavelike muscular contractions.

PH: Measure of the acidity or alkalinity of a solution; potential of hydrogen.

PHYSIOLOGY: The biological science of life processes, activities and functions.

PITOCIN: An oxytocic often used to induce labor artificially; may be used after the birth to reduce blood loss.

PKU: Phenylketonuria; PKU test is done sometime between the second and fourth day of the baby's life to screen for phenylketonuria, a heredity disease characterized by an inability to utilize one specific amino acid —the disease can cause severe mental retardation if it is not detected in the newborn.

PLACENTA: The circular, flat, vascular structure through which the fetus is nourished in utero, and through which the fetal waste products are expelled; attached to the wall of the uterus; connected to the fetus by the umbilical cord.

PLACENTA PREVIA: Placenta which is attached in the lower uterus; normally the placenta attaches in the upper part of the uterus.

POSTERIOR PRESENTATION: Presentation in which the fetus is coming down the birth canal head-first, but with its face toward the mother's stomach rather than toward the mother's back.

POSTPARTUM: After the birth; literally, after the separation; postpartum period often considered to be the 4 to 6 weeks following the birth during which the mother's reproductive organs return to their normal, non-pregnant state, but the postpartum adjustments to living with the baby take much longer.

PRECIPITOUS LABOR: Rapid labor.

PREECLAMPSIA: Condition of pregnancy characterized by hypertension, edema and albumin in the urine, often accompanied by headaches, blurred vision, sharp abdominal pain and sudden rapid weight gain; can lead to eclampsia.

PREGNANCY: The period of time during which one has a developing embryo or fetus within the body.

PREMATURE: An infant which weighs 5 pounds 8 ounces or less at birth.

PRENATAL: Before the birth.

PREP: The procedures that the medical staff completes when admitting a woman to the labor room in the hospital, often includes an enema, blood test, urinalysis, vaginal or rectal examination, shaving of the pubic hair;

often used to refer to just the shaving of the pubic hair, i.e., a "full prep" is the shaving of all of the pubic hair, including the front hair, a "mini prep" is the shaving of just the hair around the vaginal opening.

PREPUCE: The foreskin on the penis.

PRESENTATION: The part of the fetus which lies over the cervical os and which is the part of the fetal body that will lead the way down the birth canal.

PRIMIGRAVIDA: Woman who is pregnant for the first time.

PRIMIPARA: Woman who has given birth once; often used to refer to woman who is giving birth for the first time.

PROGESTERONE: The hormone which prepares the uterine lining for reception and development of a fertilized egg.

PROLAPSE OF CORD: Condition whereby the umbilical cord is expelled before the baby is born.

PUBIC BONE: The bone forming the front of the pelvis; the pubic symphysis.

PUBOCOCCYGEUS MUSCLE: Muscle of the pelvic floor that surrounds and contracts the vagina and the urethra; Kegel muscle.

PUDENDAL: Anesthetic injected into nerves of the vagina.

PUERPERIUM: The interval between the birth and the return of the reproductive organs to their normal position and condition.

QUICKENING: When the mother first perceives the movements of the fetus.

RECTUM: Lower end of large intestine.

REGIONAL ANESTHESIA: Loss of sensation in a particular area of the body, more widespread than local infiltration anesthesia.

RESPIRATION: Breathing.

RH FACTOR: The presence or absence of a particular antigen in the blood.

RHOGAM: A drug administered to prevent an Rh− mother who has carried an RH+ fetus from producing antibodies against the baby's RH+ antigens, the RhoGAM is a protection for the future RH+ fetuses; not all Rh− mothers can accept RhoGAM.

RIPE: The condition of the cervix when it has softened in anticipation of labor.

SACRUM: Bony triangle between the coccyx and the lower vertebrae at the small of the back.

SADDLE BLOCK: Anesthetic injected into the spinal fluid.

SECOND STAGE OF LABOR: The part of labor during which the baby is born; the labor between the time when the cervix is completely dilated (10 centimeters) until the baby is born.

SEDATIVE: A drug which has a calming, quieting effect on the mother and can reduce tension and anxiety; causes drowsiness.

SEMEN: The fluid secreted by the male reproductive organs which carries the sperm.

SHOW: The blood and mucus, including the mucus plug, which is discharged from the vagina either before or during labor; often called "bloody" show or "pink" show.

SPECULUM: An instrument which is inserted into the vagina to facilitate examination of the cervix.

SPERM: The reproductive cells of the male which travel in the semen.

SPINAL: Anesthetic injected into the spinal fluid.

SPONTANEOUS BIRTH: When the baby is born without the aid of forceps, vacuum extractor, etc.

SPOTTING: Small amount of blood from the vagina; some women have spotting throughout the pregnancy at the time when the menstrual period would normally occur.

STATION: Measurement of the progress of the fetus down through the mother's pelvis; the station indicates how far the baby has descended; minus station indicates the baby is still above the ischial spines, plus station is below the ischial spines and closer to the vaginal opening.

STERILE: Unable to reproduce; free from germs.

STERILITY: Inability to reproduce.

STILLBORN: Baby that is born dead.

STRIAE GRAVIDARUM: Stretch marks that some women develop on the abdomen during pregnancy.

STRIPPING OF MEMBRANES: Separation of the amniotic sac from the cervix by the medical caretaker, done by inserting a finger into the cervix and running it around the edge of the cervix; rimming the cervix.

SUTURE: Surgical stitch.

TERM: The time when the pregnancy is expected to be complete; a term infant is one who has remained in the uterus for 38 weeks (266 days).

TESTES: Plural of testicle.

TESTICLE: One of the two glands contained in the male scrotum.

THIRD STAGE OF LABOR: The part of labor during which the placenta is expelled.

TOXEMIA: Advanced preeclampsia.

TRANQUILIZER: Drug used to calm the mother.

TRANSITION: The part of first stage labor during which the cervix dilates from approximately 7 centimeters to 10 centimeters (full dilatation); the most difficult phase of labor.

TRANSVERSE PRESENTATION: Presentation in which the upper back or the shoulder area is over the opening of the cervix.

TRIMESTER: A three-month period of time in pregnancy; the first trimester is months 1, 2 and 3, the second trimester is months 4, 5 and 6, and the third trimester is months 7, 8 and 9.

UMBILICAL CORD: The cord-like structure which connects the fetus and the placenta, the umbilical cord contains 2 arteries and 1 vein surrounded by Wharton's jelly.

UMBILICUS: The place where the umbilical cord is attached to the body of the fetus; the navel; the "belly button."

URETHRA: The tube through which urine is carried from the bladder to the outside of the body.

URGE TO PUSH: The physical desire to bear down and expel the fetus.

URINALYSIS: A laboratory analysis of urine.

UTERUS: The hollow, pear-shaped organ in the female in which the fetus develops until birth; the womb.

VAGINA: The canal which extends from the uterus to the outside of the body; the birth canal.

VARICOSE VEINS: Distended, enlarged veins.

VASCULAR SPIDERS: Small, bright red spots that may appear on pregnant woman's body.

VERNIX CASEOSA: The layer of thick, white oily material which covers and protects the body of the fetus in utero.

VERSION: Turning of the fetus in utero to change the presentation to one more favorable for delivery.

VERTEX: The crown of the head.

VERTEX PRESENTATION: When the crown of the head leads the way down the birth canal.

VIABLE: A term meaning the baby is able or likely to live outside of the uterus.

VULVA: External genitals of the female.

WATERS: The amniotic fluid.

WHARTON'S JELLY: The jelly-like tissue which surrounds the blood vessels in the umbilical cord.

WITCHES MILK: Fluid secreted from the breasts of some newborns; caused by female hormones which have passed from the mother to the baby.

WOMB: Uterus.

DILATATION OF THE CERVIX

Actual size
centimeters

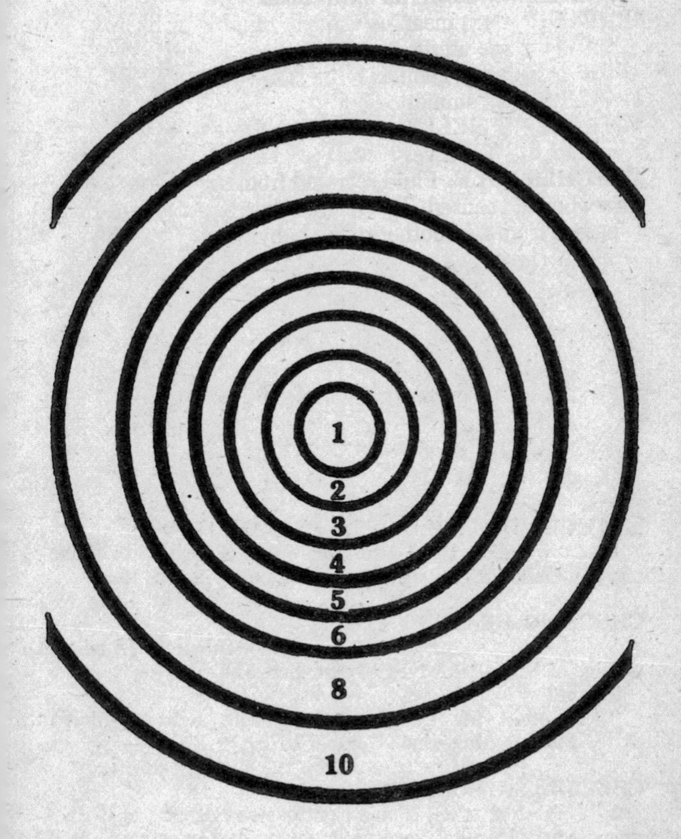

Appendix B: Notes

METHODS OF CHILDBIRTH PREPARATION

1) Doris Haire, **The Cultural Warping of Childbirth** (International Childbirth Education Association, 1972), p. 15.

CHOOSING HEALTH CARE

1) ...., **What is a Nurse-Midwife?** (American College of Nurse-Midwives, Washington, D.C.).

2) **Ibid.**

3) Dorothea M. Lang, "The Midwife Returns—Modern Style," **Parents' Magazine** (October 1972).

CHOOSING A HOSPITAL

1) H. Gezon, et al., "Some Controversial Aspects in the Epidemiology of Hospital Nursery Staphylococcal Infections," **Amer. J. of Public Health,** 50:473-484, 1960.

2) R. Ravenholt and G. LaVeck, "Staphylococcal Disease—An Obstetric Pediatric and Community Problem," **Amer. J. of Public Health,** 46:1287-1296, 1956.

3) L. Dahm and L. James, "Newborn Temperature: Heat Loss in Delivery Room," **Pediatrics** 49:504-513, 1972.

4) L. Salk, "The Critical Nature of the Post-Partum Period

in the Human for the Establishment of the Mother-Infant Bond: A Controlled Study," Dis. Nerv. Sys., 31:Suppl: 110-116.

5) M. Klaus, et al., "Maternal Attachment—Importance of the First Postpartum Days," **N.E.J. of Med.** 286:460-463, March 2, 1972.

PREGNANCY

1) Elise Fitzpatrick, Sharon R. Reeder, Luigi Mastroianni, **Maternity Nursing** (Philadelphia: J.B. Lippincott Company, 1971) 12th edition, p. 86.

2) ...., **Perinatal Mortality, Clinical Obstetrics and Gynecology** (Medical Department of Harper and Row), Vol. 13, #1, March 1970.

3) Margaret F. Myles, **Textbook for Midwives** (London: Churchill Livingstone, 1971), 7th edition, p. 76.

4) Lanie Black and Connie Jackson, **An Act of Love** (San Pedro, CA: Caligraphics Printing and Publishing, 1974), p. 35.

5) Peg Beals, ed., **ICEA Parents' Guide to the Childbearing Year** (ICEA Publication Distribution Center, P.O. Box 9316 Midtown Plaza Post Office, Rochester, NY 14604: The International Childbirth Education Association, 1975), 5th edition, p. 3.

6) Black and Johnson, **An Act of Love**, p. 25.

LABOR: SECOND STAGE (BIRTH OF BABY) AND THIRD STAGE (EXPULSION OF PLACENTA)

1) Haire, **The Cultural Warping of Childbirth**, p. 21.

2) **Ibid.**, p. 21.

3) **Ibid.**, p. 21.

4) **Ibid.**, p. 21.

5) A Blankfield, "The Optimum Position for Childbirth," **Med. J. Australia**, 2:666-668, 1965.

6) Myles, **Textbook for Midwives**, p. 303.

7) Black and Jackson, **An Act of Love**, p. 56.

8) Haire, **The Cultural Warping of Childbirth**, p. 24.

9) **Ibid.**, p. 24.

10) Black and Jackson, **An Act of Love**, p. 56.

11) Haire, **The Cultural Warping of Childbirth**, p. 24.

12) M. Klaus, et al., "Maternal Attachment—Importance of the First Post-Partum Days."

13) L. Salk, "The Critical Nature of the Post-Partum Period in the Human for the Establishment of the Mother-Infant Bond: A Controlled Study."

14) Fitzpatrick, Reeder, and Mastroianni, **Maternity Nursing**, p. 264.

15) N. Cooperman, F. Rubovits, and F. Hesser, "Oxygen

Saturation in the Newborn Infant," **Am. J. Obstet. & Gynec.,** 81:385-394, 1961.

16) P. Hubinont, et al., "Effects of Vacuum Extractor and Obstetrical Forceps on the Fetus and Newborn—A Comparison," V World Congress Gynec. & Obstet., Sydney, Australia, 1967.

17) N. Butler, "A National Long Term Study of Perinatal Hazards," Sixth World Congress, Fed. Int'l. Gynec. & Obstet., 1970.

SPECIAL LABORS AND BIRTHS

1) Myles, **Textbook for Midwives,** p. 76.
2) **Ibid.,** p. 76.
3) **Ibid.,** p. 76.
4) **Ibid.,** p. 76.
5) **Ibid.,** p. 76.
6) **Ibid.,** p. 76.
7) Haire, **The Cultural Warping of Childbirth,** p. 19.
8) P. Boylan, "Oxytocin and Neonatal Jaundice," **Br. Med. J.,** 2:564-5, Sept. 1976.

MEDICATIONS USED IN CHILDBIRTH

1) T. Berry Brazelton, M.D., "What Childbirth Drugs Can Do to Your Child," **Redbook Magazine** (February 1971), Vol. 130, No. 4, p. 65.
2) **Ibid.,** p. 65.
3) John J. Bonica, M.D., ed., **Obstetric Analgesia and Anesthesia** (New York: Springer-Verlag, 1972), p. 29.
4) **Ibid.,** p. 16.
5) **Ibid.,** p. 46.
6) **Ibid.,** p. 46.
7) **Ibid.,** p. 77.
8) **Ibid.,** p. 25.
9) **Ibid.,** p. 61.
10) **Ibid.,** p. 61.
11) **Ibid.,** p. 61.
12) **Ibid.,** p. 25.
13) **Ibid.,** p. 25.
14) **Ibid.,** p. 25.
15) **Ibid.,** p. 26.
16) **Ibid.,** p. 26.

THE NEWBORN

1) Geraldine Lux Flanagan, **The First Nine Months of Life** (New York: Pocket Books, 1965), p. 132.
2) **Ibid.,** p. 134.
3) Fitzpatrick, Reeder, and Mastroianni, **Maternity Nursing,** p. 347.

4) **Ibid.**, p. 347.
5) **Ibid.**, p. 355.
Circumcision information from **Patient Care** (July 15, 1971) pp. 51-73.

BREASTFEEDING
1) Karen Pryor, **Nursing Your Baby** (New York: Pocket Books, 1973), p. 61.
2) Beals, **ICEA Parents' Guide to the Childbearing Year,** p. 69.

Appendix C: Sources of Information and Support

CHILDBIRTH EDUCATION CLASSES, SUPPORTIVE PHYSICIANS, SUPPORTIVE HOSPITALS

American Academy of Husband-Coached Childbirth
P.O. Box 5224
Sherman Oaks, California 91403

American Society for Psychoprophylaxis in Obstetrics (ASPO)
1411 K Street, Northwest
Washington, D.C. 20005

Childbirth Without Pain Education League
3940-11th Street
Riverside, California 92501

International Childbirth Education Association (ICEA)
P.O. Box 20852
Milwaukee, Wisconsin 53220

Maternity Center Association
48 East 92nd Street
New York, New York 10028

Preparation for Expectant Parents
P.O. Box 33532
Seattle, Washington 98133

The Birthplace
19316-3rd Avenue N.W.
Seattle, Washington 98177

BREASTFEEDING

La Leche League International, Inc.
9616 Minneapolis Avenue
Franklin Park, Illinois 60131

CESAREAN CHILDBIRTH

Dee Giles
1530 West Encanto Boulevard
Phoenix, Arizona 85007

Priscilla Schragl
5557 Somerset Drive
Santa Barbara, California 93111

Cesarean Birth Education Group
1290 Coven Street
Boulder, Colorado 80303

CIG
49 Trapstone Drive
Danbury, Connecticut 06708

Cesarean Birth Counseling
1516 Willow Wick
Tallahassee, Florida 32303

PACES Cesarean Group
138 Park
River Forest, Illinois 60305

Cesarean Support Group
Ann Lealy
Porters Landing
Freeport, Maine 04032

Maryland Cesarean Section Association
303 Townleigh
Reisterstown, Maryland 21136

Cesareans/Support, Education, Concern (C/SEC)
132 Adams Street Room 6
Newton, Massachusetts 02158

Kalamazoo Association for Prepared Childbirth
C-Section Birth Committee
626 East Bridge
Plainwell, Michigan 49080

Cesarean Birth
Childbirth Education Association
1513 West 26th Street
Minneapolis, Minnesota 55405

Childbirth Education of Mississippi
Cesarean Section Division
101 Holly Train
Brandon, Mississippi 39042

Cesarean Support Group
6042 Sutherland
St. Louis, Missouri 63109

Our Section
2808 T Street
Lincoln, Nebraska 68503

Upper Valley Cesarean Birth Association
16 West Park
Claremont, New Hampshire 03743

Cesarean Support Group of New Jersey
184 Elm
Teaneck, New Jersey 07066

Cesarean Birth Association
133-29 122nd Street
South Ozone Park, New York 14221

Cesarean Birth Association
998 Amelia Avenue
Akron, Ohio 44302

Cesarean Committee of Childbirth and Family Life
1224 South Del Place
Tulsa, Oklahoma 74104

Operation Childbirth
2215 Monterey Lane
Eugene, Oregon 97401

Cesarean Support Group
1850-23rd N.E.
Salem, Oregon 97303

Caesarean Mothers Group
418 Carsonia Avenue
Reading, Pennsylvania 19606

Cesarean Birth of Rhode Island
46 Emeline Street
Providence, Rhode Island 02906

Cesarean Mothers Group
Route 3 Box 347A
Clinton, Tennessee 37716

Cesarean Awareness
1817 Leicester
Garland, Texas 75042

Bennington Cesarean Childbirth Association
P.O. Box 188
Shaftsbury, Vermont 05262

Child and Parent of Fredericksburg
1020 Mannings Drive
Falmouth, Virginia 22401

Cesarean Birth Support
P.O. Box 33532
Seattle, Washington 98133

CCMA
Route 2 Box 96A
Marshfield, Wisconsin 54449

SPARC of British Columbia
2210 West 12th Avenue
Vancouver, British Columbia
CANADA V6K 2N6

MULTIPLE BIRTH

National Organization of Mothers of Twins Clubs, Inc.
512 Wallace Drive
Wayne, Pennsylvania 19087

NURSE-MIDWIVES

American College of Nurse-Midwives
Suite 801
1012 14th St., N.W.
Washington, D.C. 20005

Maternity Center Association
48 East 92nd Street
New York, New York 10028

PATIENTS' RIGHTS

For a free copy of the Pregnant Patient's Bill of Rights and Responsibilities, mail a stamped, self-addressed envelope to:

Committee on Patient's Rights
Box 1900
New York, New York 10001

BOOKS

ICEA Supplies Center
P.O. Box 70258
Seattle, Washington 98107

ICEA Publication/Distribution Center
P.O. Box 9316 Midtown Plaza
Rochester, New York 14604

SUDDEN INFANT DEATH SYNDROME

National Sudden Infant Death Syndrome Foundation
310 South Michigan Avenue
Chicago, Illinois 60604

Index

ABOUT THE AUTHOR

VICKI WALTON is a childbirth educator and a frequent public speaker to high school and college classes on the subject of childbirth. She and her husband, Philip, have shared the births of their three daughters, Alisa, Ami and Tria. Ms. Walton holds a degree in communications and is a free-lance writer and photographer.